The Impact of
Biology on
Modern Psychiatry

The Impact of Biology on Modern Psychiatry

Proceedings of a Symposium Honoring the 80th Anniversary of the Jerusalem
Mental Health Center Ezrath Nashim held in Jerusalem, Israel, December 9—10, 1975

Edited by

Elliot S. Gershon, M. D.
National Institute of Mental Health
Bethesda, Maryland

Robert H. Belmaker, M. D.
Jerusalem Mental Health Center Ezrath Nashim
Jerusalem, Israel

Seymour S. Kety, M. D.
Harvard Medical School
Boston, Massachusetts

and

Milton Rosenbaum, M. D.
Jerusalem Mental Health Center Ezrath Nashim
Jerusalem, Israel

PLENUM PRESS · NEW YORK AND LONDON

Library of Congress Cataloging in Publication Data

Main entry under title:

The Impact of biology on modern psychiatry.

"Proceedings of a symposium honoring the 80th anniversary of the
Jerusalem Mental Health Center Ezrath Nashim held in Jerusalem, Israel,
December 9-10, 1975."
Includes index.
1. Mental illness—Physiological aspects—Congresses. 2. Mental illness—
Genetic aspects—Congresses. I. Gershon, Elliot S. II. Ezrat nashim, bet
holim le-hole nefesh.
RC455.4.B5I46   616.8'9'042   76-49665

ISBN-13: 978-1-4684-0780-8   e-ISBN-13: 978-1-4684-0778-5
DOI: 10.1007/978-1-4684-0778-5

Proceedings of a Symposium Honoring the 80th Anniversary of the
Jerusalem Mental Health Center Ezrath Nashim held in Jerusalem, Israel,
December 9-10, 1975
Softcover reprint of the hardcover 1st edition 1975
© 1977 Plenum Press, New York
A Division of Plenum Publishing Corporation
227 West 17th Street, New York, N.Y. 10011

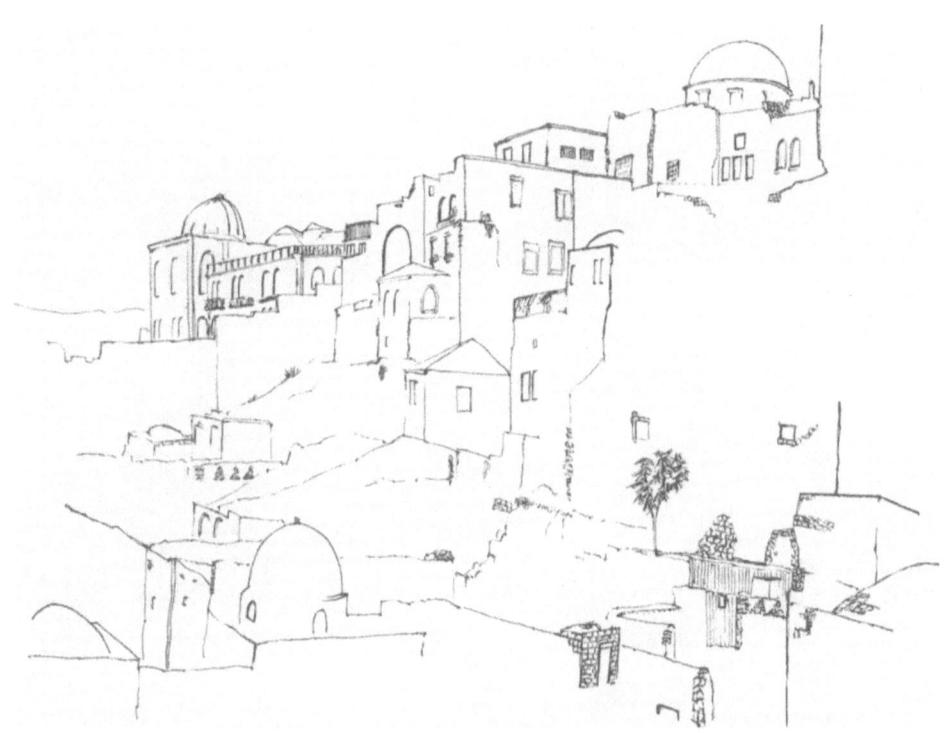

Jerusalem
(Drawing by Paul B. Ruttkay)

Introduction

The Jerusalem Mental Health Center - Ezrath Nashim was founded
in 1895 as a voluntary effort by a charitable women's society to
provide a refuge for the homeless and incurably ill of Jerusalem.
Gradually it evolved into a psychiatric hospital, but the outlook
was still based on providing custodial care for the most hopeless
of all people, the incurably insane. As with mental hospitals all
over the world, this perspective has changed dramatically over the
past two decades, largely because of the development of effective
psychopharmacologic treatments for the major psychiatric illnesses.
In the case of Ezrath Nashim, these decades have coincided with a
period of national rebuilding and rejuvenation, so that this 80th
anniversary symposium is taking place in a most modern institution
whose role in psychiatry in Israel and in the world has become an
important one. If this were the 8th anniversary instead of the 80th,
the entire institution would be found in two small rooms within the
walls of the Old City.

It is a tribute to the founders and philanthrophic supporters
of this institution that even under the most adverse of circumstances, this hospital has maintained a devotion to the goals of
excellence and progress in psychiatry. Recognizing the opportunity
offered by the new biological and pharmacologic advances in psychiatry, Ezrath Nashim has in the past few years radically expanded
the range and comprehensiveness of the services it offers, and
also established the first research laboratories and clinical research facility in psychiatry in Israel. By their presence here,
the participants in this symposium are giving recognition to the
fruitfulness of these efforts to participate in and to contribute
to the progress of the biological advances in modern psychiatry.
The most important events in the development of biological research
in psychiatry were the dicoveries of the effectiveness of certain
drugs in the treatment of the two major psychotic disorders -
schizophrenia and the manic-depressive psychoses. Interestingly
enough, the introduction of these drugs came from clinical observations by nonpsychiatrists and not by planned studies. Only now,
two decades after the introduction of these drugs, are scientists

beginning to understand their action, as will be brought out in
this symposium.

During this same period another development took place in
psychiatry, namely, social and community psychiatry, interpreted
by some, incorrectly, in my opinion, as the antitheses of the
biological approach. The whole area of the delivery of mental
health services, which quickly became more of a political and
social issue than a medical one, led to confusion, disillusionment,
despair, and also soul-searching by psychiatrists and other mental
health professionals. The remarkable Pablo Picasso said, "the
development of photography freed the artist to express his own
creativity." I have paraphrased Picasso's insightful remark,
namely, "the development of biology and social and community
psychiatry should free the psychiatrist to express his own creativity as a physician." It should allow him to regain his basic medical identity. As his medical identity becomes paramount, then the
pejorative classification of psychiatrists into those "organically-
oriented" and those "dynamically-oriented" will no longer be valid.
The psychiatrist, like his medical colleague, must be concerned
with the psychological, psychosocial, biological, and technical
aspects of psychiatry.

The strengthening and development of the medical identity of
the psychiatrist imposes increased responsibilities on him and on
psychiatry as a medical discipline. On the one hand, he will have
to become more of a neuro-bi.   gist and, on the other, more of a
behavioral scientist. He will also have to continue his expertise
in psycho-dynamics, regardless of whether or not he limits his
practice to psychotherapy. The psychiatrist's diagnostic skills
will have to be sharpened. Because of the advances in the biological
areas of psychiatry, he must not be permitted to throw out the baby
with the bath-water by eliminating the role of psychological and
psychosocial determinates in the major psychiatric disorders. He
will have to become more involved with the psychological aspects of
medicine, which involves not only psychosomatic but also somatic-
psychological factors.

Our task would be easier if we would accept the fact that the
so-called problems of living, which include much of the neuroses,
personality disorders and behavioral problems of children and
adults, should not be the primary concern of the psychiatrist but
of his mental health colleagues and associates. The primary concern
of the psychiatrist would then be the psychoses, the psychosomatic
disorders, the consultation and liaison services in general hospitals
and psychiatric hospitals, and in basic and clinical research. In
the community mental health centers the psychiatrist will function
as a supervisor, a consultant, a diagnostician, but not necessarily
as the administrator or executive officer, although he must play

an important role in decision and policy making and standard
setting.

For advances to continue through the study of brain and
behavior, it will be most important to strengthen the ties between
the clinic and the research laboratory. Despite all the advances
in biology, clinical observations have and will continue to have
their place in medicine and a proper flow of information between
the wards of the hospital and the research laboratories will enrich
as well as enlighten both the clinician and the investigator. This
is why we are sponsoring this symposium, to have Israeli psychiatrists sit next to basic scientists, and to present as models those
clinicians who have made a synthesis between the clinical and
biological. And this is why, in our own research division, the
laboratories and the wards are fully intergrated.

A warning is in order. The temptation will be to pursue the
reductionistic view that the study of the brain itself will be
sufficient to solve the riddle of behavior and its relation to
disease. Nothing could be more sterile. As important as the contributions of the basic scientists are, the clinician must not under-
estimate the opportunities of his unique role. It is he who has
the widest access to the life history, the trials and tribulations,
the successes and triumphs, the losses and tragedies, and the whole
developmental span of the life of many human beings. It is also
he who must be ever aware of what Arthur Mirsky's called the
"3 P's", namely, predisposition, precipitation and perpetuation,
in approaching and understanding his patients. In the final analysis,
it is the clinical psychiatrist together with his laboratory-orien-
ted colleague who will make the impact of biology a progressive
force in psychiatry.

Milton Rosenbaum
Jerusalem Mental Health Center
Jerusalem, Israel

Contents

THE SIGNIFICANCE OF THE CEREBRAL DOPAMINE METABOLISM IN THE PATHOGENESIS AND TREATMENT OF PSYCHOTIC DISORDERS

H.M. van Praag

Department of Biological Psychiatry

State University Grŏningen, The Netherlands

RESEARCH INTO BIOLOGICAL DETERMINANTS OF SCHIZOPHRENIC PSYCHOSES

For many years, well into the Sixties, research into the biological determinants of schizophrenic psychoses has suffered from
a dearth of more or less well-founded and testable working hypotheses. Without much system, efforts were made to find abnormal
metabolites in a wide variety of body fluids. Strange people,
strange substances: not a very powerful research strategy. It has
recently dawned, however, that neuroleptics could serve as the pace-
maker of biological psychosis research (Matthysse 1973; Snyder,
1974; Van Praag 1975), much as the antidepressants are the pace-
maker of biological depression research (Van Praag 1976a). I shall
briefly discuss the arguments which have led to this conclusion.

NEUROLEPTICS AND CENTRAL CATECHOLAMINE METABOLISM

All known neuroleptics exert an influence on the central catecholamine (CA) metabolism; they do this in two different ways (re-
views by Anden et al. 1970; Nybäck and Sedvall, 1970; O'Keefe et al.
1970; Randrup and Munkvad 1970; Westerink and Korf 1975a; Seeman and
Lee 1975; Wiesel and Sedvall 1975; Iversen 1975; Van Praag 1976b).

a. Neuroleptics of the Receptor-Blocking Type

The first group, the so-called neuroleptics of the receptor-
blocking type, comprises the phenothiazines (e.g. chlorpromazine;
Largactil) and the butyrophenones (e.g. haloperidol; Serenase) as
well as chemically related groups of thioxanthenes (e.g. clopenthixol;

1

Sordinol) and of diphenylbutylpiperidines (pimozide; Orap). In
animals given such a compound the concentration of CA metabolites
in the brain increases, whereas that of CA proper remains unchanged.
This suggests an increased degradation of CA in combination with
increased CA synthesis, which compensates for the loss of CA. In
other words: it indicates an increased CA turnover. With the aid
of isotope kinetics (administration of radioactive CA precursors)
and by the method of synthesis inhibition (with subsequent determination of the rate of disappearance of the amine), this hypothesis was verified and confirmed.

Functionally, an increased turnover can have two entirely
different implications: increased transmission activity in CA-ergic
synapses or, alternatively, transmission block in CA-ergic synapses.
The latter process leads to an increased impulse flow in the presynaptic element and, probably via this way, to increased CA synthesis. A logical inference is that a compensatory mechanism is
involved which aims at breaking the block.

In the case of the abovementioned neuroleptics, the increased
turnover is presumably secondary to transmission block. This pre-
sumption is based on the following arguments.
1) At the behaviour level, neuroleptics antagonize symptoms of
   CA-ergic hyperactivity, e.g. the motor hyperactivity provoked
   by amphetamines.
2) Neuroleptics cause reduction of motor activity. Motor hypoactivity is a constant symptom when CA-ergic activity is
   suppressed, e.g. by inhibition of CA synthesis or via destruction
   of CA-ergic neuronal systems.
3) Neuroleptics inhibit adenylcyclase, an enzyme involved in the
   synthesis of cyclic AMP. This compound is needed for activation
   of postsynaptic CA receptors, and inhibition of its synthesis
   indicates or leads to reduced transmission activity.

Receptors are probably located at two sites in a CA-ergic
synapse: not only in the postsynaptic but also in the presynaptic
membrane. The former bring the postsynaptic element to a state of
excitation. The task of the latter is believed to be regulation of
the rate of CA synthesis, guided by the amount of CA available in
the synaptic cleft. Neuroleptics are presumed to block both receptor types. Block of the postsynaptic receptors inhibits transmission,
while block of the presynaptic receptors is believed to contribute
to the increased turnover of transmitter substance due to abolition
of the feedback inhibition.

Another important point is that the extent to which neuroleptics
of this type block dopamine (DA) and noradrenaline (NA) receptors
varies from one compound to the other; and that the classification
of neuroleptics on the basis of this ratio is completely at odds
with their classification according to chemical structure.

Finally, there are indications that these neuroleptics inhibit the release of DA in the synaptic cleft which is normally effected by excitation of the axon. This mechanism, like that of receptor block, leads to diminished transmission activity.

b. Neuroleptics of the Store-Depleting Type

Neuroleptics of this second type interfere with the uptake of CA into the stores (synaptic vesicles), causing these compounds to accumulate in the cytoplasm where they are degraded by monoamine oxidase (MAO), so that their concentration decreases. Neuroleptics of this category include reserpine (Serpasil), which depletes the DA, NA and serotonin (5-HT) stores, and the indole derivative oxypertine (Opertil), which shows some predilection for NA stores.

c. Conclusions

Neuroleptics differ widely in chemical structure, but show unmistakable similarities in their net effect on the central CA metabolism. Neuroleptics of the phenothiazine and the butyrophenone type are believed to block presynaptic and postsynaptic CA receptors, and possibly also the release of DA in the synaptic cleft following nerve stimulation. The ratio DA receptor-blocking and NA receptor-blocking capacity differs from one neuroleptic to the next. Reserpine and oxypertine interfere with the storage of CA in the intraneuronal stores, causing the CA degradation to increase and their concentration to decrease.

Neuroleptics reduce transmission in DA-ergic and NA-ergic neurons, but to different extents and via different mechanisms. This seems to be a group characteristic.

RESEARCH STRATEGY

Neuroleptics are compounds of diverse chemical structure, but they show two similarities.

In biochemical terms: they reduce transmission in CA-ergic systems either by inhibition of postsynaptic receptors or by reduction of the amount of transmitter available. In psychopathological terms: they alleviate motor unrest, anxiety and psychotic disorders of thinking and experiencing.

These data logically prompt a number of closely interrelated questions.

1) Do neuroleptics also reduce transmission in human central CA-ergic neurons?
2) If so, is there a correlation between this effect and: a) the therapeutic, and b) the extrapyramidal (side) effects of neuroleptics?
3) Is the ratio between DA receptor-blocking and NA receptor-blocking capacity predictive of the therapeutic action profile of a neuroleptic? In this respect I note that their chemical structure is of little assistance.
4) Is the activity in central CA-ergic neurons increased in (schizophrenic) psychoses?

    In the past few years these questions have provided us with a research strategy in the biological study of psychotic disorders (Van Praag 1967, 1975). The principal results will be summarized in the following sections which, for brevity's sake, are largely confined to studies of the DA metabolism.

DO NEUROLEPTICS REDUCE HUMAN CENTRAL DA-ERGIC TRANSMISSION?

    This question has two components: 1) are there indications that neuroleptics of the phenothiazine and the butyrophenone type increase the human central DA turnover and, if so, 2) is this associated, as it is in test animals, with decreased activity in the postsynaptic DA receptors?

a.   Neuroleptics and Central DA Turnover

    Methodology. An impression of the DA turnover in the human CNS can be gained in two ways. The first method is determination of the baseline concentration of homovanillic acid (HVA) in the CSF; and determination of the HVA accumulation in the CSF after administration of probenecid. HVA is the principal metabolite of DA in the CNS. The second method is considerably more reliable than the first, and in this paper I shall confine myself to results obtained by this method.

    Probenecid is a compound which inhibits transport of HVA (and of 5-hydroxyindole acetic acid (5-HIAA), the principal 5-HT metabolite) from the CNS to the blood stream (Goodwin et al. 1973; Van Praag et al. 1973; Bowers 1972; Sjöström and Roos 1972). As a result, HVA accumulates in the brain as well as in the CSF. Since probenecid does not influence the rate of HVA synthesis, the rate of HVA accumulation is an index of the rate of HVA production and, therefore, of the rate of degradation of the mother substance DA. Under steady state conditions the rate of degradation and the rate of synthesis of DA are equal. The probenecid-induced accumulation

of HVA in test animals thus provides an index of the turnover rate
of central DA. Human studies must confine themselves to the CSF.
Ethical considerations, moreover, preclude the construction of an
accumulation curve in the CSF. In actual practice, two HVA deter-
minations must suffice: one before and one after the probenecid
load. The difference between the two HVA concentrations provides
an overall index of the DA turnover in the entire CNS. A strong
HVA response indicates a large production of this metabolite, therefore a high degradation and therefore a higher turnover of DA.
Inversely, a low HVA response is indicative of a small HVA production and therefore of a low DA turnover. For the sake of brevity,
I shall henceforth not refer every time to 'probenecid-induced
accumulation of HVA in lumbar CSF', but simply mention DA turnover.
In reality, however, the probenecid technique gives no more than
a general impression of the DA degradation in the CNS.

In the CNS, DA is concentrated mainly in three systems: the
nigrostriatal system, the mesolimbic and mesocortical system, and
the tuberoinfundibular system. Very little DA is present in the
spinal cord. Lumbar HVA chiefly originates from the first-mentioned
system.

Background, limitations and procedure of the probenecid technique have elsewhere been described in detail (Van Praag 1976a).
5-HIAA and HVA were determined in the CSF according to Korf et al.
(1973) and Westerink and Korf (1975b), respectively. In all CSF
samples the probenecid concentration was determined as well (Korf
and Van Praag 1971). None of the findings to be discussed here could
be explained by variations in the probenecid concentration.

Design. In 33 patients with acute schizophrenic psychoses
hospitalized in the research unit of the Department of Biological
Psychiatry in Groningen, we studied the influence of neuroleptics
of various types on the probenecid-induced accumulation of HVA in
lumbar CSF (Van Praag and Korf 1975a). The following neuroleptics
were tested.
1) Chlorpromazine (Largactil) at a daily dosage of 150-300 or
   400-600 mg (n = 12).
2) Haloperidol (Serenase) at a daily dosage of 3-4.5 or 9-12 mg
   (n = 10).
3) Oxypertine (Opertil) at a daily dosage of 50-100 or 200-450 mg
   (n = 11).

The first two are neuroleptics of the receptor-blocking type,
while the last-mentioned is a store-depleting neuroleptic with a
certain predilection for NA stores (Hassler et al., 1970).

Results. Haloperidol caused an unmistakable increase in HVA
accumulation after probenecid. In large doses, it tripled the response; in small doses it doubled the response. This means that the

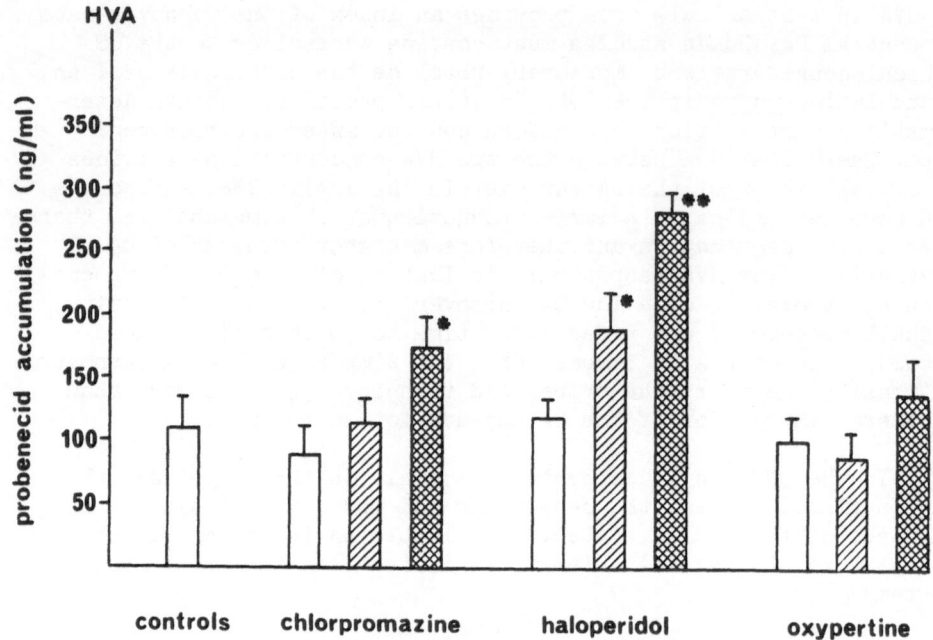

Fig. 1.   Increase of homovanillic acid (HVA) accumulation in the
           CSF in response to probenecid during treatment with
           neuroleptics in various doses. (Open columns = prior to
           medication; hatched columns = during low-dosage medication;
           cross-hatched columns = during high-dosage medication).
           * P $<$ 0.05 (Student's t-test); ** P $<$ 0.01 (Student's
           t-test).

response is dose-dependent (Fig. 1).

The effect of chlorpromazine was less pronounced, but again
dose-dependent. The largest dose doubled the HVA response, which
remained uninfluenced by oxypertine.

None of the neuroleptics affected the 5-HIAA accumulation
(Van Praag and Korf 1975a); this corresponds with the observation
that they exert no influence on 5-HT turnover in animal experiments.

Conclusion. Chlorpromazine and haloperidol increase the central
DA turnover, haloperidol having the more marked effect. Their effects
are dose-dependent. Other authors have likewise reported an increase
in post-probenecid HVA accumulation caused by neuroleptics (Chase
1972; Bowers, 1972, 1973). Oxypertine has no demonstrable effect

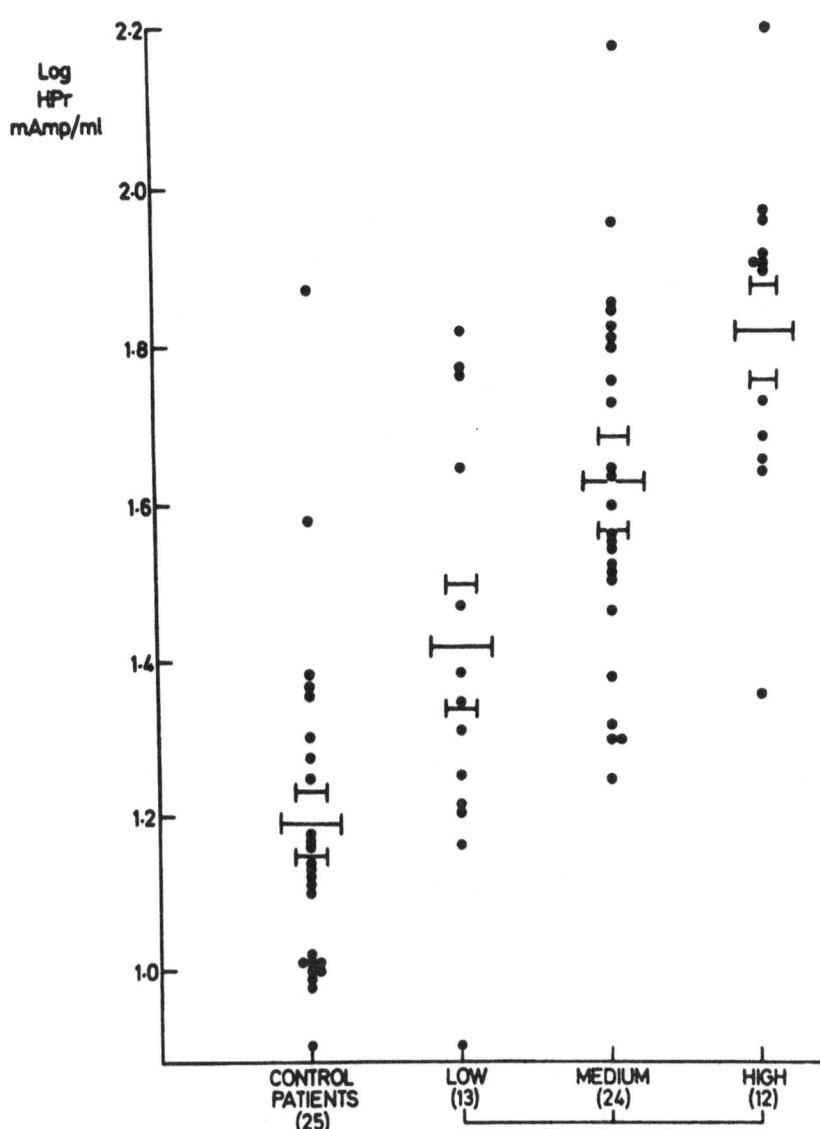

Fig. 2.   Plasma prolactin in control women and those receiving
          thioridazine. The difference between control and low
          (20-30 mg.) and medium (40-80 mg.), and between medium
          and high ($>$ 80 mg.) dose groups were significant.
          (From Wilson et al., 1975).

on DA turnover. These results are in agreement with what could be
expected on the basis of animal experiments.

b. Neuroleptics and Activity of Postsynaptic DA receptors

The prolactin concentrations in blood and CSF provide an index
of the activity of postsynaptic DA receptors. Prolactin (luteotropin)
is a hormone produced exclusively in the anterior lobe of the
hypophysis, whose production and release are regulated by the so-
called prolactin-inhibiting factor (PIF). PIF is a peptide produced
in the hypothalamus, whose production is influenced by DA-ergic
neurons of the tuberoinfundibular system. Increased DA-ergic
activity increases the PIF production, as a result of which the
production and release of prolactin diminish and its concentration
in blood and CSF decreases. The reverse is observed when DA-ergic
activity diminishes. Whenever a substance reduces the activity of
postsynaptic DA receptors, therefore, an increased prolactin concentration in blood and CSF is to be expected. This effect indeed
presents itself in response to neuroleptics of the phenothiazine
type (Fig. 2), and this is a strong argument that transmission in
central DA-ergic neurons does in fact diminish (Wilson et al. 1975;
Meltzer et al. 1975).

c. Conclusion

Neuroleptics of the phenothiazine and the butyrophenone type
increase the human central DA turnover, Since in addition they
increase the prolactin concentration in blood and CSF, this effect
is probably based on inhibited transmission in DA-ergic neurons,
and not on increased DA-ergic transmission.

IS THERE A CORRELATION BETWEEN REDUCED DA-ERGIC TRANSMISSION AND THE CLINICAL EFFECTS OF NEUROLEPTICS?

a. Therapeutic Effects

Design. In 32 patients hospitalized in the research unit of
the Department of Biological Psychiatry in Groningen for acute
schizophrenic psychoses, probenecid-induced HVA accumulation was
determined before medication (drug-free) and after 10-14 days'
neuroleptic medication (Van Praag and Korf 1975b, 1976). The patients'
clinical condition was regularly assessed by two evaluators: a
research nurse and a physician, using a 10-item 5-point rating
scale.

The patients were treated with chlorpromazine (Largactil; n = 12), haloperidol (Serenase; n = 10) or perphenazine (Trilafon; n = 10), the dosage being kept flexible in that thrice daily a capsule was given which contained a varying quantity of the neuroleptic prescribed. The capsules were of identical appearance. The dosage was determined daily by the psychiatrist not involved in the scoring, who aimed at an optimal therapeutic efficacy. The mean daily dose was 425 mg chlorpromazine, 10 mg haloperidol and 20 mg perphenazine.

Results. Fig. 3 shows the correlation between the percentual increase in HVA response due to neuroleptics on the one hand, and the improvement scores on the other. The term 'improvement score' denotes the difference between the pretherapeutic total scores and those during the second week of medication. A positive correlation was found (p $<$ 0.03), which means that the therapeutic effect was as much more marked as the increase in HVA response compared with the pretherapeutic value was more marked.

This correlation is not mainly based on the sedative action component of the neuroleptics (Fig. 4). When the percentual increase in HVA response is plotted against the improvement scores for the three prototypical psychotic symptoms delusion, hallucination and anxiety, the positive correlation persists (p $<$ 0.05).

b. Hypokinetic-Rigid Symptoms

In the same group of patients used in the preceding study, an effort was made to establish whether the increase in HVA response correlates with the occurrence of hypokinetic-rigid symptoms, if any.

Fig. 5 demonstrates the fact that such a correlation exists. In the total group of patients who developed hypokinetic-rigid symptoms during neuroleptic medication, the HVA response showed a more marked increase than that in the patients without these motor symptoms (p $<$ 0.05).

A second study was devoted to a possible correlation between DA turnover and hypokinetic-rigid symptoms. The reasoning behind it was: if inhibition of transmission in DA-ergic systems underlies neuroleptic parkinsonism, then it is to be expected that patients with a low pretherapeutic DA turnover are most susceptible to this side effect. We tested this hypothesis in 43 patients treated with various doses of chlorpromazine or haloperidol (Van Praag and Korf 1976). In the 11 patients who developed hypokinetic-rigid symptoms during neuroleptic medication, the pretherapeutic HVA response was significantly lower than that in the group without motor disorders (p $<$ 0.05).

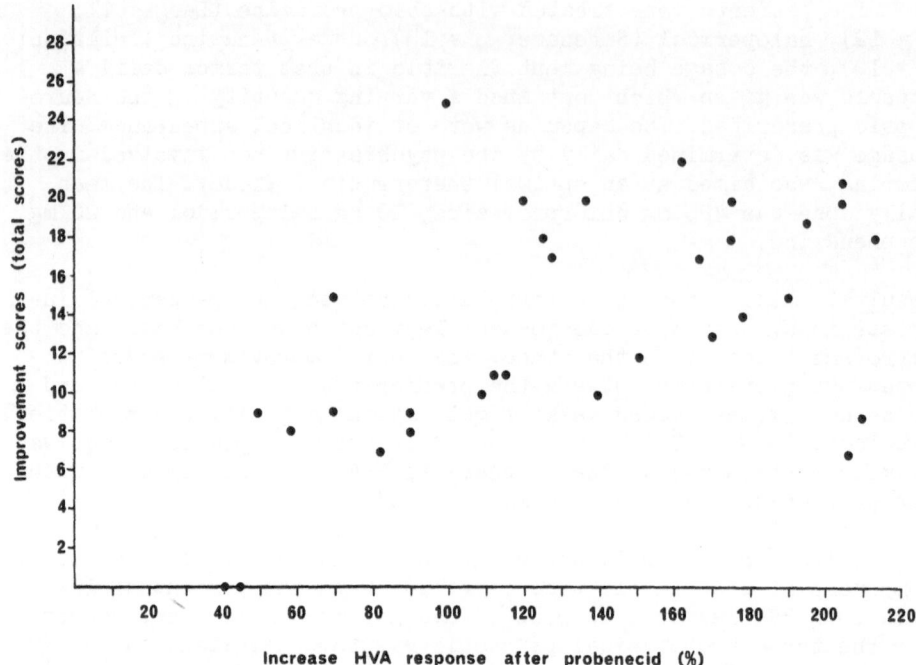

Fig. 3.   Correlation between increase in HVA response to probenecid
          and overall clinical improvement.
          x-axis: percentage increase of HVA response at end of
                   first week of medication in relation to prethera-
                   peutic response.
          y-axis: difference between pretherapeutic total score and
                   total score at end of first week of medication
                   with chlorpromazine, haloperidol or perphenazine.

                              c. Conclusion

     The increased DA turnover in the CNS (viewed as an index of
the inhibition of transmission in DA-ergic systems) shows a significant correlation with the therapeutic effect of neuroleptics
and with the occurrence of parkinson-like symptoms. Moreover, patients
with a low pretherapeutic DA turnover proved to be particularly susceptible to these side effects. These are strong, direct indications
that the clinical effects of neuroleptics are indeed correlated with
changes in DA-ergic transmission.

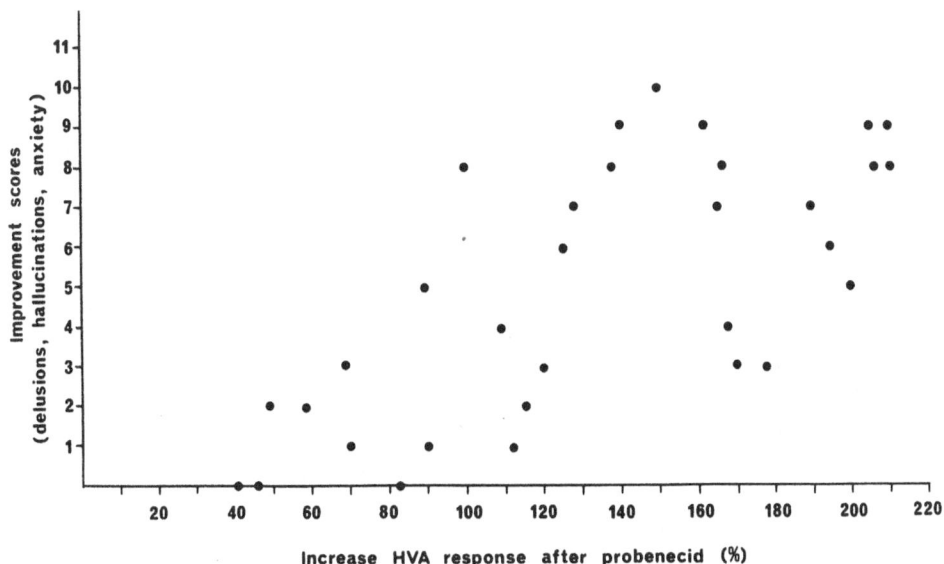

Fig. 4.   Correlation between increase of HVA response to probenecid
and clinical improvement of some prototypically psychotic symptoms.
x-axis: as in figure 3.
y-axis: difference between pretherapeutic score and score at end
          of first week of medication for items delusion, halluci-
          nation and anxiety.

THE PREDICTIVE VALUE OF THE BIOCHEMICAL ACTION
PROFILE OF NEUROLEPTICS

     The chemical structure of a compound determines whether it is
able to act as a neuroleptic (Horn and Snyder, 1971; Horn et al.,
1975). The term "neuroleptics", however, is a collective noun for
drugs with sedative and antipsychotic properties, and gives no
precise information on the pattern of therapeutic actions and side
effects that one can expect of a given compound. Its informative
value is of the same order of magnitude as that of the term "heart
drugs" as a collective noun for drugs in use for heart diseases.
Considering the limited extent wherein the chemical structure of a
neuroleptic is predictive of its profile of clinical actions, we
raised the question whether their biochemical actions, specifically
the extent to which they block DA-ergic or NA-ergic transmission,
have a higher predictive value. With respect to this question we
have so far carried out two studies.

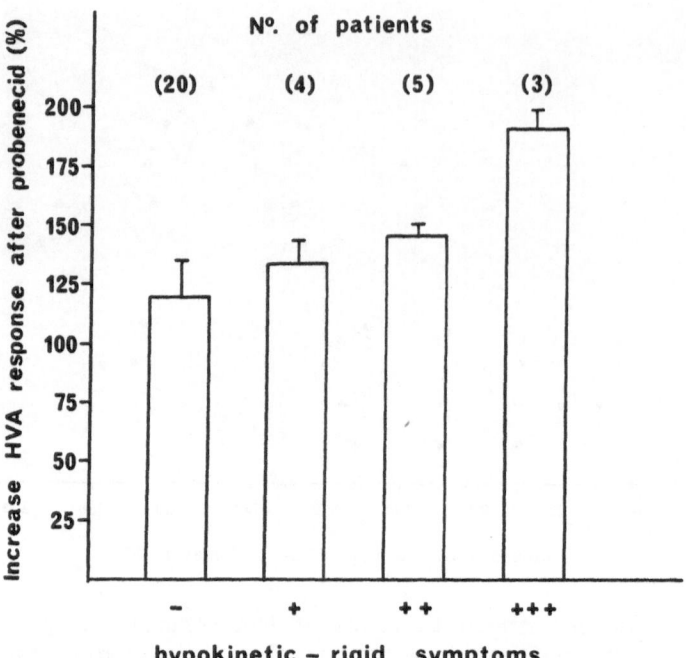

Fig. 5.   Increase of HVA response to probenecid in % of prethera-
          peutic response, in patients who during medication with
          chlorpromazine, haloperidol or perphenazine developed no
          (-), mild (+), moderate (++) or severe (+++) hypokinetic-
          rigid symptoms.

                    a.   Chlorpromazine versus oxypertine

Problem definition. First of all we made a comparative study of the
clinical efficacy of chlorpromazine (Largactil) and oxypertine
(Opertil) in patients with acute psychoses of diverse aetiology
and symptomatology (Van Praag et al. 1975b). The choice of these
two compounds was determined by biochemical considerations.

     Chlorpromazine increases the turnover of DA and NA in the brain
in test animals: an indication that DA as well as NA receptors are
blocked (Anden et al. 1970). The human central DA turnover also increases, but the NA metabolism is not demonstrably influenced; this,
however, may be due to the method used (Van Praag and Korf 1975a).
Because probenecid does not inhibit transport of 3-methoxy-4-hydroxy-
phenylglycol (MHPG) from the CNS (Korf et al. 1971), we must rely on
determination of the baseline concentration of MHPG in the CSF for

information on the central NA metabolism; and baseline concentrations of MA metabolites are a less faithful reflection of the metabolism of the mother amines than the postprobenecid concentrations (Van Praag 1976a). We note in passing that MHPG is the principal NA metabolite in the CNS.

Oxypertine is a neuroleptic of a different type (Hassler et al. 1970). It does not block CA receptors but causes depletion of intraneuronal CA stores, and in this respect it is fairly selective. Within a given dosage range, oxypertine has a predilection for NA stores: the NA concentration decreases, that of the NA metabolites increases, but the DA metabolism is hardly influenced. Its activity in human individuals is probably similar (Van Praag and Korf 1975a). A substance which more or less selectively blocks central NA receptors was not available at the time and still is not. The two compounds were selected because chlorpromazine reduces both DA-ergic and NA-ergic transmission, while oxypertine reduces mainly NA-ergic transmission. On the basis of the biochemical action of these neuroleptics, the following hypotheses were tested.

1. Chlorpromazine is superior to oxypertine as overall therapeutic agent in psychoses. The difference is based on a more pronounced therapeutic effect of chlorpromazine on delusions and hallucinations.

Motivation: an increase in central DA-ergic activity may be a psychosis-provoking factor. The principal indication that this is so is that amphetamines and l-DOPA can induce psychotic symptoms in normal individuals and cause exacerbation of these symptoms in psychotic patients; and both drugs increase central DA-ergic activity, be it via different routes (Snyder et al. 1970; Snyder 1973). In addition, fusaric acid, an inhibitor of DA-β-hydroxylase, was found to be detrimental in patients with psychoses of the manic type (Sacks and Goodwin, 1975), and after inhibition of this enzyme reduced NA production goes hand in hand with increased DA production (all available DOPA now being converted to DA). In the context of this hypothesis, a neuroleptic with a low anti-DA effect must be expected to have a relatively small antipsychotic effect.

2. Chlorpromazine and oxypertine are equivalent in sedative effect, but oxypertine is superior in cases in which loss of initiative is the predominant symptom.

Motivation: in test animals, both reduction of central DA concentration and reduction of central NA concentration lead to a decrease in motor activity (Svensson and Waldeck 1970). Nothing is known with certainty about the distribution of tasks between DA-ergic and NA-ergic systems. According to Barbeau (1972a, 1972b), DA is essential for starting movements (the so-called set), while NA is more involved in maintaining a state of motor activity (the so-called drive). Reduction of both the set component and the drive

component of motor activity clinically leads to hypokinesia. In
agreement with Barbeau's view, it is particularly the starting of
movements that is impeded in Parkinson's disease with its typical
defects in the DA-ergic system. By Barbeau's reasoning oxypertine,
with its limited effect on the DA system, can be expected to cause
little or no inertia.

3. Chlorpromazine exerts a stronger influence on extrapyramidal
motor functions than does oxypertine.

     Motivation: a decrease in DA-ergic activity leads to hypomoti-
lity in test animals, and to hypokinetic-rigid symptoms in human
subjects (Hornykiewicz 1966). A limited influence on the DA-ergic
system therefore warrants the expectation that parkinsonoid symptoms
in response to such a neuroleptic will be slight.

Results. I mention only the conclusions drawn from this study. In
agreement with the first hypothesis, the overall therapeutic effect
of oxypertine was less than that of chlorpromazine. The difference
was based on two factors. To begin with, the influence of chlorpromazine on delusions exceeded that of oxypertine. Hallucinations were
favourably influenced by chlorpromazine, whereas oxypertine was ineffective in this respect; this difference, however, did not attain
a statistically significant level. Secondly, chlorpromazine exerted
a favourable influence on motor unrest and anxiety, whereas oxypertine did not; in fact the latter was found capable of inducing these
symptoms. Of the second hypothesis, postulating that chlorpromazine
and oxypertine are equivalent in sedative effect but assigning superiority to oxypertine in the treatment of loss of initiative, only
the second term was confirmed, not the first. Chlorpromazine had no
therapeutic effect on inertia, and in a few patients induced this
symptom. Oxypertine, however, proved to be a psychomotor stimulant;
in no patient did it induce inertia. In inert patients with motor
retardation, this effect resulted in an improved clinical condition;
but in patients with anxious agitation it caused clinical deterioration due to an increased level of anxiety. Chlorpromazine, finally,
exerted a significantly stronger influence on the extrapyramidal
system than oxypertine; and this confirms the third starting-hypo-
thesis.

            b. Perphenazine Versus Clozapine

     In a second study of this type, the therapeutic potency of
clozapine (Leponex) was compared with that of perphenazine (Trilafon).
The former exerts a less marked influence on central DA turnover
than the latter, both in test animals and in patients (Van Praag
et al. 1976; Westerink and Korf 1975a). On the basis of this fact
it was expected that perphenazine would be superior to clozapine
in antipsychotic effect. This hypothesis was confirmed. Clozapine

was unmistakably superior in sedative effect - a difference which
could be based on a more pronounced suppression of NA-ergic transmission.

In any case, the data discussed would seem to suggest that the
biochemical action profile of neuroleptics is probably more predictive of their clinical effects than their chemical structure. Apart
from the practical importance of this observation, it enhances the
plausibility of the hypothesis that changes in central CA metabolism
caused by neuroleptics are of essential importance for their clinical
efficacy.

c. Conclusions

The factor 'chemical structure' has only limited importance in
explaining differences in clinical efficacy between different neuroleptics. Neuroleptics also differ in the ratio DA:NA receptor-blocking
potency, and their classification on the basis of this criterion is
at odds with the classification based on chemical structure. The
question arises whether this biochemical property is a better pre-
dictor of clinical efficacy than the chemical structure. In view
of the only two experiments so far made in this context, this conclusion is in fact justifiable. The theoretical importance of this
observation is that it enhances the plausibility of the hypothesis
that reduction of central DA-ergic and NA-ergic activity is of essential importance for the clinical effects of neuroleptics.

THE DA METABOLISM IN ACUTE SCHIZOPHRENIC PSYCHOSES

Neuroleptics - a group of compounds heterogeneous in terms of
chemical structure - all have the ability to suppress transmission
in central DA-ergic neurons. Non-neuroleptic phenothiazines differ
from their therapeutically active counterparts by lack of DA-anta-
gonistic potency (Matthysse, 1973). This observation warrants the
question whether hyperactivity in central DA-ergic systems is or
can be involved in syndromes which show a favourable response to
neuroleptics, such as psychoses.

a. Design

In the group of 33 patients with acute types of schizophrenia
already mentioned in section 4, we analysed the results of the pretherapeutic probenecid test (Van Praag et al. 1975a; Van Praag and
Korf 1975a). According to two independent evaluators, all patients
showed manifest delusions and hallucinations. This selection was
made, firstly in order to avoid discussion of the question whether
or not the patients were psychotic, and secondly in order to achieve

optimal demarcation of the group from that of the depressions. In this way, 'contamination' could only be caused by patients suffering from melancholia, i.e. deep vital depression with delusions of guilt, sin and poverty. Such patients can be identified with relative ease, however, and were excluded from this study. The group was heterogeneous in terms of aetiology, but comprised mainly psychogenic psychoses and psychoses diagnosed as schizophrenia (Van Praag 1976c).

b. Results

The postprobenecid HVA response in the CSF was slightly higher in the group of psychoses than in the control group, the difference being hardly spectacular and not significant. The situation changed, however, when the group was divided into three subgroups on the basis of independent evaluations made by the research nurse and attending physician concerning the items motor activity and anxiety (Fig. 6), as follows:
1) Patients assessed as: severely agitated. All these patients also scored a high degree of anxiety (n = 10).
2) Patients showing severe anxiety and tension but no or only slight motor unrest (n = 8).
3) Patients who, in spite of delusions and/or hallucinations, showed neither motor unrest nor any serious degree of anxiety (n = 15).

In this division the first subgroup stands out in that the HVA response was significantly increased - a finding indicative of hyperactivity of DA-ergic neuronal systems. In the second sub-group the HVA accumulation was slightly but not significantly increased. In the third subgroup it was quite normal. No correlation was found between the aetiology of the psychoses and the increase or non-increase of the postprobenecid HVA accumulation.

c. Conclusion

An increased DA turnover can exist in psychoses, but this phenomenon seems less dependent on the factor aetiology of the psychosis or the presence of 'true' psychotic symptoms (delusion and hallucination) than on the presence or absence of motor unrest.

In a group of acute schizophrenics Post et al. (1975) also found a normal HVA response to probenecid. Bowers (1974) and Kirstein et al. (1976) reported decreased postprobenecid HVA values in one study, and increased values in another. The variability of his results likewise raises the suspicion that the disorders of the DA metabolism are not so much related to the syndrome schizophrenia or the disease entity schizophrenia as to a particular component (or to a particular subgroup, as yet unidentified in psychopathological terms). The serum prolactin level, a peripheral indicator

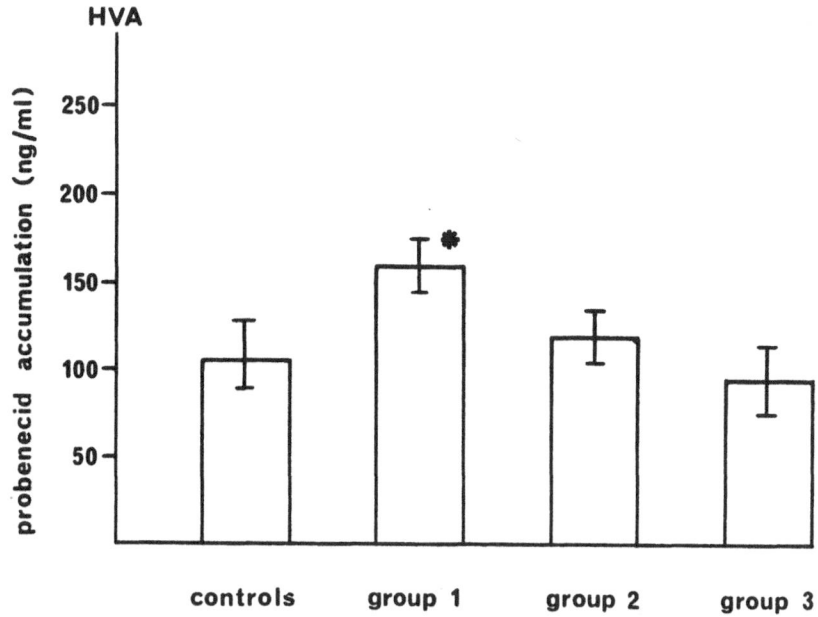

Fig. 6.   HVA accumulation in the CSF after probenecid administration
          in psychotic patients with maifest delusions and/or hallu-
          cinations. Group 1 = Marked motor agitation and anxiety;
          group 2 = Marked anxiety but no or no pronounced motor
          agitation; group 3 = No or no pronounced motor agitation
          or anxiety.   *P $<$ 0.05 (Student's t-test).

of central DA-ergic activity, is normal in schizophrenic patients
(Meltzer et al. 1974; Fig. 7).

    In all, there are no indications that hyperactivity in DA-ergic
systems plays a decisive role in the pathogenesis of acute schizophrenic psychoses.

CONCLUSIONS

a.   DA and Clinical Effects of Neuroleptics

    Neuroleptics are substances of diverse chemical structure which
nevertheless have two similarities in common: they reduce transmission in central CA-ergic systems and they have a therapeutic
effect on psychoses. This warrants the question whether these two
characteristics of neuroleptics are correlated. Such a correlation
is indeed plausible, at least so far as disturbed DA-ergic trans-

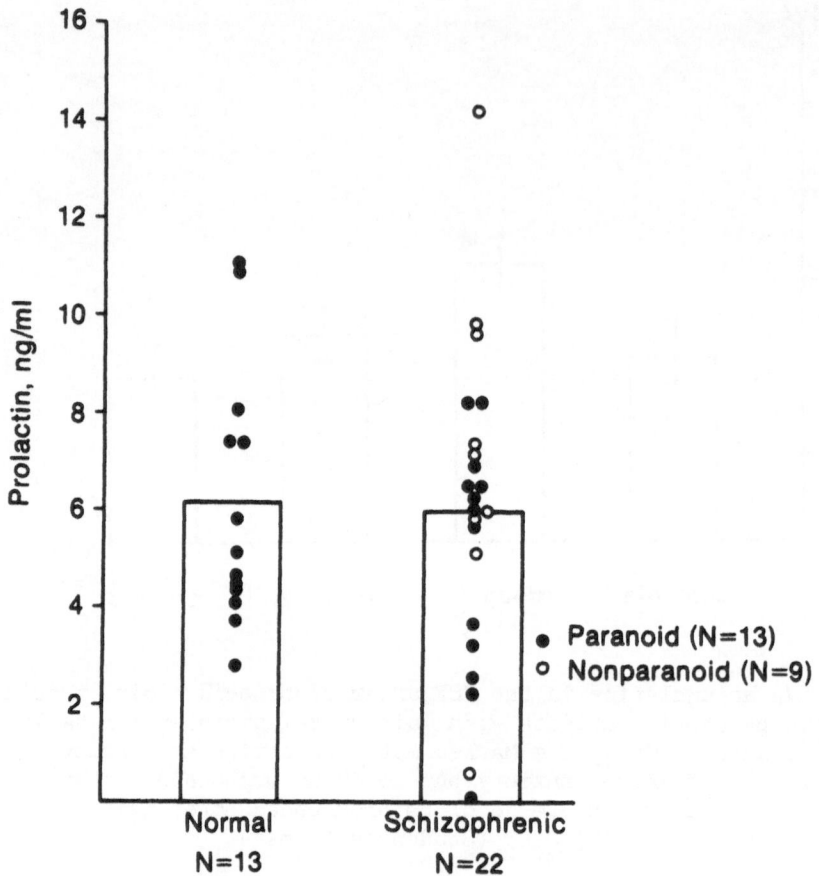

Fig. 7.   Serum prolactin levels in controls and schizophrenic
          patients at admission to the hospital (From Meltzer et
          al., 1974).

mission is concerned:

1) Neuroleptics of the receptor-blocking type increase the probenecid-induced accumulation of HVA in lumbar CSF - a phenomenon
accepted as an indicator of increased DA turnover in the CNS.

2) Since these compounds increase the prolactin concentration in
blood and CSF, the increased DA turnover is probably secondary to
inhibition of transmission, and not an expression of increased
transmission activity.

3) A positive correlation exists between the degree of increase

in DA turnover during neuroleptic medication and the strength of
the therapeutic effect; this is an indication that the two factors
are correlated. There is likewise a positive correlation between
the increase in DA turnover and the occurrence of hypokinetic-
rigid symptoms. Moreover, the risk that these side effects occur
is greater at a low than at a high pretherapeutic DA turnover.
This fact also indicates that DA turnover and neuroleptic parkinsonism are indeed related.

4) There are indications that the ratio DA-ergic: NA-ergic transmission inhibition exerts an influence on the clinical action profile of a neuroleptic. Such a correlation would be unlikely if
suppression of CA-ergic activity had nothing to do with the clinical
effects of neuroleptics.

     Neuroleptics of the receptor-blocking type block not only DA-
ergic but also NA-ergic transmission. The significance of this fact
for their clinical effects is not entirely understood. There are
indications that propranolol, a β-blocker which centrally blocks
postsynaptic NA receptors but leaves DA receptors uninfluenced,
can have a therapeutic effect on schizophrenic psychoses (Atsmon
et al. 1971, 1972; Steiner et al. 1973; Yorkston et al. 1975)
although this work still needs confirmation in a controlled trial.
In view of this, there are sound reasons for further investigation
of the NA-ergic system in its relation to the clinical effects of
neuroleptics.

          b.   DA and the Pathogenesis of Schizophrenic Psychoses

     If transmission inhibition in DA neurons and antipsychotic
effects of neuroleptics are related, then it is an obvious inference
that increased transmission activity in DA neurons plays a role in
the pathogenesis of (schizophrenic) psychoses. There are only indirect arguments in favour of this hypothesis. Drugs which can be
expected to increase activity in DA-ergic systems, particularly
amphetamines and 1-DOPA, are psychosis-provoking and intensify
schizophrenic symptoms (Snyder 1973; Randrup and Munkvad 1972;
Munkvad 1975). Compounds which inhibit synthesis of DA (and NA)
potentiate the therapeutic effect of neuroleptics (Carlsson et al.
1972, 1973). However, there are no direct arguments to support the
above hypothesis: the central DA turnover can be increased in schizophrenic (and other) psychoses, but this corresponds with increased
motor activity rather than with the presence of prototypical psychotic symptoms such as delusion and hallucination. The normal serum
prolactin level, too, is no indication of increased central DA
activity.

     A possible explanation of the negativity of these findings is
that the HVA concentration in CSF reflects mainly the DA metabolism

in the nigrostriatal DA system, whereas serum prolactin is a function of the DA activity in the tuberoinfundibular DA system. There
are no methods which supply information on the human limbic DA system, and it may be precisely this system that is involved in the
pathogenesis of psychotic symptoms.

Moreover, it is of course to be borne in mind that the mechanism
of action of a therapeutically active drug does not necessarily co-
incide with or is located near the substrate of the symptoms controlled with the aid of this drug. Example: anticholinergic drugs
are effective antiparkinson drugs. Nevertheless, it is not the
cholinergic but the DA-ergic system which plays the principal role
in many cases of Parkinson's disease.

c. Aetiology and Pathogenesis

The preceding subsection discusses the pathogenesis of schizophrenic psychoses. In this context I define pathogenesis as the
complex of cerebral functional disorders which is instrumental in
disturbing behaviour. This is not a euphemistic version of the view
that 'schizophrenia is a biochemical disease'. Numerous factors can
contribute to a disorder of behaviour. Not only acquired or hereditary imperfections in the cerebral machinery, of course, but
equally such factors as intrapsychic conflicts and tensions in
human relations. However, I presume that these factors - which I
call aetiological factors - do not affect behaviour directly, via
some sort of vacuum, but via functional changes in the cerebral
machinery; and these changes collectively constitute the cerebral
substrate of the behaviour disorders. Speaking of schizophrenia:
biochemical changes in the brain enable this complex of behaviour
disorders to occur. In this sense schizophrenia, like any other
disorder of behaviour, is a biochemical disease. A different
question is how schizophrenic behaviour disorders, including the
cerebral substrate which generates them, are causes: mainly by
psychosocial factors, by somatic factors (acquired or hereditary),
or by a combination of these. This is a problem or a different order,
and subject to differences of opinion (Van Praag, 1976c).

In my view the discussion of the causation of behaviour disorders would be well-served if investigators would not simply refer
to 'causes' but would clearly differentiate between aetiological
and pathogenetic factors (Van Praag 1971).

SUMMARY

Animal experiments have demonstrated the likelihood that all
known neuroleptics inhibit transmission in central CA-ergic systems,
regardless of their chemical structure and via different mechanisms.

For clinical psychiatry this fact prompts a number of questions:
1) is this phenomenon also to be found in human individuals;
2) if so, is it of importance for the clinical (side) effects of
neuroleptics; 3) do patients with (schizophrenic) psychoses show
signs of central CA-ergic hyperactivity. This article presents a
survey of clinical research focused on these questions which, for
the sake of brevity, is confined to DA metabolism. The available
data indicate the plausibility of a correlation between inhibition
of DA-ergic transmission on the one hand, and on the other hand the
therapeutic effects of neuroleptics and the occurrence of hypokinetic
-rigid symptoms. The hypothesis that DA-ergic hyperactivity is an
important pathogenetic mechanism in schizophrenic psychoses can be
based only on indirect arguments; direct studies of the DA metabolism have so far failed to reveal supporting evidence. The possible
causes of this failure are discussed. The final section stresses
the importance of differentiating between aetiological and pathogenetic factors in discussing the origin of behaviour disorders.

REFERENCES

ANDEN, N.E., BUTCHER, S.G., CORRODI, H., FUXE, K., UNGERSTEDT, U.:
    Receptor activity and turnover of dopamine and noradrenaline
    after neuroleptics. J. Pharmacol. 11: 303-314, 1970.

ATSMON, A., BLUM, I., MAOZ, B., STEINER, M., ZEIGELMAN, G.,
WIJSENBEEK, H.: The short-term effects of adrenergic blocking agents
    in a small group of psychotic patients: preliminary clinical
    observations. Psychiatr. Neurol. Neurochir. 74: 251-258, 1971.

ATSMON, A., BLUM, I., STEINER, M., LATZ, A., WIJSENBEEK, H.: Further
    studies with propranolol in psychotic patients. Psychopharma-
    cologia 27: 249-254, 1972.

BARBEAU, A.: Dopamine and mental function. In: L-DOPA and behavior
    (ed) S. Malitz, Raven Press, New York, 1972a.

BARBEAU, A.: Role of dopamine in the nervous system. Monographs in
    Human Genetics. 6: 114-130, 1972b.

BOWERS, M.B. Jr.: Acute psychosis induced by psychomimetic drug
    abuse. II. Neurochemical findings. Arch. Gen. Psychiatry.
    27: 440-442, 1972.

BOWERS, M.B. Jr.: Clinical measurements of central dopamine and
    5-hydroxytryptamine metabolism: reliability and interpretation
    of cerebrospinal fluid acid monoamine metabolite measures.
    Neuropharmacology 11: 101-111, 1972.

BOWERS, M.B., Jr.: 5-Hydroxyindoleacetic acid (5-HIAA) and homo-
    vanillic acid (HVA) following probenecid in acute psychotic
    patients treated with phenothiazines. Psychopharmacologia
    28: 309-318, 1973.

BOWERS, M.B., Jr.: Central dopamine turnover in schizophrenic syn-
    dromes. Arch. Gen. Psychiatry. 31: 50-54, 1974.

CARLSSON, A., PERSSON, T., ROOS, B-E., WÅLINDER, J.: Potentiation
    of phenothiazines by α-methyl-tyrosine in treatment of chronic
    schizophrenia. J. Neural. Transm. 33: 83-90, 1972.

CARLSSON, A., ROOS, B-E., WÅLINDER, J., SKOTT, A.: Further studies
    on the mechanism of antipsychotic action: potentiation by
    α-methyl-tyrosine of thioridazine effects in chronic schizo-
    phrenia. J. Neural. Transm. 34: 125-132, 1973.

CHASE, T.N.: Drug-induced extrapyramidal disorders. In: Neurotrans-
    mitters (ed) I.J. Kopin, Williams and Wilkins, Baltimore,
    448-471, 1972.

GOODWIN, F.K., POST, R.M., DUNNER, D.L. and GORDON, E.K.: Cerebro-
    spinal fluid amine metabolism in affective illness: the pro-
    benecid technique. Amer. J. Psychiatry 130: 73-79, 1973.

HASSLER, R., BAK, I.J., KIM, J.S.: Unterschiedliche Entleerung der
    Speicherorte für Noradrenalin, Dopamin und Serotonin als
    Wirkungsprinzip des Oxypertins. Nervenartz 41: 105-118, 1970.

HORN, A.S., POST, M.L. and KENNARD, O.: Dopamine receptor blockade
    and the neuroleptics, a crystallographic study. J. Pharm.
    Pharmacol. 27: 553-563, 1975.

HORN, A.S. and SNYDER, S.H.: Chlorpromazine and dopamine. Confor-
    mational similarities that correlate with the antischizophrenic
    activity of phenothiazine drugs. Proc. Nat. Ac. Sc. 68:
    2325-2328, 1971.

HORNYKIEWICZ, O: Dopamine (3-hydroxytyramine) and brain function.
    Pharmacol. Rev. 18: 925-964, 1966.

IVERSEN, L.L.: Dopamine receptors in the brain. Science 188:
    1084-1089, 1975.

KIRSTEIN, A., BOWERS, M,: CSF amine metabolites, clinical symptoms
    and body movement in psychiatric patients. Biol. Psychiatry,
    1976.

KORF, J., PRAAG, H.M. van: Amine metabolism in human brain: further
    evaluation of the probenecid test. Brain Res. 35: 221-230, 1971.

KORF,J., PRAAG, H.M. VAN, SEBENS, J.B.: Effect of intravenously administered probenecid in humans on the levels of 5-hydroxy-indoleacetic acid, homovanillic acid and 3-methoxy-4-hydroxy-phenyl-glycol in cerebrospinal fluid. Biochem. Pharmacol. 20: 659-668, 1971.

KORF, J., SCHUTTE, H.H., VENEMA, K.: A semi-automated fluorometric determination of 5-hydroxyindoles in the nanogram range. Anal. Biochem. 53: 146-153, 1973.

MATTHYSSE, I.: Antipsychotic drug actions: a clue to the neuro-pathology of schizophrenia? Feder. Proc. 32: 200-205, 1973.

MELTZER, H., SACHAR, E.J., FRANTZ, A.G.: Serum prolactin levels in unmedicated schizophrenic patients. Arch. Gen. Psychiatry. 31: 564-569, 1974.

MELTZER, H., SACHAR, E.J., FRANTZ, A.G.: Dopamine antagonism by thioridazine in schizophrenia. Biol. Psychiatry. 10: 53-57, 197, 1975.

MUNKVAD, I., FOG, R., RANDRUP, A.: Amphetamine psychosis: A useful model of schizophrenia? In: On the origin of schizophrenic psychoses. (ed) H.M van Praag, De Erven Bohn B.V. Amsterdam, 1975.

NYBÄCK, H., SEDVALL, G.: Further studies on the accumulation and disappearance of catecholamines formed from ^{14}C in mouse brain. Effect of some phenothiazine analogues. Eur. J. Pharmacol. 10: 193-205, 1970.

O'KEEFE, R., SHARMAN, D.F., VOGT, M.: Effect of drugs used in psy-choses on cerebral dopamine metabolism. Br. J. Pharmacol. 38: 287-304, 1970.

POST, R.M., FINK, E., CARPENTER, W.T., GOODWIN, F.K.: Cerebrospinal fluid amine metabolites in acute schizophrenia. Arch. Gen. Psychiatry 32: 1063-1069, 1975.

PRAAG, H.M. VAN.: The possible significance of cerebral dopamine for neurology and psychiatry. Psychiatr. Neurol. Neurochir. 70: 361-379, 1967.

PRAAG, H.M. VAN.: The position of biological psychiatry among the psychiatric disciplines. Compr. Psychiatry. 12: 1-7, 1971.

PRAAG, H.M. VAN., KORF, J., SCHUT, T.: Cerebral monoamines and depression. An investigation into their correlation with the aid of the probenecid technique. Arch. Gen. Psychiatry. 28: 827-831, 1973.

PRAAG, H.M. VAN, KORF, J., LAKKE, J.P.W.F., SCHUT, T.: Dopamine
    metabolism in depressions, psychoses and parkinson's disease:
    the problem of the specificity of biological variables in
    behavior disorders. Psychol. Med. 5: 138-146, 1975a.

PRAAG, H.M. VAN., DOLS, L.C.W., SCHUT, T.: Biochemical versus
    psychopathological action profile of neuroleptics: A compara-
    tive study of chlorpromazine and oxypertine in acute psychotic
    disorders. Compr. Psychiatry. 16: 255-263, 1975b.

PRAAG, H.M. VAN.: Neuroleptics as a guideline to biological research
    in psychotic disorders. Compr. Psychiatry. 16: 7-22, 1975.

PRAAG. H.M. VAN., KORF, J.: Neuroleptics, catecholamines and psy-
    chotic disorders. A study of their interrelation. Amer. J.
    Psychiatry 132: 593-597, 1975a.

PRAAG, H.M. VAN., KORF, J.: The importance in the pathogenesis of
    psychosis and the actions of antipsychotic (neuroleptic) drugs.
    Proceedings of the Sixth International Congress of Pharmacology,
    Helsinki, 1975b (in press).

PRAAG, H.M. VAN.: Monoamine metabolism in affective disorders. In:
    Current developments in psychopharmacology (eds) W.B. Essman
    and L. Valzelli, Vol. 4, Spectrum Publications, New York, 1976b.

PRAAG, H.M. VAN.: Monoamine metabolism in schizophrenic psychosis.
    In: Current Developments in psychopharmacology (eds) W.B.
    Essman and L. Valzelli, Vol. 4, Spectrum Publication, New York,
    1976b.

PRAAG, H.M. VAN., KORF, J.: Importance of the dopamine metabolism
    for the clinical effects and side effects of neuroleptics.
    Amer. J. Psychiatry. 1976.

PRAAG, H.M. VAN.: About the impossible concept of schizophrenia.
    Compr. Psychiatry (in press), 1976c.

PRAAG, H.M. VAN., KORF, J., DOLS, L.C.W.: A comparative investiga-
    tion of the biochemical and clinical effects of clozapine and
    perphenazine in acute psychotic patients (in press) 1976.

RANDRUP, A., MUNKVAD, I.: Biochemical anatomical and psychological
    investigations of stereotyped behavior induced by amphetamines.
    In: Amphetamines and related compounds. (eds) E. Costa and
    S. Garattini, Raven Press, New York, 695-713, 1970.

RANDRUP, A., MUNKVAD, I.: Evidence indicating an association between
    schizophrenia and dopaminergic hyperactivity in the brain.
    Orthomolecul. Psychiatry. 1: 2-27, 1972.

SACK, R.L. AND GOODWIN, F.K.: Inhibition of dopamine- β -hydroxy-
    lase in manic patients. Arch. Gen. Psychiat. 31: 649-654, 1974.

SEEMAN, P., LEE, T.: Antipsychotic drugs: direct correlation between
    clinical potency and presynaptic action on dopamine neurons.
    Science 188: 1217-1219, 1975.

SJÖSTRÖM, R., ROOS, B-E.: 5-Hydroxyindoleacetic acid and homovanillic
    acid in cerebrospinal fluid in manic-depressive psychosis.
    Europ. J. Pharmacol. 4: 170-176, 1972.

SNYDER, S.H., TAYLOR, K.M., COYLE, J.R., MEYERHOFF, J.L.: The role
    of brain dopamine in behavioural regulation and the actions
    of psychotropic drugs. Amer. J. Psychiatry. 127: 199-207, 1970.

SNYDER, S.H.: Amphetamine psychosis: a "model" schizophrenia medi-
    ated by catecholamines. Amer. J. Psychiatry. 130: 61-66, 1973.

SNYDER, S.H., BANERJEE, S.P., YAMAMURA, H.I., GREENBERG, D.: Drugs,
    neurotransmitters and schizophrenia. Science 184: 1243-1253,
    1974.

STEINER, M., LATZ, A., BLUM, I., ATSMON, A., WIJSENBEEK, H.: Pro-
    pranolol versus chlorpromazine in the treatment of psychoses
    associated with childbearing. Psychiatr. Neurol. Neurochir.
    76: 421-426, 1973.

SVENSSON, T.H., WALDECK, B.: On the role of brain catecholamines
    in motor activity: experiments with inhibitors of synthesis
    and monoamine oxidase. Psychopharmacologia 18: 357-365, 1970.

WESTERINK, B.H.C., KORF, J.: Influence of drugs on striatal and
    limbic homovanillic acid concentration in the rat brain.
    Europ. J. Pharmacol. 33: 31-40, 1975a.

WESTERINK, B.H.C., KORF, J.: Determination of nanogram amounts of
    homovanillic acid in the central nervous system with a rapid
    semi-automated fluorometric method. Biochem. Med. 12: 106-114,
    1975b.

WIESEL, F.A, SEDVALL, G.: Effect of antipsychotic drugs on homo-
    vanillic acid levels in striatum and olfactory tubercle of
    the rat. Europ. J. Pharmacol. 30: 364-367, 1975.

WILSON, R.G., HAMILTON, J.R., BOYD, W.D., FORREST, A.P.M., COLE, E.N.,
    BOYNS, A.R., GRIFFITHS, K.: The effect of long-term pheno-
    thiazine therapy on plasma prolactin. Brit. J. Psychiatry.
    127: 71-74, 1975.

YORKSTON, N.J., ZAKI, S.A., MALIK, M.K.U., MORRISON, R.C., HARVARD,
    C.W.H.: Propranolol in the control of schizophrenic symptoms.
    Brit. Med. J. 4: 633-635, 1974.

A COMPARISON OF THE EFFECT OF LITHIUM AND HALOPERIDOL ON

HUMAN PERIPHERAL β-ADRENERGIC ADENYLATE CYCLASE

Richard P. Ebstein and Robert H. Belmaker

The Jerusalem Mental Health Center

P.O.B. 140, Jerusalem, Israel

Lithium (Li) is an effective therapy in the treatment and prevention of the manic phase of manic-depressive illness (1). Lithium influences a number of physiological systems including biogenic amines (2,3), membrane transport (4-6), amino acid metabolism (7,8) protein synthesis (9-11), endocrine secretion (12) and some kinds of behaviour (13-15). Although the involvement of Li in cellular processes appears to be ubiquitous, no specific mechanism has been identified for Li's therapeutic efficacy in manic-depressive illness.

In addition to the aforementioned effects of Li, this drug also affects the metabolism of cyclic AMP. The action of Li on the so-called "second messenger" is most likely mediated by its effect on adenylate cyclase since this drug inhibits the ADH-sensitive cyclase in the kidney (16,17), the TSH-stimulated adenylate cyclase in the thyroid (18,19), the prostaglandin-activated adenylate cyclase in human platelets (20,21), and the norepinephrine-sensitive adenylate cyclase in rat brain (22,23). These reports suggest the possibility that a primary physiological site of Li action is hormone-stimulated adenylate cyclase (24).

The postulated role of Li as an inhibitor of adenylate cyclase activity suggests that therapeutic concentrations of this drug in man may inhibit adenylate cyclase activity. Ball et al (25) have shown that administration of β-adrenergic agonists in healthy volunteers leads to a rise in plasma AMP levels. Plasma cyclic AMP is derived from intracellular cyclic AMP of several tissues including liver, muscle, and adipose tissue, but the rise in plasma cyclic AMP after β-adrenergic stimulation seems to result largely from stimulation of receptors other than these in the liver or adipose tissue (26). The report of Ball et al (25) suggested to us an experimental approach to examine the effect of Li in therapeutic doses on adenylate cyclase activity in man. We therefore measured the epinephrine-induced rise in plasma cyclic AMP in subjects on and off Li therapy.

The effect of epinephrine on plasma cyclic AMP levels for a group of Li-treated and control subjects is shown in Fig. 1. In the control subjects there is a rise in plasma cyclic AMP levels which commences at 10 minutes after epinephrine injection, reaches a peak at 40 minutes, and by 70 minutes almost returns to base line. Li-treated subjects show no increase in plasma cyclic AMP levels after epinephrine administration. The individual plasma cyclic AMP levels are given in Table 1 (control) and 2 (Li-treated). Examination of these individual responses reveals a marked inhibitory effect of Li on epinephrine-stimulated adenylate cyclase activity, despite considerable individual variation. Every one of the control subjects (Table 1) shows a rise in plasma cyclic AMP levels after epinephrine and the magnitude of the maximum response varies from 38 to 233%. In contrast, 5 out of 9 Li subjects (Table 2) show no rise whatsoever in plasma cyclic AMP levels, and the remaining 4 only a small increase. It should be noted that there appears to be no effect of Li on the static levels of plasma cyclic AMP suggesting that there is no effect of Li on basal adenylate cyclase activity but only on the activation of this enzyme by the hormone. Similar results have been reported for the ADH-sensitive adenylate cyclase in the kidney (16).

Table 1 reveals no relationship between clinical state or diagnosis and the degree of response to the epinephrine. Moreover, Fig. 2 shows that two normal individuals (R.E. and H.B.) who respond to epinephrine with a rise in plasma cyclic AMP levels, cease to show a response when the test is repeated after 3 days of Li treatment. This suggests that the effect of Li on epinephrine-stimulated adenylate cyclase is a pharmacologic effect of the drug and is not dependent on pre-existing pathology.

The results of this study demonstrate in vivo inhibition by therapeutic doses of Li on β-adrenergic-stimulated adenylate cyclase in humans. These findings are consistent with previous observations in vitro that Li inhibits the hormone-stimulated activity of adenylate cyclase (16-24). In addition to a direct effect of Li on adenylate cyclase, it has recently been proposed that this drug may also act at a site more distal to the synthesis of cyclic AMP (29, 30). However, the demonstration that Li blocks the epinephrine-induced rise in plasma cyclic AMP levels suggests that a more distal action of Li need not to be postulated in order to explain Li's effect on the adrenergic system.

TABLE 1. The Effect of Epinephrine on Plasma Cyclic AMP Levels

Patient, Age, Sex	Diagnosis	Clinical State	Minutes after epinephrine injection (Values in picomoles cAMP/ml plasma $\pm$ SEM)								% Maximum Increase
			0	10	20	30	40	50	60	70	
A. 28 M	Normal	------	16	13	24	36	39	39	32	26	143
B. 27 M	Normal	------	12	12	15	18	19	16	18	--	58
C. 26 M	Normal	------	12	15	19	16	19	21	15	17	75
D. 27 M	Normal	------	13	16	25	33	31	21	18	18	153
E. 32 M	Normal	------	18*	18*	18		36*	28*			100
F. 47 F	M-D	Hypomanic	9	10	19	30	24	23	20	13	233
G. 33 M	U-D	Depressed	16	15	14	16	25	26	27	20	68
H. 52 M	M-D	Euthymic	15	16	21	17	20	21	22	23	40
I. 29 M	S-A	Agitated	24	22	28	33	29	24	24	21	38
			14.6 ±1.6	14.8 ±1.3	21.0 ±1.6	24.9 ±3.1	26.7 ±2.6	23.9 ±2.4	22.0 ±2.0	19.7 ±1.6	100

Abbreviations used: M-D, Manic-depressive; S-A, Schizo-affective; U-D, Unipolar-depressive

* These values not included in the calculated mean since this subject was sampled at 15 min rather than 10 min intervals. All subjects were physically healthy, with no evidence of renal, cardio-vascular or hepatic disease.

TABLE 2.   The Effect of Lithium on the Plasma Cyclic AMP response to Epinephrine

Patient, Age, Sex	Diagnosis	Clinical State	meq/L plasma Lithium level	Minutes after epinephrine injection (Values in picomoles cAMP/ml plasma ± SEM)								% Max. Increase
				0	10	20	30	40	50	60	70	
J. 24 M	M-D	Euthymic	1.15	18	21	21	18	25	22	21	23	39
K. 45 F	M-D	Euthymic	0.90	8	7	6	8	8	6	8	8	N.C.
L. 31 F	M-D	Hypomanic	1.10	14	16	18	16	12	12	16	11	29
H. 52 M	M-D	Euthymic	0.32	16	17	17	16	15	17	19	17	N.C.
M. 55 M	S-A	Euthymic	0.94	15	14	11	11	13	13	12	13	N.C.
N. 42 M	M-D	Euthymic	0.49	18	15	18	18	16	15	17	19	N.C.
O. 37 F	U-D	Euthymic	0.25	13	14	14	14	11	12	15	19	N.C.
A. 28 M	Normal	------	0.66	14	17	16	17	17	18	17	17	21
E. 32 M	Normal	------	0.60	15	15	18	15	17	20	19	18	20
				14.6 ±1.0	15.1 ±1.2	15.4 ±1.5	14.8 ±1.1	14.9 ±1.6	15.0 ±1.6	16.0 ±1.3	16.1 ±1.5	

Abbreviations used: M-D, Manic-depressive;   S-A, Schizo-affective;   U-D, Unipolar-depressive; N.C. No change.

All subjects were physically healthy with no evidence of renal, cardio-vascular or hepatic disease.

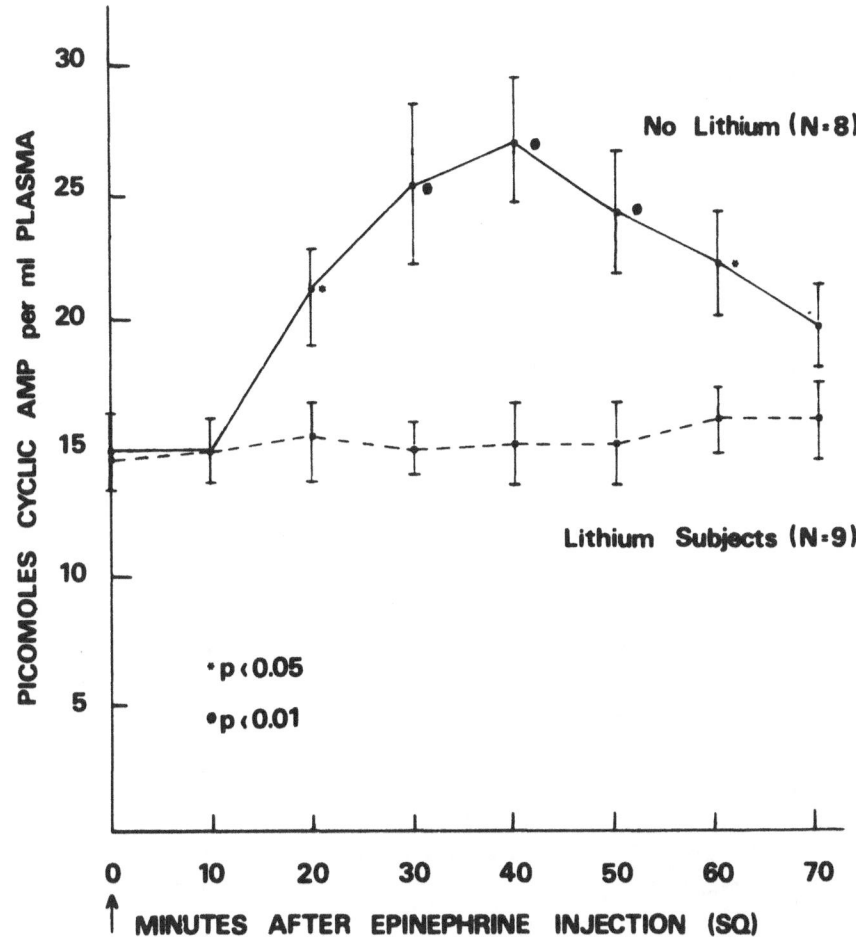

Fig. 1.   The effect of Li on plasma CAMP response
          to epinephrine administration. Subjects
          receive 0.5 mg of epinephrine subcutaneously
          at time 0 and blood was drawn every ten
          minutes using an indwelling catheter in the
          antecubital vein. Subcutaneous epinephrine
          injection was chosen rather than intravenous
          injection on grounds of greater clinical
          safety, despite the possibility of increased
          variability. Samples were collected into
          plastic test tubes containing heparin and
          theophylline. Cyclic AMP was determined by
          the protein binding method of Brown et al(27)
          as modified for plasma by Lattner and
          Prudhoe (28).

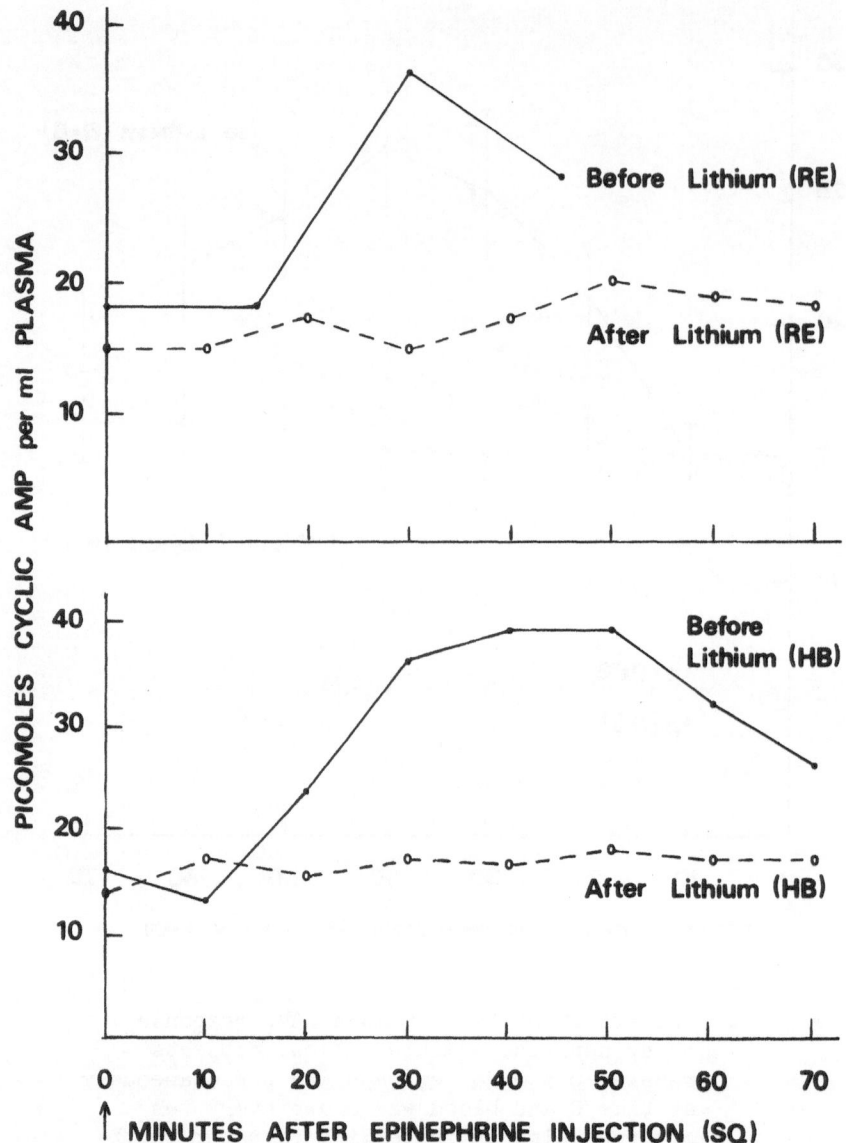

Fig. 2. The response of plasma CAMP to epinephrine before
         and after Li treatment in two normal subjects.
         After initially testing the response of plasma
         CAMP to epinephrine (SQ) in the absence of Li,
         both subjects were given Li for three days until
         a blood level of 0.60 meq/L (RE), and 0.66 (HB)
         was attained. The test was then repeated. The ex-
         perimental procedure is the same as described in
         the legend to Fig. 1.

Li's marked effect on β-adrenergic adenylate cyclase contrasts with the paucity of reports of Li effects on the peripheral cardiovascular system. Intracellular levels of cyclic AMP after receptor stimulation are probably many times greater than those occurring in extracellular fluids (26). It is possible that intracellular cyclic AMP responses, even after Li administration, are adequate to maintain homeostatic integrity. Fann et al. (31) have shown, however, that Li does decrease the pressor response to infused norepinephrine by 22%.

The catecholamine hypothesis of affective disorders postulates that mania is characterized by a functional excess of norepinephrine at a site in the central nervous system (32). We have shown that in man therapeutic doses of Li inhibit the peripheral β-adrenergic-stimulated adenylate cyclase. The brain norepinephrine-stimulated adenylate cyclase and the peripheral β-adrenergic-stimulated adenylate cyclase may be related since both synthesize cyclic AMP after hormonal stimulation. This is in contrast to stimulation of the peripheral α-adrenergic receptor, by either epinephrine or norepinephrine, which leads to a rise in plasma cyclic GMP levels (25). Segel (1974) has shown that Li applied iontophoretically inhibits firing of noradrenergic neurons in the rat hippocampus in a manner consistent with an effect on cyclic AMP metabolism (33). It is therefore possible that the antimanic efficacy of Li is directly related to an effect on brain norepinephrine-stimulated adenylate cyclase. If so, perhaps other drugs that are efficacious in the treatment of mania have the same effect. Snyder (34), and also van Praag (35), have suggested a pharmacological strategy for understanding mental illness. These authors have proposed that if several drugs are effective in a given mental abnormality, the biochemical nature of that abnormality must be affected by a common property of all the efficacious drugs. Thus Snyder (34) advanced the dopamine hypothesis of schizophrenia partly on grounds that all antischizophrenic drugs block dopamine transmission in the brain. He found, moreover, that related compounds ineffective clinically in schizophrenia were poor dopamine blockers, and that clinical efficacy on a per mgm basis correlated with the effectiveness of antischizophrenic drugs as dopamine blockers in vitro (34).

Clinical practice has long accepted phenothiazines and more recently haloperidol as effective in the treatment of mania (36). Following the strategy of Snyder (34) and van Praag (35), we wished to see if this class of drug also affected the peripheral β-adrenergic adenylate cyclase in our model. Haloperidol was chosen as a representative of the "dopamine-blocking" or "antischizophrenic" drugs for two reasons. Firstly, some clinicians consider it the most effective against mania of this class (37) and secondly, it has minimal cardio-vascular side effects mediated by α-adrenergic blocking (38). Chlorpromazine, by contrast, has strong α-adrenergic blocking effects that could conceivably also effect the β-receptors in our model (38). Blocking by chlorpromazine in our model might

TABLE 3. The Effect of Haloperidol on the Plasma Cyclic AMP response to Epinephrine

Patient, Age, Sex	Diagnosis	Clinical State	Dose (mg/day)	Minutes after epinephrine injection (Values in picomoles cAMP/ml plasma $\pm$ SEM)								% Maximum Increase
				0	10	20	30	40	50	60	70	
P. 40 M	M–D	Euthymic	30	15	22	22	17	31	16	12	12	106
Q. 28 M	S–A	Excited	80	11	18	15	35	33	28	15	15	218
R. 50 M	M–D	Hypomanic	90	13	17	14	20	18	23	17	10	76
L. 31 F	M–D	Euthymic	30	16	20	18	21	21	24	30	26	88
S. 27 F	S	Remission	60	10	10	21	20	33	22	28	11	230
T. 24 M	S	"	30	10	11	4	11	20	11	12	22	100
U. 26 M	S	"	20	12	12	10	12	11	10	12	12	N.C.
V. 45 F	S	"	30	10	20	19	18	27	21	24	22	170
W. 43 F	S	"	30	13	13	14	19	18	18	14	14	46
X. 25 M	M–D	Euthymic	50	12	10	8	10	10	12	21	14	75
			45	12.2	15.3	14.5	18.3	22.2	18.5	18.5	15.8	111

Abbreviations used: M–D, Manic-depressive, S–A, Schizo-affective S, Schizophrenic

All subjects were physically healthy with no evidence of renal, cardiovascular or hepatic disease.

only be related to this side effect. To truly test our hypothesis
according to the strategy described above, we chose a good antimanic agent (haloperidol) with little reason to expect an effect
on β-adrenergic adenylate cyclase on the basis of side effects
alone.

The effect of haloperidol on the epinephrine-stimulated rise
in plasma cyclic AMP levels is given in Table 3. Except for one
patient, all the haloperidol-treated patients show a rise in plasma
cyclic AMP levels. As in the Li-treated and untreated subjects, no
relationship is evident between clinical state or diagnosis and the
degree of response to epinephrine. The average maximum increase for
all 10 individuals was 111%. Almost identical results were obtained
for the non-drug treated individuals (100%). This is marked contrast
to Li-treated subjects where the plasma cyclic AMP response to
epinephrine stimulation is completely abolished.

The lack of inhibition by haloperidol of the peripheral
β-adrenergic adenylate cyclase may be understood in several ways.
First, of course, is the possibility that the effect of Li on the
cyclase is unrelated to its therapeutic efficacy and thus not an
essential property of other antimanic agents. Clinical literature,
however, suggests an alternative explanation. Shopsin et al (37)
found Li and haloperidol to be equally effective in the treatment
of acute mania, according to their double-blind rating scales, but
elaborate in their discussion on their clinical impression of Li's
qualitative superiority. Clinicians have suggested that Li acts
differently than the neuroleptic agents in mania, in that Li first
normalizes mood while phenothiazines or haloperidol first reduce
motor hyperactivity (39). It is possible that several systems are
disturbed in mania, and that improvement in one of them leads
gradually to improved function of the other disturbances. Thus the
clinical impression of differences between Li and haloperidol in
mania may find reflection in our finding of biochemical differences.
Li's effect on β-adrenergic adenylate cyclase may be the biochemical
basis of its unique effect on the mood component of mania.

A number of animal experiments support this concept. Originally
Dousa and Hechter (40) reported that relatively high levels of Li
(25-50 mM) inhibited the fluoride as well as epinephrine-stimulated
adenylate cyclase in rat brain. Although high levels of Li were
required, the brain adenylate cyclase was particularly sensitive
to the inhibitory action of Li. Uzonov and Weiss (41) were able to
demonstrate that Li in vivo (after acute i.p. administration)
prevented the post-mortem rise in cyclic AMP levels in rat cere-
bellum presumably by inhibiting the noradrenergic-sensitive adenylate cyclase in this region (41). Using concentrations of Li in the
therapeutic range Forn and Valdecasas (42) showed that 2 mM Li
inhibited (by 26%) the norepinephrine-stimulated rise in cyclic AMP
levels in rat cortical slices. Similar results were obtained by

Palmer et al (43) who reported that 1 mM Li significantly inhibited the norepinephrine-induced rise in cyclic AMP in rat hypothalamic slices. The inhibitory action of Li appears to be specific to the norepinephrine-stimulated adenylate cyclase since Walker using 0.5 mM Li found no effect of this drug on the dopamine-sensitive adenylate cyclase in the caudate nucleus but an equivalent dose inhibited the noradrenergic cyclase (45). It should be noted that none of these animal experiments employed chronic Li administration which of course, is the normal therapeutic treatment schedule in man. Demonstration of Li inhibition of β-adrenergic adenylate cyclase in vivo in humans complements the reports of work in animal brain, and overcomes the objection that Li effects on adenylate cyclase in vitro derive from in vitro changes in the cyclase's properties (24,41,42). The absence of an effect of haloperidol on human peripheral β-adrenergic adenylate cyclase is also paralleled by work in animal brain. Palmer et al (43,44) reported that halo- peridol did not inhibit hypothalamic norepinephrine-stimulated adenylate cyclase (though an effect on brain stem cyclase was observed).

A possible biochemical mechanism for the action of Li on adenylate cyclase may be related to the inhibitory action of Li on a number of Mg^{++} dependent enzymes (46,47). A recent report suggests that Li inhibits adenylate cyclase by forming a Mg-Li- nucleotide complex which interferes with the formation of the Mg-ATP substrate required for enzyme activity (48). These reports (40-48) suggest that Li may act in mania by inhibiting the brain norepinephrine-sensitive adenylate cyclase. Experiments are under- way in our laboratory to further elucidate the differential effect of Li both in vitro and after chronic administration, on the rat brain dopamine and norepinephrine-sensitive adenylate cyclases.

In summary, our results show that Li inhibits the peripheral β-adrenergic-stimulated adenylate cyclase in man. This action of Li and the results from a number of animal experiments (see above discussion) provide a basis for a theory of Li action in mania. It is suggested that the clinically effective role of Li is to inhibit the brain norepinephrine-sensitive adenylate cyclase. How- ever, haloperidol, an effective drug in the treatment of acute mania, does not reduce the rise in plasma cyclic AMP levels after epinephrine injection. The failure of haloperidol to act in our model system may be related to the clinically different pattern by which haloperidol and Li appear to control mania (49,50).

REFERENCES

1. SCHOU, M. and THOMSEN, K.: Lithium Research and Therapy, (ed. Johnson, F.N.), 63-84, Academic Press, N.Y., 1975.

2. SCHILDKRAUT, J.: <u>Lithium, Its Role in Psychiatric Research and</u>
    <u>Treatment</u>. (ed. Gershon S.   and Shopsin, B.), 51-73
    Plenum Press, N.Y. 1973.

3. SHAW, D.M.: <u>Lithium Research and Therapy</u>, (ed. Johnston, F.N.),
    411-423, Academic Press, N.Y., 1975.

4. COLBURN, R.W., GOODWIN, F.K., BUNNEY, W.E. Jr., and DAVIS, J.M.
    <u>Nature</u>, 215, 1395-1397, 1967.

5. MURPHY,D.L., COLBURN, R.W., DAVIS, J.M., and BUNNEY, E.W. Jr.:
    <u>Life Sci</u>.,8, 1187-1193, 1969.

6. RADOMSKI, M.W. and WATSON, W.J.: <u>Aerospace Med</u>., 44, 387-392,
    1973.

7. GOTTESFELD, Z., EBSTEIN, B.S.and SAMUEL, D.: <u>Nature New Biology</u>,
    234, 124-125, 1971.

8. BERL, S. and CLARKE, D.D.: <u>Brain Res</u>., 36, 203-213, 1972.

9. SUZUKA, I. and KAJA, A.: <u>J. Biol. Chem</u>. 243, 3136-3141, 1968.

10. TURKINGTON, R.W.: <u>Experientia,</u> 24, 226-228, 1968.

11. VOLM, M., SCHWARTZ, V. and WAYSS, K.: <u>Naturwiss,</u> 57, 250, 1970.

12. BERENS, S.C. and WOLFF, J.: <u>Lithium Research and Therapy</u>
    (ed. Johnson, F.N.), 443-472, (Academic Press, N.Y. 1975).

13. JOHNSON, F.N.: <u>Experientia,</u> <u>28</u>,533-535, 1972.

14. JOHNSON, F.N. and WORMINGTON, S.: <u>Nature New Biology</u>, <u>235</u>,
    159-160, 1972.

15. CADE, J.F.: <u>Med. J. of Austra</u>., <u>36</u>, 349-352, 1949.

16. GEISLER, A., WRASE, O. and OLESEN VENDELIN, OLE.: <u>Acta Pharmacol</u>.
    <u>et Toxicol</u>., 31, 203-208, 1972.

17. DOUSA, T., and HECHTER, O.: <u>Life Sci</u>., 9, 765-770, 1970.

18. WOLFF, J., BERENS S.C. and JONES, A.B.: <u>Biochem, Biophys. Res</u>.
    Comm., 39, 77-82, 1970.

19. BURKE, G.:<u>Biochem. Biophys. Acta</u>. 220, 30-41, 1970.

20. MURPHY, D.L., DONNELLY, C. and MOSKOWITZ, J.: <u>Clin. Pharmac</u>.
    <u>Therapeut</u>., 14, 810-814, 1973.

21. WANG, Y.C., PANDEY, G.N., MENDELS, J. and FRAZER, A.:
        Biochem. Pharmacol., 23, 845-855, 1974.

22. WALKER, J.B.: Biol. Psychiat., 8, 245-251,1974.

23. FORN, J. and VALDECASAS.: Biochem. Pharmacol., 20, 2773-2779,
        1971.

24. FORN, J.: Lithium Research and Psychotherapy, (ed. Johnson,
        F.N.), 485-497, (Academic Press, N.Y., 1975).

25. BALL, J.H., KAMINSKY, N.I., HARDMAN, J.G., BROADUS, A.E.,
        SUTHERLAND, E.W. and GRANT, W.L.: J. of Clin. Invest., 51,
        2124-2129, 1972.

26. STRANGE, R.C. and MJOS, O.D.: Europ. J. Clin. Invest., 5,
        147-152, 1975.

27. BROWN, B.L., ALBANO, J.D.M., EKINS, R.P., SGHERZI, A.M.:
        Biochem. J., 121, 561-562, 1971.

28. LATNER, A.L. and PRUDHOE, K.: Clin. Chim. Acta, 48, 353-357,
        1973.

29. FORREST, J.N.: New Engl. J. of Med., 292, 423-424, 1975.

30. COX, M. and SINGER, I.: New Engl. J. of Med., 293, 46-47, 1975.

31. FANN, W.E., DAVIS, J.M., JANOWSKY, D.S, CAVANANGH, J.H.,
        KAUFMANN, J.S., GRIFFITH, J.D., and OATES, J.D., Clin. Pharm.
        Ther. 13, 71-77, 1971.

32. SCHILDKRAUT, J.J.: Am. J. Psychiat. 122, 509-522, 1965.

33. SEGAL, M.: Nature, 250, 71-73, 1974.

34. SNYDER, S.H., BANERJEE, S.P., YAMAMURA, H.I. and GREENBERG, D.:
        Science, 184, 1243-1253, 1974.

35. PRAAG, H.M. VAN: Comprehens Psychiat. 16, 7-22, 1975.

36. KLEIN, D.K. and DAVIS, J.M.: Diagnosis and Drug Treatment of
        Psychiatric Disorders. (Williams and Wilkins, Baltimore,
        1969).

37. SHOPSIN, B., GERSHON, S., THOMPSON, H. and COLLINS, P.:
        Archiv. Gen. Psych. 32, 34-42, 1975.

38. SHADER, R.I. and DIMASCIO, A.: Psychotropic Drug Side Effects
        (Williams and Wilkins, Baltimore, 1970.)

39. TAKASHI, R., SAKUMA, A., ITOH, K., ITOH, H., KURIHARA, M.,
     SAITO, M., and WATANABE, M.: Archiv. Gen. Psych. 32, 1310-1318,
         1975.

40. DOUSA, T. and HECHTER, O.: Lancet I, 834-835, 1970.

41. UZONOV, P. and WEISS, B.: Advances in Cyclic Nucleotide
         Research, (ed. Greengard, P. and Robinson, G.A.), 435-453,
         (Raven Press, N.Y. 1972).

42. FORN, J. and VALDECASAS, F.G.: Biochem, Pharmacol. 20, 2773-2779,
         1971.

43. PALMER, G.C., ROBINSON, G.A., MAMAN, A.A. and SULSER, F.:
         Psychopharmacol. 23, 201-211, 1972.

44. PALMER, G.C., ROBINSON, G.A. and SULSER,F.: Biochem. Pharmacol.
         20, 236-239, 1972.

45. WALKER, J.B.,: Biological Psychiat. 8, 245-251, 1974.

46. KADIS, B.: Lancet II, 1209, 1974.

47. LAZARUS, L.H. and KITRON, N.: Lancet II, 225-226, 1974.

48. BIRCH, N.J. and GOULDING, I.: Anal. Biochem. 66, 293-297, 1975.

49. EBSTEIN, R., BELMAKER, R., GRUNHAUS, L. AND RIMON, R.: Nature,
         259, 411-413, 1976.

50. BELMAKER, R., EBSTEIN, R., SCHOENFELD, H., AND RIMON, R.:
         Psychopharmacologia, in press.

CENTRAL BIOCHEMICAL CORRELATES TO ANTIPSYCHOTIC DRUG ACTION IN MAN

G. Sedvall, G. Alfredsson, L. Bjerkenstedt, P. Eneroth,
B. Fyrö, C. Härnryd and B. Wode-Helgodt

Departments of Pharmacology and Psychiatry
Karolinska Institutet, S-104 01 Stockholm, Sweden

The present paper summarizes work carried out at the
Karolinska Institute, Stockholm, Sweden, over the last few years.
The studies deal with the possibility of finding chemical parameters useful for the selection of drugs and their dosage to treat
psychotic patients.

Every psychiatrist is aware of the difficulty in selecting
the right drug and dose for the individual patient only on the
basis of clinical data. Often therapeutic failures or toxic
reactions will follow from an inappropriate dose selection. This
can at least partly be explained by two factors (Table I). One
represents the variation in the <u>pharmacokinetics</u> of the drug, i.e.
the fate of the compound and its metabolism in the individual
patient. Since most psychoactive drugs are metabolized at rates
which vary more than tenfold in a group of patients it should
be of great value if the pharmacokinetic parameters could be
optimally adjusted in each patient. The other factor represents
the <u>pharmacodynamics</u>, i.e. the effect of the drug on the patient.
So far we have analysed the pharmacodynamic effect exclusively by
studying the influence of the drug on the psychopathology of the
patient as evaluated from conventional clinical and psychological
data. In all probability the action of any drug on psychopathology
is mediated by effects on brain chemistry. Therefore information
on the effect of the drug on central chemical parameters that are
related to the antipsychotic effect may be of value not only for
the selection of optimal drug dosage for the individual patient.
This knowledge may also be of importance for our understanding of
the neurochemistry of psychosis.

TABLE I

PRINCIPLES OF PSYCHOACTIVE DRUG TREATMENT

Pharmacotherapy ———— Medication

Pharmacokinetics ———— Fate of drug in patient

Pharmacodynamics < Effect of drug on brain chemistry

Effect of drug on psychopathology

RELATIONS BETWEEN PHARMACOKINETIC AND CLINICAL PARAMETERS IN DRUG TREATED PSYCHOTIC PATIENTS

During the last decade attempts to find relations between concentrations of chlorpromazine and other antipsychotic drugs in plasma and clinical outcome in psychotic patients were not conclusive. This may partly be due to the difficulty in finding appropriate chemical methods for the determination of the very low drug concentrations obtained in the body fluids after administration of therapeutic doses. Recently highly specific and sensitive mass fragmentographic methods for the determination of small organic molecules in tissues and body fluids were developed (Sweeley et al. 1966). The technique of mass fragmentography is based on the principle that a mass spectrometer is used as an ion specific detector for the effluent from a gas chromatography column. Recently such a method was developed for the determination of chlorpromazine concentrations in plasma and cerebrospinal fluid (Alfredsson and Sedvall 1975, Alfredsson et al. 1976). Figure 1 demonstrates the quantification of chlorpromazine concentrations in plasma as well as in cerebrospinal fluid (CSF) of patients in relation to administration of ordinary therapeutic doses.

In a preliminary study on chlorpromazine treated psychotic women given fixed doses of the drug during 4 weeks we have examined the possible relation between the clinical therapeutic effect and the chlorpromazine concentration in the CSF (Wode-Helgodt et al., to be published 1976). The clinical state of the patients was independently evaluated by two psychiatrists before as well as after treatment for 4 weeks. The interrater reliability between the scores rated by the two psychiatrists was 0.84, $p < 0.001$. When the global score at the end of treatment was related to the concentration of chlorpromazine in lumbar CSF a significant negative correlation was found (Fig. 2). Patients with a high chlorpromazine concentration in CSF exhibited the lowest global score, i.e. they were markedly improved. The relation found in figure 2 indicates that in psychotic

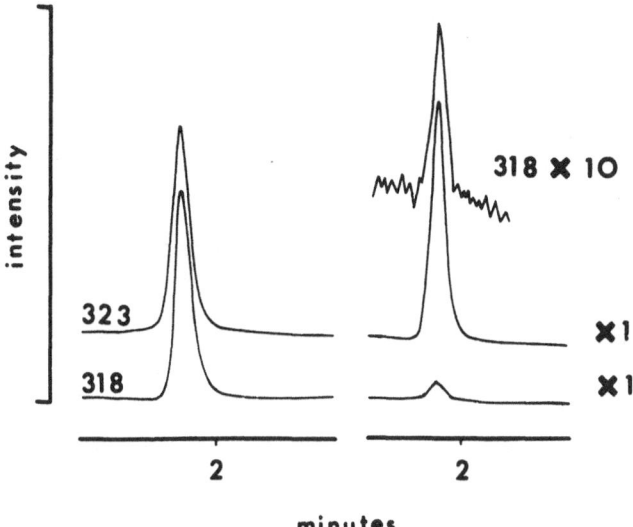

Fig. 1. Mass fragmentographic analysis of
chlorpromazine in plasma and CSF

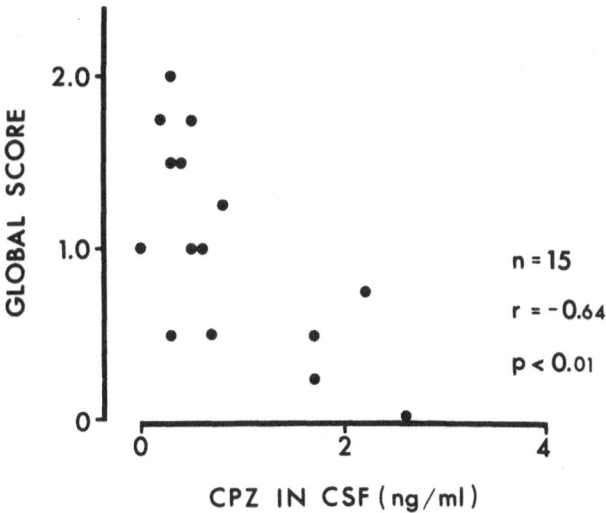

Fig. 2. Relation between global score and
chlorpromazine in CSF of psychotic
women treated for 4 weeks with chlorpromazine

women the chlorpromazine concentration in CSF should be above 1 ng
per ml for the achievement of an optimal antipsychotic effect.
Interestingly enough the patients who had the highest chlorpromazine
concentrations in CSF were not always those given the highest doses
of the drug. Thus the chlorpromazine concentration in CSF appears
to be better related to clinical outcome than the dose of the drug
given to the patient. This is in all probability due to the great
variation in the rate of chlorpromazine metabolism in different
patients. The relationship found in this study points to the possibility of using a specific pharmacokinetic parameter i.e. the drug
concentration in CSF for the design of an optimal drug therapy in
psychosis.

RELATIONS BETWEEN CENTRAL BIOCHEMICAL PARAMETERS AND
THERAPEUTIC EFFECTS IN DRUG TREATED PSYCHOTIC PATIENTS

It is now fairly well established that antipsychotic drugs
exert profound effects on the metabolism of the monoaminergic
transmitters in the central nervous system (c.f. Sedvall 1975).
In our search for chemical parameters related to antipsychotic
drug action we have therefore focused our interest on biochemical
parameters related to transmission from dopamine, noradrenaline
and serotonin neurons in the brain. The major metabolites of these
transmitter systems are homovanillic acic (HVA), methoxyphenyl-
ethylene glycol (MOPEG) and 5-hydroxyindoleacetic acid (5-HIAA)
(Table II). The levels of these three major monoamine metabolites
can be determined in small volumes of human lumbar CSF by mass
fragmentography (Fig. 3).

The levels of the monoamine metabolites in all probability
reflect the release of the metabolites from pre-synaptic monoaminergic neurons in the central nervous system. The levels of
these three transmitter metabolites should therefore reflect
predominantly pre-synaptic events in the monoaminergic synapses.

TABLE II

CENTRAL TRANSMITTER SYSTEMS OF POSSIBLE
RELEVANCE FOR THE MECHANISM OF ACTION
OF ANTIPSYCHOTIC DRUGS

Transmitter		Metabolite
1. Dopamine	———	HVA
2. Noradrenaline	———	MOPEG
3. Serotonin	———	5-HIAA

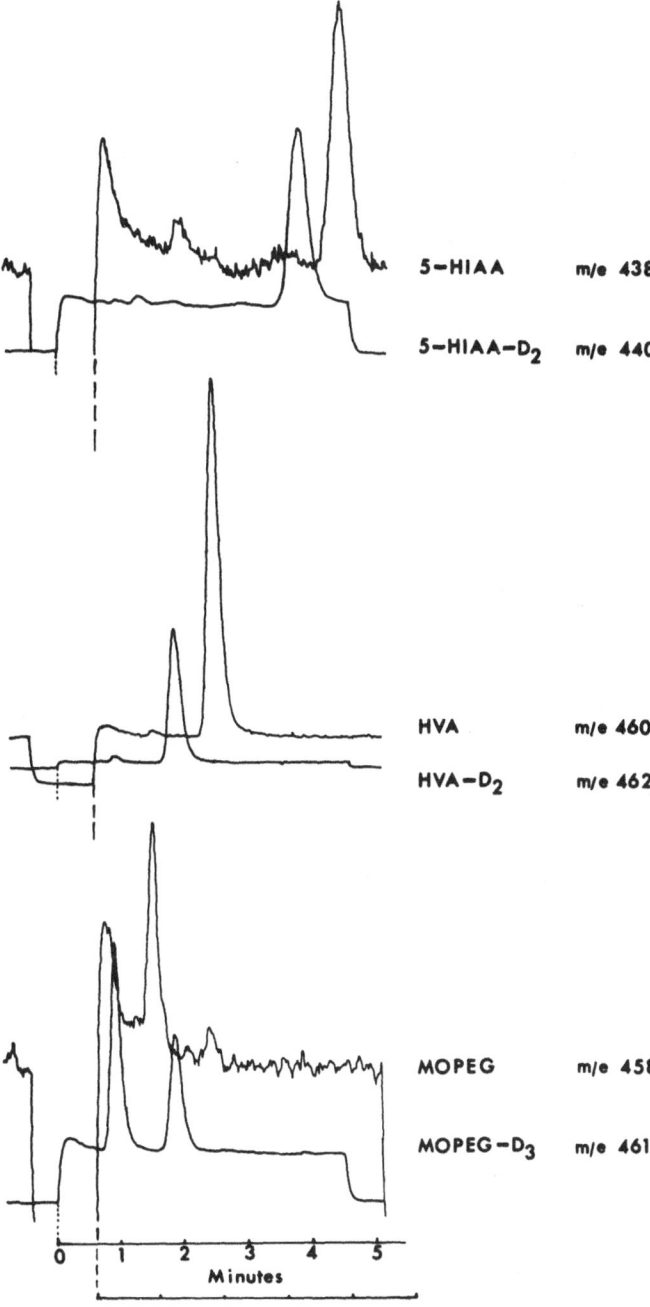

Fig. 3. Simultaneous mass fragmentographic
determination of monoamine metabolites in lumbar CSF

It is generally assumed on the basis of animal experiments that the antipsychotic properties of neuroleptic drugs are related to their ability to block postsynaptic dopamine receptors in the central nervous system (c.f. Sedvall 1975). Clinical data demonstrating such a relation has hitherto not been available. Dopamine neurons in the hypothalamus are involved in the release of prolactin from the pituitary gland (Frantz 1973). Prolactin release from the pituitary gland is under the influence of prolactin releasing factor (PRF) and prolactin inhibitory factor (PIF) (Fig. 4).

Dopamine in the hypothalamus is either identical with PIF or stimulates the release of this hypothetical compound. During the administration of chlorpromazine the influence of the released dopamine which mediates inhibition of prolactin release is removed and thereby prolactin release from the pituitary gland is markedly augmented. We therefore also examined whether the prolactin level as determined in plasma and cerebrospinal fluid can be used as a biochemical index of postsynaptic events in central dopaminergic synapses (Sedvall et al. 1975 a). The prolactin level was determined by a homologous radioimmunoassay. The pre- and postsynaptic biochemical parameters analysed are summarized in Table III.

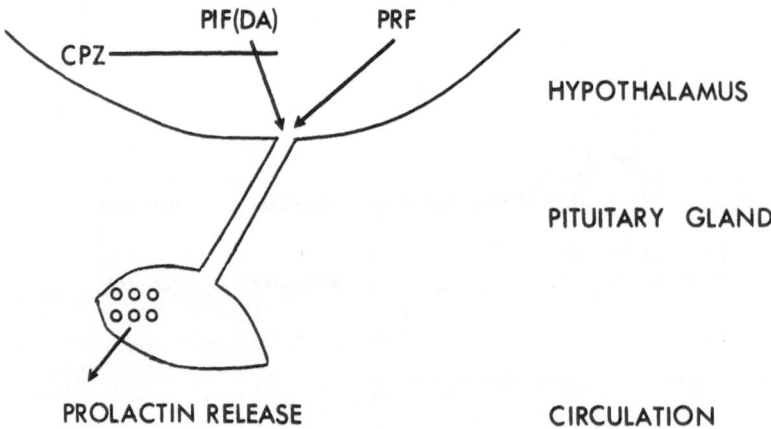

Fig. 4.   Hypothalamic factors affecting
          prolactin release

TABLE III

PARAMETERS ANALYSED

Biochemical

1. Presynaptic events
    HVA
    MOPEG
    5-HIAA

2. Postsynaptic events
    Prolactin   CSF
    Prolactin   Plasma

In the clinical studies we have used chemically different types of antipsychotic compounds as tools. The well-known, non-sedative thioxanthene derivative thiothixene is used in one study (Bjerkenstedt et al., to be published 1976). In another study, chlorpromazine, the first and still most commonly used neuroleptic drug is used (Wode-Helgodt et al., to be published 1976). Psychotic patients selected according to specific inclusion criteria were treated with fixed doses of the drugs for 4 weeks. Before as well as after treatment for 2 and 4 weeks clinical ratings and CSF samples were obtained. The design of the investigations was approved by the Ethical Committee of the Karolinska Institute. Figure 5 illustrates the changes in the levels of the three monoamine metabolites in CSF in relation to treatment.

During thiothixene treatment the level of the major dopamine metabolite homovanillic acid is markedly elevated. The level remains high for at least 4 weeks. During thiothixene treatment there is no significant alteration of the MOPEG or the 5-HIAA level. Thus the change in the major dopamine metabolite appears to be a selective biochemical change during thiothixene treatment. Figure 6 shows data obtained during chlorpromazine treatment. As can be seen there is here about the same elevation of the HVA level as during thiothixene treatment. On the other hand during chlorpromazine treatment there is also a marked and highly significant alteration of the concentration of MOPEG, the major noradrenaline metabolite. The MOPEG level is changed in the opposite direction to that of HVA, i.e. a reduction to about 50% of the control level is obtained. Chlorpromazine treatment also caused a slight but significant reduction of the 5-HIAA level.

To what extent are those biochemical effects related to the clinical antipsychotic effect of the drug. In the thiothixene treated patients the elevation of the HVA level in CSF was plotted against the global clinical improvement after 4 weeks resulting in

G. SEDVALL ET AL.

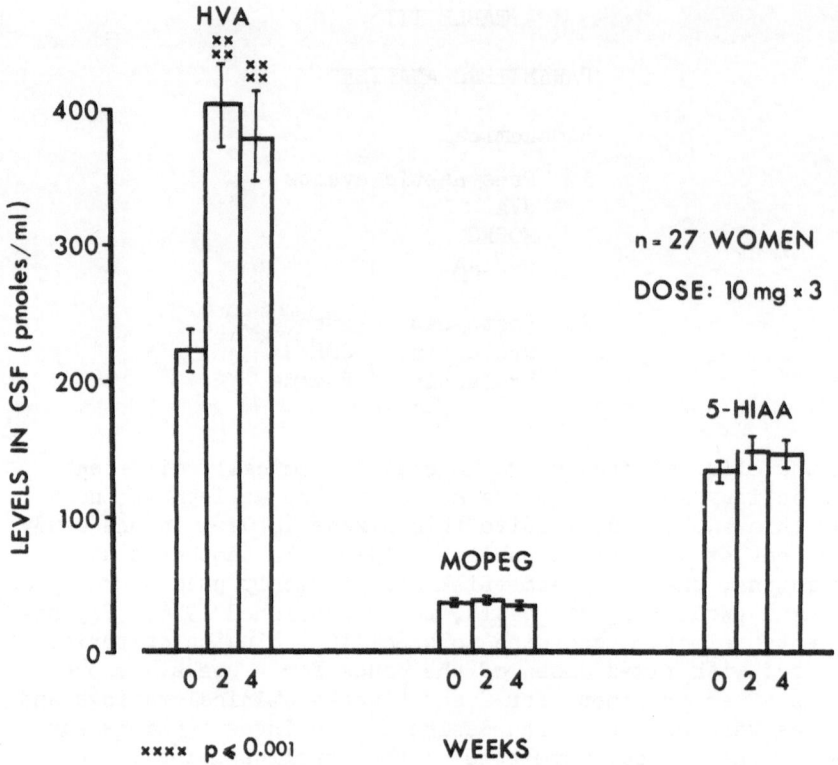

Fig. 5.   Levels of monoamine metabolites in
           CSF during thiothixene treatment

the relation presented in figure 7. Even if there is a considerable
scatter between the values a significant positive Spearman's rank
correlation was obtained (r=0.06, p < 0.01). The greater the change
in the HVA level the more the patients tended to improve. When a
similar plot was made for the chlorpromazine treated patients a
positive but lower correlation coefficient was obtained. However,
it was not significant in this preliminary study.

However, when the reduction of the MOPEG level in the chlorpromazine treated patients was plotted against the change in the clinical
condition a highly significant relationship was found. The greater
the reduction of the MOPEG level the more the patients improved
Fig. 8. On the other hand, such a relation was not at hand for the
thiothixene treated patients.

Since it was found, with the two drugs investigated, that both
the elevation of the HVA level as well as the reduction of the MOPEG
level was significantly correlated to clinical improvement and since

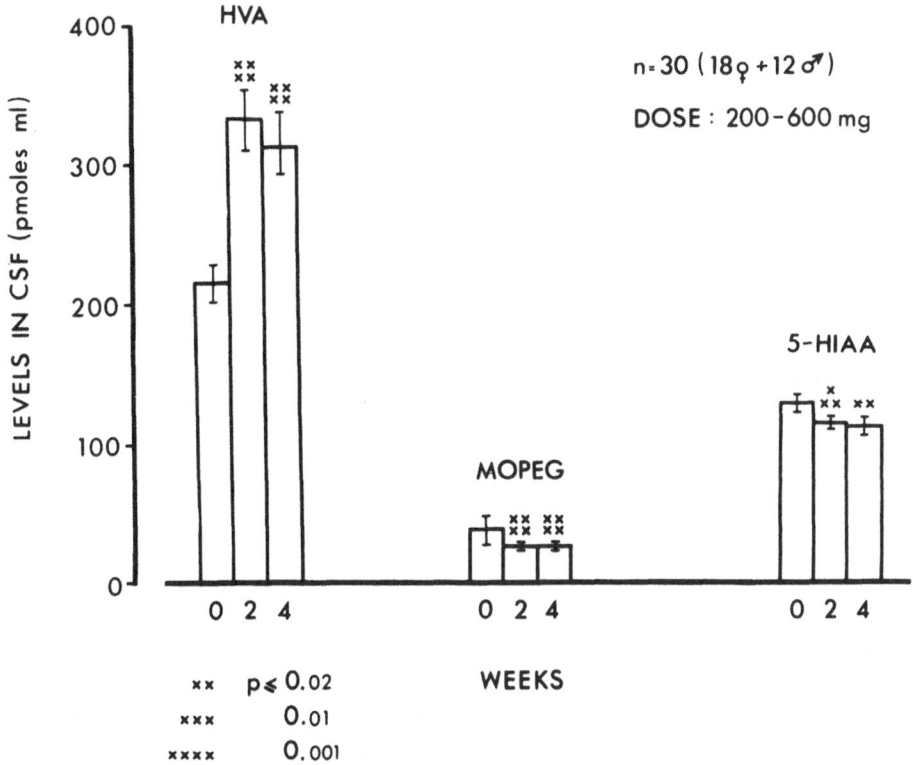

Fig. 6.   Levels of monoamine metabolites in
          CSF during chlorpromazine treatment.

chlorpromazine exerted both effects, it seemed possible that both
the dopamine and the norepinephrine systems may be involved in the
mechanism of action of the drugs. For this reason we calculated for
each patient the ratio between the HVA and the MOPEG levels in CSF.
When the change in the HVA/MOPEG ratio was plotted against clinical
improvement it was found that a significant positive correlation
was found in the thiothixene (Fig. 9) as well as the chlorpromazine
treated patients. The more the patients improved the greater was
the change in the HVA/MOPEG ratio.

With 3 types of chemically different antipsychotic drugs, we
have analysed so far, the HVA/MOPEG ratio in CSF is increased during
treatment (Bjerkenstedt et al. to be published 1976, Wode-Helgodt
et al., to be published 1976). For all these drugs we have found
that the change in the HVA/MOPEG ratio is significantly correlated
to the clinical improvement. The data are compatible with the view
that the antipsychotic action of neuroleptic drugs is related to
their interaction with central dopaminergic as well as noradrenergic
mechanisms.

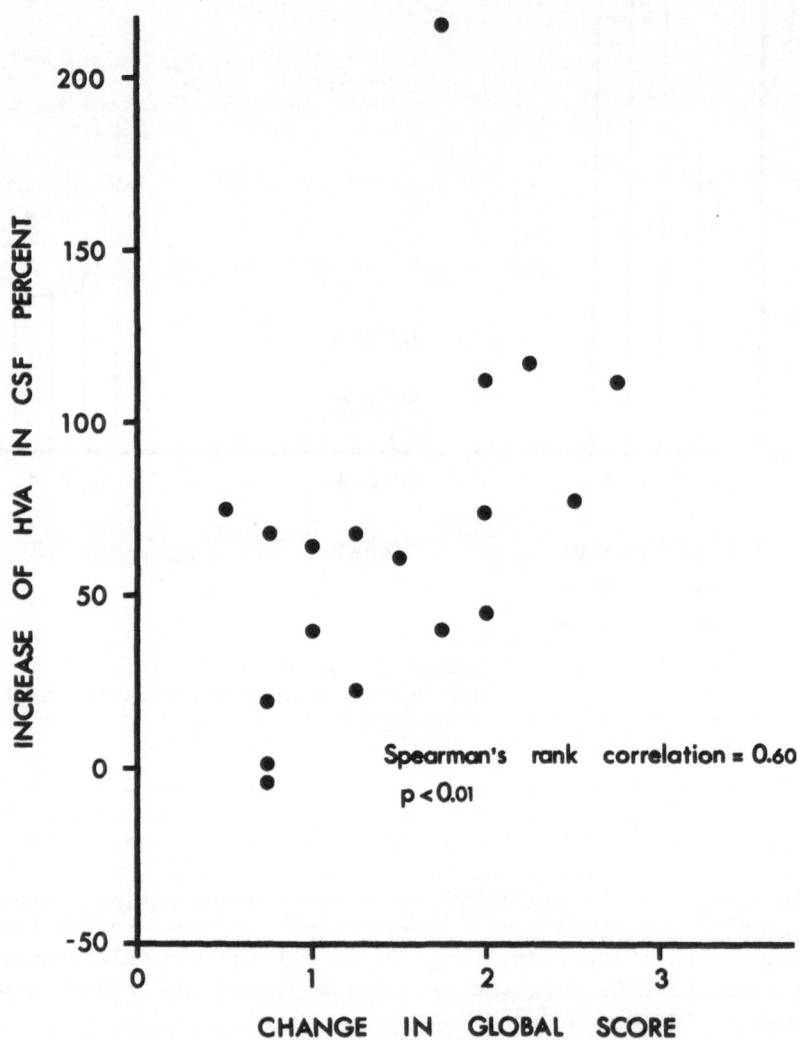

Fig. 7.   Relation between change in HVA and
          clinical effect in thiothixene treated
          patients.

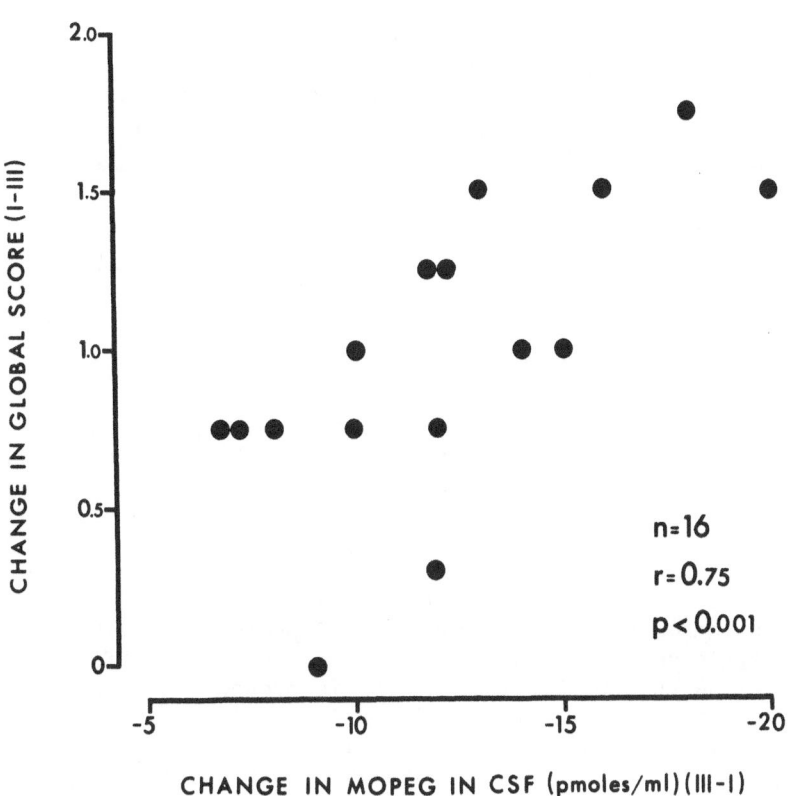

Fig. 8. Relation between change in global score and MOPEG
in CSF of psychotic women treated with chlorpromazine.

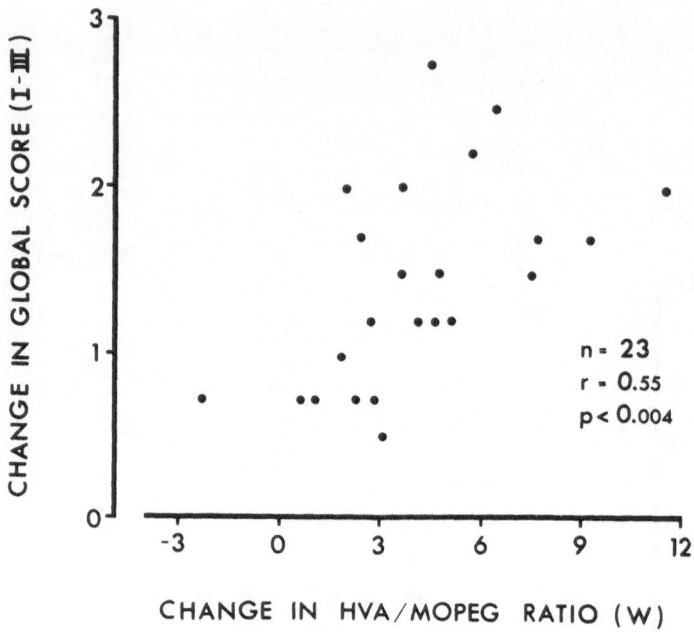

Fig. 9.   Relation between changes in global
          score and HVA/MOPEG ratio in thiothixene
          treated psychotic women.

PROLACTIN LEVELS AS A BIOCHEMICAL CORRELATE TO ANTIPSYCHOTIC EFFECT

     As mentioned earlier the secretion of prolactin may be related
to postsynaptic dopamine receptor blockade. Recently we found that
radioimmunoassayable prolactin activity is present in cerebrospinal
fluid as well as plasma of psychotic patients (Sedvall et al. 1975 b).
In men as well as women there is a significant elevation of the prolactin like material in CSF during treatment with chlorpromazine.
This effect remains relatively unchanged during treatment for at
least 4 weeks. In a preliminary study we have analysed whether the
change in the prolactin concentration in CSF in chlorpromazine treated
patients is related to the clinical change. The women exhibited the
most marked change of the prolactin level in CSF during treatment but
there was a large scatter between the values. A positive correlation
coefficient was found between the elevation of the prolactin level
and the change in the clinical condition, but it is so far not significant. On the other hand in a small sample of chlorpromazine treated
psychotic men we found a significant positive correlation between the
change in the clinical condition and the prolactin elevation in CSF
(Fig. 10).

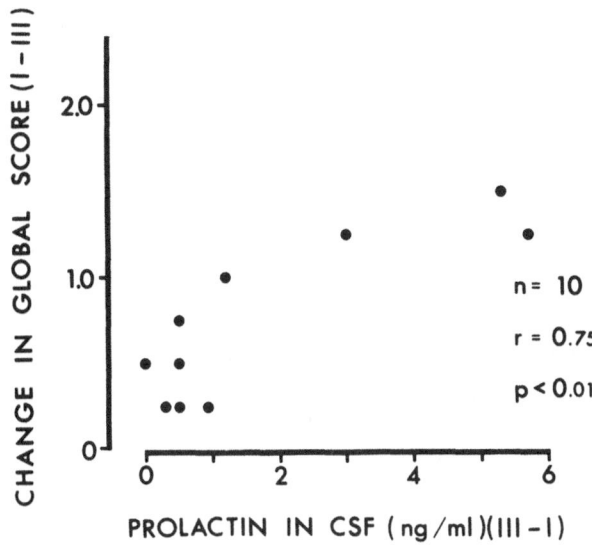

Fig. 10. Relation between change in global
          score and prolactin in CSF of psy-
          chotic men treated with chlorpro-
          mazine.

SUMMARY

The results presented indicate that by the analysis of pharmacokinetic data and biochemical pharmacodynamic parameters related to
dopaminergic and noradrenergic mechanisms in the central nervous
system it is possible to find chemical correlates to changes in
psychopathology. The demonstration of such relationships may be of
value not only for the selection of optimal drug dosage in psychotic
patients but also for an understanding of the pathophysiological
mechanisms involved in psychotic states. Drug treatment of psychosis
is accordingly an area in which biochemistry may have a considerable
impact on the development of psychiatry in the future.

ACKNOWLEDGMENTS

The present study was supported by grants from the Swedish
Medical Research Council (No. 40X-3560, 14X-2381), the National
Institute of Mental Health, Bethesda, Maryland, USA (MH 15755-06),
Magnus Bergvalls Stiftelse, Karolinska Institutet, F. Hoffmann-La
Roche & Co., Basle, Switzerland.

REFERENCES

ALFREDSSON, G. and G. SEDVALL, Mass fragmentographic analysis of
    chlorpromazine in human plasma. In: Antipsychotic Drugs,
    Pharmacodynamics and Pharmacokinetics. Eds. G. Sedvall, B. Uvnäs
    and Y. Zotterman. Pergamon Press, Oxford, 1975, in press.

ALFREDSSON, G., B. WODE-HELGODT and G. SEDVALL, A mass fragmento-
    graphic method for the determination of chlorpromazine and two
    of its active metabolites in human plasma and CSF. Psychophar-
    macologia, 1976, in press

FRANTZ, A.G., Catecholamines and the control of prolactin secretion
    in humans. Progr. in Brain Res. 39, 311.-322, 1973

SEDVALL, G., Receptor feedback and dopamine turnover in CNS. In:
    Handbook of Psychopharmacology, vol. 6. Eds. L.L. Iversen,
    S.D. Iversen and S.H. Snyder. Plenum Publ. Corp., New York, 1975

SEDVALL, G., G. ALFREDSSON, L. BJERKENSTEDT, P. ENEROTH, B. FYRÖ, C.
    HÄRNRYD, C.-G. SWAHN, F.-A. WIESEL and B. WODE-HELGODT, Selective
    effects of psychoactive drugs on levels of monoamine metabolites
    and prolactin in cerebrospinal fluid of psychiatric patients.
    In: Proc. VI International Congress of Pharmacology. Pergamon
    Press, Oxford, 1975 a

SEDVALL, G., L. BJERKENSTEDT, P. ENEROTH, B. FYRÖ, C. HÄRNRYD and
    B. WODE-HELGODT, Prolactin levels in plasma and cerebrospinal
    fluid of psychiatric patients in relation to treatment with
    psycho-active drugs. Europ. J. Clin. Pharmacol., 1975 b, in press

SWEELEY, C.C., W.H. ELLIOT, I. FRIES and R. RYHAGE, Mass spectrometric
    determination of unresolved components in gas chromatographic
    effluents. Analyt. Chem. 38, 1549-1553, 1966

INTRA/EXTRA RED BLOOD CELL LITHIUM AND ELECTROLYTE DISTRIBUTIONS

AS CORRELATES OF NEUROTOXIC REACTIONS DURING LITHIUM THERAPY

Avner Elizur, Eran Graff[*], Meir Steiner, Shamai Davidson

Shalvata Psychiatric Center, Tel-Aviv University, Israel

[*] "Ichilov" General Hospital, Tel-Aviv, Israel

A major contribution to the investigation of electrolyte metabolism in affective disorders was the successful use of lithium
(Li) in the treatment of manic-depressed patients. It was found to
be effective in the treatment of the manic phase (Gershon 1960)
and in the prophylaxis of manic and depressive episodes (Bastrup
1967). Lithium also shows a mild anti-depressive action, but this
is still a controversial issue (Mendels 1972).

Such clinical data have led to interest in the effect of
lithium on electrolyte metabolism. The metabolic impact may be
mediated via Na and K in view of the similarity in the ionic charge,
via magnesium owing to the similarity in ionic radius (1.33 Å and
1.36 Å respectively), and/or via calcium due to the similarity in
polarizing power (2.8 and 2.05 respectively) (Stern 1959).

Evidence is accumulating regarding the effects of lithium on
the distribution and metabolism of electrolytes in experimental
animals and in human beings with and without affective disorders
(Coppen 1966; Baer 1970; Birch 1973; and Carman 1974). Coppen (1965)
suggested that there might be a relative elevation in intracellular
sodium in depression and that intracellular potassium is lower than
normal in depression and elevated upon recovery. His results with
Li "responders" suggested that Li has an effect on the Na^+ distri
bution in affective illness. Coppen's technique used a radioactive
measurement of the distribution of whole body electrolytes. An
alternative experimental approach was the measurement of intra-
erythrocyte electrolyte values. Mendels (1972) reported a low level
of sodium in red blood cells of both depressed and manic patients.
However, Naylor (1970) failed to demonstrate a difference between
psychotic depressives and controls in the RBC Na concentration.

More recently, changes in the intra- and extra-cellular values of
calcium (Ca) and magnesium (Mg) have been reported by Flack (1964)
Birch (1973), Glen (1973) and Carman (1974) after Li treatment.
While requiring further confirmation, such results have theoretical
significance since these cations participate in the energic process
of the "sodium pump", and since Li has an effect on the Mg-Na-K
ATP-ase activity in several tissues.

On the basis of these data Singer (1973) and Glen (1973) suggested that lithium acts therapeutically in two ways:

1)   As an imperfect substitute for the cations in processes of
      ionic transfer, i.e., as an external, potassium-like cation,
      providing immediate and readily reversible stimulation of the
      sodium pump; and as an internal cation, in competition with
      sodium itself in the pump mechanism.

2)   As a possible vital constituent of the cellular micro-environ-
      ment that determines the basic spatial structure, energy supply
      and time course of the cellular process via its effect on Ca-
      and Mg-activated ATP-ase.

In view of the above, we have begun to investigate the distribution of Li and other electrolytes across the RBC membrane in
manic and depressed patients. This investigation deals with the
relationship between the electrolyte distribution, the clinical
diagnosis, and the therapeutic outcome. In this paper we present
preliminary data regarding changes which occurred during lithium
neurotoxicity. Based on our previous findings of high RBC Li concentration in toxic patients (Elizur 1972), and on our present data
it seems that the intra/extra RBC lithium and electrolyte distributions may have direct implications for the following issues:

a)   The prediction of impending lithium neurotoxicity even when
      lithium plasma (Pl) levels are within therapeutic range.

b)   The identification of the drug responsible for toxic side
      effects in cases of combined lithium and tricyclic anti-
      depressant drug therapy.

c)   The mechanisms of lithium action during neurotoxicity.

                           Clinical Material

Four women out of an original sample of 20 manic-depressive
patients under investigation at our clinical research unit reacted
to lithium therapy with severe, acute, reversible neurotoxicity.
All four were diagnosed as bipolar manic-depressive psychosis,
depressed type. Their age, duration of illness, treatment, maximum

dose on day of toxic reaction and duration of treatment are shown in Table 1. Prior to lithium treatment, all the patients had been somatically healthy and the treatment had been started after an initial observation period of four-seven days. The method for the measurement of RBC Li and electrolytes is based on the technique described by Solomon (1952) and Frazer (1972).

Results

The four neurotoxic patients did not show any clinical improvement prior to, during or after the toxic episode. In all of them the neurotoxic reaction had a sudden onset. No prior gastro-intestinal or peripheral autonomic manifestations were observed. The most striking symptoms in all cases were tremor, ataxic, dysarthria and difficulties in coordination. One patient had myoclonic carpal and facial convulsions and finally became stuporous. In three patients confusional state and difficulty in concentration were evident.

The EEGs showed bilateral irregular slow waves and irregular diffuse α, δ, σ waves with bitemporal accentuation. The ECGs showed flattening of the T waves in all leads. All other laboratory results revealed no pathology. Medication was discontinued immediately and within two-five days all toxic manifestations disappeared. The EEG as well as the ECG returned to normal following recovery.

The lithium and electrolyte levels in the toxic phase as compared with the non-toxic phase are presented in Table II. The non-toxic levels chosen for presentation above are those which were observed on the day of maximum lithium plasma level - in the absence of discernible side effects. Changes in the toxic phase may be summarized as follows: The plasma K levels showed a decrease in three patients. The plasma Mg levels were normal in the non-toxic phase but pretoxic as well as toxic elevations are evident. The RBC Na levels increased in all while the RBC K levels decreased in all patients. The RBC Mg levels showed pretoxic as well as toxic elevation.

In all patients, the RBC/pl Li ratio during the non-toxic phase was 40-50%. During the toxic phase, however, the RBC/pl Li ratio in three of the patients exceeded 60%. In one patient the RBC/pl ratio during the toxic phase was 45%. In this case, Li blood levels were carried out after four hours from the last lithium ingestion instead of the usual 12 hour interval.

The changes in RBC/pl ratio and RBC Na/K ratio as a function of the plasma Li levels are presented in Figure 1. For comparison purposes, the RBC/pl Li and RBC Na/K ratios of one Li-treated non-responder who did not show any toxic side effects are presented in

TABLE I.   The Neurotoxic Subjects

PAT.	AGE	DURATION OF ILLNESS	TREATMENT	MAX. DOSE ON DAY OF TOXIC REACTION	DAYS OF TREATMENT
A	50	15 y.	Lithium	2.5 gr.	15
B	60	10 y.	Lithium	2.25 gr.	15
C	64	12 y.	Lithium + Nortriptylin	1.5 gr. 150 mg.	8
D	45	18 y.	Lithium + Imipramine	1.75 gr. 300 mg.	30

Figure 1 as well. While there appears to be a close relationship between the change in the RBC/pl Li and the RBC Na/K ratios, no relationship is evident between the former and the plasma Na/K ratio in any of the patients.

The plasma and RBC levels of Na and K during the tricyclic anti-depressant therapy were stable and did not change after recovery. Those levels were similar to those during baseline. In comparison, the RBC Na levels during the combined lithium and tricyclic antidepressant therapy decreased and the RBC K levels increased.

Discussion

Acute lithium neurotoxicity is usually observed when lithium plasma levels exceed 1.5 meq/l, and it is accompanied by EEG and ECG abnormalities (Gershon 1971). However, in many cases, neurotoxicity has been observed to develop even when lithium plasma levels are within the therapeutic range. In such cases we have suggested (Elizur 1972), and this was confirmed in the Zakowska-Dobrowska study (1973), that the RBC/pl ratio is more closely related to neurotoxicity than the Li plasma level alone. With regard to our two Li-only patients, while a Li plasma level of 1.8 meq/l was "toxic" for patient A, a roughly equivalent level was "non-toxic" for patient B, whose "toxic" value was 2.3 meq/l. On

TABLE II. Lithium and Electrolyte Values Prior To and During the Toxic Phase

TREATMENT	LITHIUM ONLY				LITHIUM + TRICYCLIC ANTIDEPRESSANTS			
PATIENT	A		B		C		D	
PHASE	NON-TOXIC	TOXIC	NON-TOXIC	TOXIC	NON-TOXIC	TOXIC	NON-TOXIC	TOXIC
PLASMA								
Na	138	138	138	147	147	143	145	140
K	4.2	3.5	4.0	3.1	4.6	5.3	4.8	3.8
Ca	11.0	11.0	10.5	10.8	9.9	10.1	10.0	9.4
Mg	1.5	2.1	1.5	1.6	1.9	2.4	2.2	2.4
Lithium	1.2	1.8	1.7	2.3	0.45	1.2	1.0	1.18
Ca/Mg	7.3	5.2	7.0	6.7	5.2	4.2	4.5	3.9
RBC								
Na	25	33.6	24	34.5	20.8	43	16	29.4
K	89.6	79.6	95	90	98	80.3	97.6	88.4
Mg	5.4	6.4	4.3	4.7	2.2	5.9	—	—
Lithium	0.58	1.1	0.73	1.5	0.24	0.8	0.37	0.53
RBC/Pl Li%	48%	61%	41%	65%	52%	68.5%	37%	45%

A. ELIZUR ET AL.

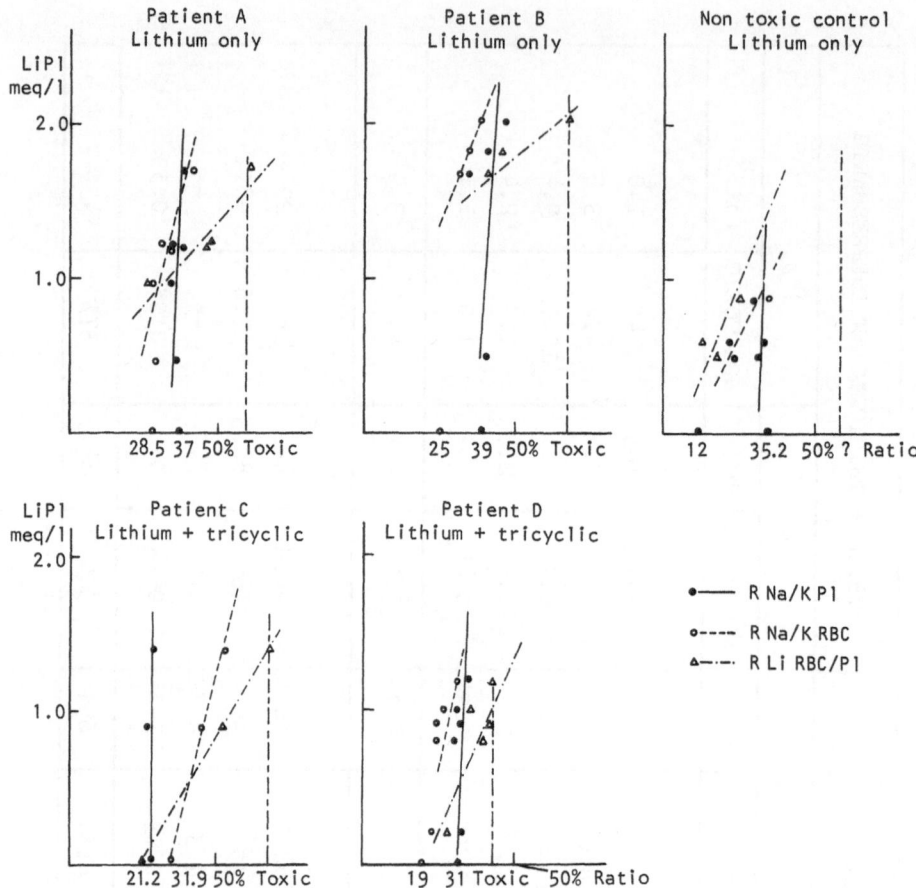

Figure 1. Lithium RBC/pl ratio, Na/K plasma ratio. Na/K ratio as
           a function of plasma lithium level. (The plasma Li
           levels on the y axis are given in meq/lit, and the
           values of the ratio on the x axis are multiplied by
           100 and presented as percentage.

the other hand, in both A and B, while the RBC/pl Li ratio in the
non-toxic phase was the usual 40-50%, the ratio during neurotoxicity
exceeded 60%. It seems that, regardless of the lithium plasma level
itself, the neurotoxic syndrome may develop whenever the RBC/pl Li
ratio exceeds a certain critical level, a level which might reflect
a turning point in the permeability and excitability of the cell
membrane.

    Since the neurotoxic syndrome which may develop in patients

treated with tricyclic antidepressants is similar in many respects
to lithium neurotoxicity (Radwan 1975; Dickson 1973; Micev 1973;
Caffey 1961), identification of the drug primarily responsible for
the side effects in combined treatment becomes potentially proble-
matic. In such cases the neurotoxic syndrome or the EEG abnormalities,
per se, do not facilitate this required identification. We suggest
that, given a high RBC/pl Li ratio (regardless of plasma lithium
levels as such), it is the lithium which is primarily responsible
for the neurotoxic side effects, rather than the antidepressants.

Our thesis is supported in case C in which the RBC/pl Li
ratio was 68%. However, it is not supported in case D where this
ratio did not exceed 45%. One possible explanation for the discrepancy is the fact that the toxic symptoms were more severe in
patients A, B and C than in patient D who presented only relatively
minor side effects. Another possibility relates to the shorter time
interval between the last Li ingestion and our blood measurements.
In the case of D, one may speculate that our measurements were ill-
timed in that they may have preceded the RBC/pl Li ratio peak, this
being related to the fact that the transport of Li into the cell is
much more efficient than in the opposite direction (Keynes and Swan
1959). Still another possibility is that there is heterogeneity in
the cases of Li toxicity; and maybe case D presents the synergistic
effect with the antidepressants.

In a previous report (Elizur 1972) we suggested that patients
in an acute manic or depressed state may be distinguished from
normal individuals or manic-depressives in the normothymic inter-
phase by the RBC/pl Li ratio. This was not confirmed by Rybakowski
(1974), nor by our present data. There is also some evidence
(Mendels 1973)that a favourable response to lithium in affective
disorders is associated with an increase in RBC Li concentration.
In our study, however, such an increase was associated with a negative response. In view of such contradictory data, it would appear
that changes in RBC Li concentration are more related to toxic
phenomena than to pathogenic processes in affective disorder, or
to the therapeutic mode of action of Li.

Several workers (Nielsen 1964 and Haavaldsen 1973) have reported
increases in plasma Mg during the initial phase of Li treatment.
This response was also observed in our patients. At the same time
the RBC Mg increased as well. According to Carman et al. (1973) an
initial increase of magnesium during the first 5 days of lithium
therapy is typical of lithium responders. This was not the case in
our patients, who did not respond to lithium therapy despite the
initial increase in magnesium plasma.

In conclusion, our clinical data provide suggestive evidence
for the importance of the intra/extra-cellular distributions of
lithium and the main electrolytes during lithium treatment of manic-

depressive patients. These distributions have predictive values
for lithium neurotoxicity, both when the lithium is administered
alone and in combination with other drugs. The intra-extra RBC
electrolyte gradient may also throw light on the toxic mode of
action of lithium.

REFERENCES

1.   BASTRUP, P.C. AND SCHOU, M.: Lithium and a Prophylactic Agent.
     Its Effect Against Recurrent Depression and Manic
     Depressive Psychosis. Arch. Gen. Psychiat. 16:162, 1967.

2.   BAER, L., DURELL, J., SUNNEY, W.E., MURPHY, D., LEVY, B.S.,
     GREENSPAN, K. AND CARDON, P.V.: Sodium Balance and
     Distribution in Lithium Carbonate Therapy. Arch. Gen.
     Psychiat. 22:40, 1970.

3.   BIRCH, N.J.: Biological Effect of Lithium Salts. The Lancet ii:
     46, 1973.

4.   BIRCH, N.J. AND FENNER, F.A.: The Distribution of Lithium and
     its Effect on the Distribution and Excretion of Other
     Ions in the Rat. Brit. J. Pharmac. 47:586, 1973.

5.   CAFFEY, C.M. et al. Side Effects and Laboratory Findings
     During Combined Drug Therapy. Dis. Nerv. Syst. 22:
     370-375, 1961.

6.   CARMAN, J.S., POST, R.M., TEPLITZ, T.A. AND GOODWIN, F.K.:
     Divalent Cation in Predicting and Antidepressant Response
     to Lithium. The Lancet.ii, 1454, 1974

7.   CARMAN, J.S., POST, R.M., TEPLITZ, T.A. AND GOODWIN, F.K.:
     Lancet ii, 1454, 1974.

8.   COPPEN, A.: Biochemistry of Affective Disorders. Experta Medica
     International Congress Series No. 150, Madrid 5-11
     Sept. 1966, p.506.

9.   DEMERS, R.G AND HENINGER, G.: Electrocardiographic Changes
     During Lithium Treatment. Dis. of Nerv. Syst. 31:667-673,
     1970.

10. DICKSON, J.: Neurological and EEG Effect of Chlorimipramine,
     J. Int. Med. Res. 1:449, 1973.

11. DYSON, W. AND MENDELS, J.: Lithium and Depression. Current
     Therapeutic Research. 10:601, 1968.

12. ELIZUR, A., SHOPSIN, B., GERSHON, S. AND EHLENBERGER, A.:
       Intra- Extra-cellular Lithium Ratio and Clinical Course
       in Affective States. Clinical Pharmacology and Thera-
       peutics. 13:947, 1972.

13. FLACH, F.F.: Calcium Metabolism in State of Depression.
       Brit. J. Psychiat. 110:583, 1964.

14. FRAZER, A. ET AL: The Prediction of Brain Lithium Concentration
       from Plasma to Erythrocyte Measures. Am. J. Psychiat.
       Res. 10(1), 1 June, 1973.

15. FRAZER, A., SECUNDA, S.R., MENDELS, J.: A Method for Deter-
       mination of Sodium, Potassium, Magnesium and Lithium
       Concentration in Erythrocytes. Clin. Chem. Acta.
       36:499-509, 1972.

16. GERSHON, S. AND YUWILER, A.: Lithium Ion: A Specific Psycho-
       pharmacilogical Approach to Treatment of Mania. J.
       Neuropsych. 1:229, 1960.

17. GERSHON, S.: Lithium in Mania. Clinical Pharmacology and
       Therapeutics 11:168, 1971.

18. GIBBONS, J.L.: Electrolytes and Depressive Illness. Postgrad.
       Med. J. 39:19, 1963.

19. GLEN, A.J.M. AND READING, H.W.: Regulatory Action of Lithium
       in Manic Depressive Illness. The Lancet ii:1239, 1973.

20. GRANACHER, R.P. AND BALDESSARINI, R.J.: Physostigmine. Arch.
       of Gen. Psychiat. 32: 375-380, 1975.

21. HAAVALDSEN, R. AND INGVALDSEN, P.: Biological Effects of
       Lithium Salts. Lancet ii:1390, 1973.

22. KEYNES, R.D. AND SWAN, R.C.: The Permeability of Frog Muscle
       Fibers to Lithium Ion. J. Physiol. 147, 626, 1959.

23. MENDELS, J., FRAZER, A. AND SECUNDA, S.K.: Intra Erythrocyte
       Sodium and Potassium in Manic Depressive Illness.
       Biological Psychiatry. Vol. 5, No. 2:165, 1972.

24. MENDELS, J., SECUNDA, S.F. AND DYSON, W.L.: A Controlled
       Study of the Antidepressant Effects of Lithium Carbonate.
       Arch. Gen. Psychiat. 26:154-157, 1972.

25. MENDELS, J. AND FRAZER, A.: Intra-cellular Lithium Concentration
       and Clinical Response Toward a Membrane Theory of De-

pression. <u>Am. J. Psychiat. Res</u>. 10(1), 1 June 1973.

26. MICEV, V., MARKET, W.K.: Undesired Effect in Slow I.V. Infusion of Chlorimipramine. <u>J. Int. Med. Res</u>. 1:451, 1973.

27. NAYLOR, G.J., MCNAMEE, H.B. AND MOODY, J.P.: Erythrocyte Sodium and Potassium in Depressive Illness. <u>J. Psycho-somat. Res</u>. 14:173, 1970.

28. NIELSEN, J.: Magnesium-Lithium Studies I. <u>Acta Psychiat. Scand</u>. 40: 190-196, 1964.

29. RADWAN, H., STEINER, M. AND DAVIDSON, S.: Syndrome Cere-belleux Disparaissant de Soi-meme Secondaire au Praitement a Chlomiparmine submitted for publication <u>Gen. De Neurol. Psychiat. and Med. Psychosom</u>. Paris.

30. RYBAKOWSKY, J. ET AL.: Red Blood Cell Lithium Index in Patients with Affective Disorders in the Course of Lithium Prophylaxis. Int. <u>Pharmacopsychiat.</u> 9:166-171, 1974.

31. SINGER, J. AND ROTENBERG, D: Mechanisms of Lithium Action. <u>The New England J. of Medicine</u> 239-254, 1973.

32. SOLOMON, A.K.: Permeability of the Human Erythrocyte to Na and K. <u>J. Gen. Physiol</u>. 36:57-110, 1952.

33. STERN, K.H., AMIS, E.S.: <u>Chem. Rev</u>. 59, 1, 1959.

34. UENO, Y., AOKI, N., YAGUKI, T. AND KURAISHI, F.: Electrolyte Metabolism in Blood and C.S.F. in Psychosis. <u>Folia. Psychiat. Nonul. Jap</u>. 15:304, 1961.

35. ZAKOWSKA-DABROWSKA, S.J. AND RYBAKOWSKY, J.: Lithium-induced EEG changes: Relation to Lithium Levels in Serum and Red Blood Cells. <u>Acta Psychiat. Scand</u>. 49:457-465, 1973.

PHARMACOLOGICAL AGENTS AS TOOLS IN PSYCHIATRIC RESEARCH

Samuel Gershon, Burton Angrist and Baron Shopsin

Neuropsychopharmacology Research Unit
Department of Psychiatry, New York University Medical
Center, New York, U.S.A.

We thought we might approach this problem by exploring the effects of pharmacologically active agents as tools in modifying behavior in the different disease states, in the hope that this might resolve questions of psychoses as either a continuum or as separate and distinct disorders. Secondly - examine these findings in regard to current theories of psychoses.

This clearly stipulates the pharmacologic aspects and the use of specific drugs as provocateurs in these studies. However, we are faced with semantic and diagnostic ambiguities and quite fundamental difficulties in dealing with the other aspect of our task - the issues of diagnosis and disease state.

We must at the outset clearly state that diagnostic vagary, semantic confusion, and looseness of criteria for diagnosis have made a definition of the populations studied exceedingly difficult. For example, between the affective disorders and the schizophrenias it is becoming increasingly difficult to reach agreement on specific criteria of dysfunction. Recent publications have taken the view that if a patient with overactivity responds to treatment with lithium he must be a manic; this view overlooks the possibilities

With permission of Gershon, S., Angrist, B. and Shopsin B. (1975): Drugs, diagnosis and disease. In: Biology of the major psychoses, ed. by D.X. Freedman, Res. Publ. Assoc. Res. Nerv. Ment. Dis. Vol. 54, Raven Press, New York.

of placebo response or natural remission. The use of drugs in this
retrospective uncontrolled fashion cannot aid us in our present task,
but on the contrary, will further aggravate clarification of such
issues. The problem is further compounded by transcultural differences in diagnostic practice that exist between the United States and
other countries, particularly Great Britain and Western Europe.
Recent research has documented the considerable differences that
exist in the criteria by which affective and schizophrenias are
diagnosed (20).

Because of these diversities, an investigator can obtain
almost any clinical response to the administration of a drug by
altering the composition of the patient population. Having stated
these problems, we will try to explore the extent to which we can
utilize drugs to perform pharmacologic dissections of diagnoses
and disease states in psychiatry.

DRUG-INDUCED SWITCHES AND PSYCHOPATHOLOGY

Although many psychoactive drugs, such as the minor tranquilizers, have similar sedative effects in most individuals,
the effects of other psychopharmacologic agents appear to depend
upon the pre-existing state of the individual. For example, whereas
imipramine leads to marked improvement in mood and motor activity
in depressed patients, but is not a euphoriant or stimulant in
normals, when given to schizophrenics, a significant incidence of
activation of schizophrenic psychopathology occurs, and in bipolar
manic-depressives a precipitation of a manic episode may result.
These pharmacologic effects upon behavior are of particular interest
when the biologic changes produced by the drug can provide evidence
concerning the biochemical mechanisms involved in the behavioral
change and can highlight any specific relationships to diagnosis
and disease state.

L-DOPA

L-DOPA (1-3, 4-dihydroxyphenylalanine) is the direct amino
acid precursor of the neurotransmitter catecholamines, dopamine
and norepinephrine. However, its indirect effects on other transmitters such as serotonin cannot be excluded.

Investigators who treated parkinsonian patients with l-DOPA
soon pointed out that psychiatric side effects occurred frequently.
Reviewing these reports, both Brogden et al (18) and Goodwin (44)
have estimated that such side effects occur in approximately 20%
of the parkinsonian patients treated with l-DOPA. The behavioral
effects most often encountered have been confusion, depression,
agitation, paranoid delusions, and hypersexuality. Impulsivity,

increased anxiety, insomnia, vivid dreams, and lethargy were also noted.

In studies in our unit, 1-DOPA was administered to six non-psychotic psychiatric inpatients in large doses (mean daily dose, 8.8 g/day). The behavioral effects noted were quite similar in quality and range to those seen in nonpsychotic parkinsonian patients: hypersexuality in one patient, dysphoric stimulation in two, toxic confusion in one patient, no psychologic effects in one, and a paranoid schizophreniform psychosis in one nonschizophrenic patient (78).

However, when 1-DOPA was administered to 10 schizophrenic patients, a clear deterioration of psychiatric status occurred in all (3). In three patients it was judged that nonspecific stimulant effects (such as those seen after low doses of amphetamine) led to more intense and inappropriate verbalization of original psychotic preoccupations. However, the remaining seven showed either a clear and dose-related intensification of original base-line psychopathology (along with superimposed stimulant effects as in the first three) or a development of de novo symptoms, such as bizarre symbolic motor mannerisms and auditory hallucinations. This change occurred at a much lower dose (mean, 5 g/day 1-DOPA) than that for which behavioral effects were noted in the nonschizophrenic patients in the prior study. The data from those two studies, as well as some biochemical data regarding cerebrospinal homovanillic acid levels (CSF HVA levels), are summarized by Angrist et al (4).

Therefore, 1-DOPA can both induce a paranoid psychosis in non-psychotics and dramatically aggravate the predrug psychopathology of schizophrenic patients. Its effect on schizophrenics was seen in lower doses than those required for effects in the non-schizophrenic group. After discontinuation of this drug, its behavioral effects gradually cleared completely after approximately 72 hr.

A second diagnostic group that shows a rather specific and predictable behavioral response to 1-DOPA is manic-depressive disorder.

A much higher incidence of one specific side effect, mania, occurs in patients with manic-depressive disorder. Bipolar manic-depressive patients (those with histories of previous manic episodes) seem especially prone to develop typical, brief, hypomanic behavioral changes that are very similar to the individual patient's spontaneous hypomanic episodes (66).

The episodes reported were characterized by a sudden, clearly defined onset of increased speech, hyperactivity, increased social interaction, intrusiveness, sleeplessness, and some euphoria and grandiosity.

l-DOPA-induced hypomania is not only behaviorally very similar
but is also associated with many of the biologic changes noted in
spontaneous episodes - (a) urinary catecholamine excretion is increased during the hypomanic episode (45); (b) urinary cyclic-AMP
excretion is increased by l-DOPA (68); (c) REM sleep is decreased
(33,95); and (d) visual-evoked EEG responses show a pattern of
augmentation during l-DOPA just as they do during mania (15).

AMPHETAMINES AND METHYLPHENIDATE

Amphetamine and methylphenidate are similar to l-DOPA in that
they both cause a schizophreniform psychosis in non-schizophrenics
and can cause dramatic exacerbation of predrug symptomatology in
schizophrenics (5, 19, 26, 48, 86).

Moreover, their capacity for inducing these effects is much
more dramatic than that of l-DOPA in terms of both milligram-for-
milligram potency and rapidity of onset. Hence, de novo psychoses
have been seen at doses of under 200 mg amphetamine and after less
than 24 hr. (For l-DOPA, a daily dose of 9 g attained after a 28-
day administration was required for a de novo psychosis.) Excerbation
of psychotic symptomatology in schizophrenics was noted after single
intravenous doses of d-amphetamine and methylphenidate of 20 and
29 mg, respectively (26), whereas the schizophrenics who showed these
effects after l-DOPA administration on our unit (3) received the
drug for a mean of 21 days at a mean daily dose of just over 5 g.

It should also be noted that the comparative potency of the
stereoisomers of amphetamine, both for inducing psychosis in non-
psychotics (7) and for exacerbating the predrug symptoms of some
schizophrenics (26), are of a comparable order.

Therefore, the dramatic clinical effects of amphetamine and
methylphenidate made them important drugs in the investigation of
psychotogenic mechanisms. An extensive body of evidence reviewed
by Snyder (85) suggests that these mechanisms are mediated by
dopamine. However, in some pharmacologic respects it appears that
there are differences among amphetamine, methylphenidate, l-DOPA
and the clinically similar central nervous system (CNS) stimulant
phenmetrazine (6,61,92).

In addition, dopamine receptor stimulants such as apomorphine
have quite different clinical effects. These dopamine receptor
stimulants cause emesis at very low doses - an effect that appears
to make aggressive investigation of their psychotogenic potency
all but impossible. Why amphetamine does not cause emesis is a
question seldom raised.

Intermediate in clinical effects between l-DOPA and apomorphine is the dopamine receptor stimulant ET-495. It can both activate schizophrenic symptoms and cause psychotic states de novo.

Hence, l-DOPA can cause a schizophreniform psychosis in some, but not all, nonschizophrenics. This parallels our experience with amphetamine (5) in which some subjects received large (over 900mg) cumulative doses of the drug without psychosis. It appears then, that among nonschizophrenics a continuum exists as to the level of pharmacologic dopaminergic stimulation that can be tolerated without psychotic effects.

In contrast, patients with manifest schizophrenia show a markedly increased sensitivity to both l-DOPA and amphetamine, but within this group as well, sensitivity to these agents varies among individuals, with some showing marked activation of psychosis at relatively low doses whereas others do not.

This suggests a continuum of sensitivity to psychosis caused by these agents in both groups, but indicates some discontinuity in this spectrum, in that schizophrenics appear clearly more vulnerable.

DOPAMINE RECEPTOR STIMULANTS

Background

Several lines of evidence suggest a relationship between some psychotic states and central dopaminergic hyperactivity. These have been reviewed by Snyder (85). Among these is the observation that amphetamine and l-DOPA can induce psychoses that can be indistinguishable from naturally occurring schizophrenia (19,3) in nonschizophrenics, and can cause marked exacerbation of symptomatology when administered to schizophrenics (26). However, amphetamine clearly effects both norepinephrine and dopamine (62). Similarly, while l-DOPA elevates brain dopamine more than norepinephrine (31), it is the precursor of both. Moreover, l-DOPA affects brain serotonin (54) and some of its pharmacologic effects may be indirectly mediated by this amine (34). In an attempt to explore the hypothesized relationship between dopamine and schizophrenia we have, in this study, examined the clinical effects of drugs that promised to be more specific dopaminergic agonists. Putative dopamine receptor stimulants theoretically qualified as such. Two such drugs were examined: ET-495 and apomorphine.

The pharmacologic properties of ET-495 were reported in 1971 (21). These included decreased dopamine turnover and induction of rotation toward the intact side in rodents with unilateral 6-hydroxy-dopamine-induced nigrostriatal lesions, suggesting direct dopamine receptor stimulation.

Creese has also shown that rats treated as neonates with
6 OH-dopamine respond behaviorally to both ET-495 and apomorphine,
but not amphetamine, further suggesting post-synaptic stimulation
of dopamine receptors (25). Subsequent trials in humans with
Parkinsonism (17) indicated some efficacy in this disorder. In
one of these trials (59) it was noted that 2 of 8 Parkinsonian
patients showed both increased confusion and disorientation and
grossly psychotic deterioration, suggesting that ET-495 might be
potentially psychotogenic.

Apomorphine also induces turning to the intact side of rodents
with unilateral nigrostriatal 6-hydroxy-dopamine lesions (90) as
well as decreasing dopamine turnover (1). Moreover, its effects
are not blocked by catecholamine synthesis inhibition (30), further
suggesting direct action on dopamine receptors. It, too, has been
used in the treatment of Parkinsonism (24,27,81). One such trial
reported effects in one case suggesting psychotogenic potential(88).
In this case, a patient under treatment with l-DOPA and a decarboxylase inhibitor developed a psychosis with "paranoid symptoms,"
"disorientation", and "sexual" coloring when apomorphine was superadded which stopped when apomorphine was decreased.

Several studies of the behavioral effects of ET-495 and apomorphine are reported. The methodology for each is specified with
each individual study. All of these studies were done with the
approval of the Human Research Committee of our medical center.
All were monitored with electrocardiograms and clinical laboratory
profiles. These revealed no abnormalities.

1. Oral Administration of ET-495 in Schizophrenic Patients

In this study, seven schizophrenic patients received no
neuroleptics for from 4 days to 3 weeks. After documentation
of status with the Brief Psychiatric Rating Scale, ET-495 was
administered at an initial dosage of 20 mg t.i.d. Dosage was
increased either daily or every other day until behavioral effects
or side effects indicated discontinuation of drug. Subsequent
ratings were done weekly or at termination.

Because of the small number of patients, and the variability
of their baseline status, analysis of the BPRS scores did not attain
statistical significance. Descriptive aspects of these patients
baseline status and the changes noted are as follows:

Pat. No. 1
A 30-year old male diagnosed as having chronic undifferentiated
schizophrenia, on admission showed depression, flat, constricted

affect, ideas of reference and feelings that others could tell by looking at him that he had molested a child in the past. These symptoms were unchanged after 6 days of treatment with neuroleptics and remained constant for 8 days while he was off neuroleptics prior to receiving ET-495. After receiving ET-495 for 14 days his original symptomatology was worse and he showed superadded irritability, somatic preoccupation and fearfulness with regard to eye contact with others.

Pat. No. 2
A small (91 lb), 26-year old female with a diagnosis of schizoaffective schizophrenia, depressed type. On admission, she was withdrawn, anxious and at times laughed to herself, while apparently alone, although she denied auditory hallucinations. Her status was unchanged after 3 weeks treatment with amitryptilene and chlorpromazine, and remained constant during 3 weeks of observation on placebo.

After receiving ET-495 for 8 days (which was terminated because of vomiting), she was irritable and somewhat hostile, laughed to herself more frequently and openly, doing so in the presence of others, although still explicitly denying hearing "voices".

Pat. No. 3.
A 37-year old male with acute paranoid schizophrenia. On admission he was hostile, markedly evasive and denied that anything was wrong with him whatsoever. He received chlorpromazine for only 1 day, then was observed off neuroleptics for 8 days before ET-495 was administered. During that period his symptomatology was unchanged. After receiving ET-495 for 8 days, he knelt praying in the middle of a day room, responded verbally to auditory hallucinations, was assaultive towards another patient and could not be brought into emotional contact with the rater. He showed occasional vomiting during the time ET-495 was administered.

Pat. No. 4
A 38-year old female diagnosed as having chronic undifferentiated schizophrenia. Her status on admission was characterized by agitation, depression, continuous vivid mental imagery and constant "tunes" which were not exactly "heard" and which changed each time she looked at another person. This did not improve after 4 days treatment with chlorpromazine and lithium and was unchanged during 4 days of observation while off all medication except chloral hydrate for agitation. After receiving ET-495 for 11 days she had become disheveled in her appearance and showed disorganization of thought so that it was more difficult to follow her trend of ideas. Insomnia developed during ET-495 administration.

Pat. No. 5

A 42-year old male diagnosed as suffering from schizoaffective schizophrenia, depressed type. His depression was accompanied by severe vegetative signs, particularly psychomotor retardation and insomnia. He had had several similar past episodes over the preceding 10-12 years during which he improved on chlorpromazine and failed to respond to tricyclic antidepressants. At least one previous hospitalization was for acute psychotic symptomatology. This occurred less than 1 year prior to his current admission when he was brought to Bellevue by police after being found agitated, half-unclothed, and throwing money away on the steps of a church claiming to have seen and spoken to God. In the hospital, he showed thought disorder, preoccupation with past homosexual experiences and diffuse paranoid ideation, and improved on chlorpromazine 900 mg daily.

His current depressive symptoms were unchanged by treatment with chlorpromazine or imipramine and remained stable while he was observed off all medications for 7 days. Administration of ET-495 for 9 days did not induce any change in his status.

Pat. No. 6

A 25-year old female, with chronic undifferentiated schizophrenia. On admission she was depressed and received imipramine in high doses. This led to a deterioration in her status and the development of diffuse paranoid ideation and almost constant incongruent giggling in response to acknowledged auditory hallucinations that she stated were sexual in nature and refused to describe further. These symptoms were unchanged by treatment with chlorpromazine for 22 days and remained constant over 10 days observation off neuroleptics. No abnormal movements were present at this time. ET-495 was then given for 18 days and failed to produce any clear cut change in her symptoms. The drug was discontinued because of the sudden development of a choreoathetoid syndrome resulting in almost continuous involuntary movement. This disappeared completely 48 hrs after the drug was discontinued.

Pat. No. 7

A 24-year old female diagnosed as having chronic undifferentiated schizophrenia. On admission, she was loud, intrusive, agitated, socially inappropriate and at times impulsively assaultive in response to auditory hallucinations. Treatment with chlorpromazine for 5 days led to minimal diminution of these symptoms. Her status remained constant during 7 days observation off all neuroleptics. All psychopathology cleared during 11 days of ET-495 administration.

2.   Oral Administration of ET-495 to Non-Schizophrenics

ET-495 was administered to three non-schizophrenic patients.

The first was a 47-year old alcoholic with endogenous depression admitted because of incipient D.T's. He was initially treated with anxiolytic drugs but was on placebo for 9 days before ET-495 was initiated. He received the drug for 23 days and attained a maximal daily dose of 280 mg. The only behavioral effects noted were a decrease in depression and subjectively noted increased feelings of irritability which were not objectively apparent. Side effects consisted of transient nausea and vomiting, increased perspiration and insomnia.

The second patient was a 33-year old glutethamide addict admitted for detoxification. When this was completed and he had received sedative-hypnotics for sleep only for 5 days, he was administered ET-495 for 28 days. A maximal daily dose of 400 mg was attained. He noted the following physical side effects which were dose-related in intensity: nausea, anorexia, with a 5 lb weight loss, palpitations, overactivity, severe insomnia in spite of drowsiness and increased perspiration. This constellation suggested CNS stimulant effects but when specifically asked he stated that his feeling tone was quite different from his past experiences of cocaine or amphetamine.

The psychological effects that he noted were: 1. Slight irritability ('I can control it") 2. Depression ("I feel like crying. That's the God's honest truth. But I don't why".) 3. Feelings of coldness toward his family (...like I don't belong there".) 4. Ideas of reference, a constant feeling of being watched. He walked out of his way to avoid passing groups of people and when he did would ("look at myself, my clothes, to see what they were looking at. I'd check myself to see if I'm walking too fast or too slow.") He feared people would think he was listening to their conversation ("when I know I'm not,") and had increased startle reactions to noise which embarrassed him because he thought others noticed him because of them. 5. Auditory hallucinations consisting of hearing his name called. These occurred only during the last two days on drug at a frequency of approximately six times a day. Upon hearing his name, he would walk to where people should be and found none. "I look. No one's playing no games. I know that."

Sensorium was clear. He was oriented and able to do serial subtraction of 7's from 100 without difficulty.

It should be specifically noted that he was receiving Dilantin 400 mg/day during the time ET-495 was administered. Psychological effects cleared 72-96 hrs after ET-495 was discontinued.

The third patient was a 53-year old male manic depressive. His first psychiatric illness was a manic episode at age 44. In a subsequent hospitalization in the same year he was treated for depression with ECT. Since that time he has had 3 manic episodes during

which he was not hospitalized, and 2 periods of depressions during
which he stayed at home and was unable to work, but was not hospitalized. In August 1974, he became depressed and was treated as an
inpatient and refractory to antidepressant treatment. It was decided
to administer ET-495 for possible antidepressant effect. He received
ET-495 for 16 days and attained a maximum dose of 240 mg daily.
This caused palpitations, irritability and insomnia and the drug
was discontinued. A second trial of ET-495 was undertaken later
(after a 10-day period off all medication except h.s. chloral
hydrate). The dosage was increased more gradually over the next
16 days to a maximum of 160 mg daily. At this point he became
intensely upset by voices (which he stated he had been hearing
from 5-6 days) and rapidly became severely agitated.

The voices consisted of another patient's particularly, as
well as voices of a psychiatrist and male nurse on the ward. All
centered around accusations of homosexuality. He heard: "He's a
faggot" all day long. At the window, he heard: "There's that cocksucker S" from the street. When alone in a ward day room, he con-
tinued to hear "Look at that cocksucker S" and "He's definitely a
faggot." He was apprehensive and appeared almost tearful when he
asked if he weren't kidding himself - i.e., was he "really" a homosexual. He absolutely refused to believe that the voices were drug
induced. Although frightened of the one patient whose voice he
heard, he was not diffusely referential with regard to other patients.
No formal thought disorder was appreciated. Affect was congruent
but somewhat constricted. Sensoria were clear. He was oriented to
day and date and able to do serial subtraction of 7's from 100
fluently.

ET-495 was discontinued and haloperidol 5 mg given intra-
muscularly. After 15 min the voices stopped for 1.5 hrs and then
reappeared. Administration of haloperidol 10 mg orally 3 x daily
for 2 days led to suppression of the voices which did not recur
after haloperidol was discontinued.

3. Intravenous Administration of ET-495 to Schizophrenics and
    Non-Schizophrenics

Three schizophrenics received 6 mg ET-495 by intravenous drip
over 70-105 min. All had transient vomiting which cleared when the
rate of administration was decreased. One developed an erection
during drug administration; a second patient noted that his hearing,
vision, and thoughts seemed "extra clear". He felt "more ambitious",
and felt that "everything has a purpose". He likened his feeling to
past experiences with cocaine. None showed worsening of psychopathology.

Two other subjects, a normal and a schizophrenic patient, were administered i.v. ET-495 using an infusion pump so that a constant rate of administration was attained. The normal received 6 mg over 80 min. He did not vomit, blood pressure and pulse were 140/100 and 96 at baseline. At termination these were 134/100 and 100. He noted that the room "seemed brighter" and appeared sleepy with constant yawning. He expressed feelings of lethargy and restlessness. At termination he was nauseated and showed mild ptosis, ataxia, and slurred speech which cleared in 15 min. The schizophrenic female received 5 mg of ET-495 over 70 min. Pulse and blood pressure were 80 and 120/80 at baseline and 82 and 110/65 at termination. She felt "a little sleepy" at termination but noted no other subjective effects.Psychopathology was not exacerbated.

4.   Intravenous Administration of Apomorphine to
      Schizophrenics and Non-Schizophrenics.

Freshly prepared apomorphine has been administered intravenously by infusion pump to 4 schizophrenics who had not received neuroleptics for at least 7 days and 3 non-schizophrenics in an ongoing study. Apomorphine administered under these conditions showed mild hypotensive effects. No schizophrenic demonstrated an exacerbation of psychopathology when apomorphine was administered.

5.   Effects of Large Dose Intravenous Administration
      of Apomorphine after Blockade of Emetic Effects.

Nymark (67) has shown that metaclopromide blocks apomorphine-emesis in the dog without antagonizing the stereotyped behavior induced by apomorphine administration. Since stereotypy is generally used as a model of the stimulant psychoses in humans (29,73,76) this finding suggested the possibility of exploring the behavioral effects of apomorphine by administering doses greater than those which produce emesis. Costall and Nylor classify metaclopromide as non-neuroleptic (22).

In this study a 55.9 kg subject received 5 mg doses of meta-clopromide intravenously. These were repeated every 2-3 min with intermittent monitoring of blood pressure. A total cumulative dose of 20 mg metaclopromide was administered without effect on cardio-vascular measurements (B.P. and Pulse rate before metaclopromide 130/80, 84; 130/96, 88 on two occasions. Blood pressure and pulse rate after 20 mg metaclopromide was 130/86, 88. He was observed for 24 min after the total cumulative dose of metaclopromide. Thereafter, apomorphine was administered intravenously in 3 mg doses approximately every 10 min (in 2 cases 1.5 mg doses were given). In this way, a cumulative dose of 24 mg apomorphine was administered in 52 min. Pulse and blood pressure at cessation were 82, 140/96.

Behavioral effects noted were hiccough, which stopped spontaneously before the study was terminated, yawning, sedation and mild ptosis. Subjectively, the subject felt lightheaded, tired, found it difficult to concentrate, and follow conversations, and felt that it was difficult to keep his eyes open. At termination he had mild nausea and described his feeling tone as "queasy, and a sick, fatigued feeling like the flu." No stimulant or euphoriant effects were noted.

DISCUSSION

Oral ET-495 was found to cause worsening in some schizophrenics and to induce a paranoid state and a syndrome of auditory hallucinosis in two non-schizophrenics. These observations are consistent with the hypothesized role of dopamine in schizophrenia (85). They also confirm the observations of Lieberman et al (59) suggesting psychotogenic potential for ET-495 in Parkinsonian patients.

Some caveats to the interpretation of these data are as follows: 1. Presynaptic events may be involved in the actions of both ET-495 (36) and apomorphine (42), 2. ET-495 apparently does affect noradrenergic mechanisms to some extent (37).

In attempting to quantitate the observed effects of ET-495, however, some problems in interpretation do arise. The worsening of schizophrenic symptomatology was not nearly as florid or consistent as was noted when l-DOPA was administered to a schizophrenic population (4). Similarly, the effects of ET-495 in schizophrenics were not as dramatic as those reported by Janowski and Davis when methylphenidate or amphetamine was administered (5) or as those we have observed. Why receptor stimulators should differ so in clinical potency from dopaminergic agonists with a predominantly presynaptic mode of action is the central problem of this paper and will be discussed further.

It should be noted, however, that the mild to moderate psychotogenic potency of ET-495 that we have noted does correlate well with its quantitative potency in two other systems, antiparkinsonian efficacy, and induction of stereotypy. Chase (17) has noted that optimal doses of l-DOPA had nearly twice the overall antiparkinsonian efficacy as ET-495. Corrodi et al (21) reported stereotypy in rats only at doses over 50 mg/kg. Van Beek and Timmerman (91) found that 100 mg/kg ET-495 was required to induce stereotyped behavior in rats equal to that caused by 200 mg/kg l-DOPA given with the decarboxylase inhibitor MK-486; and that 1.25 mg/kg apomorphine i.v. caused even stronger stereotypy.

The failure of intravenously administered ET-495 and apomorphine to cause activation of schizophrenic psychopathology is superficially at least inconsistent with the hypothesized role of dopamine in schizophrenia. Several possibilities exist which might explain this finding.

1. The emetic effects of these drugs, particularly when administered intravenously, might well be so much more potent than their psychotogenic effects that the latter might never be noted in human studies. Nymark's observations (67) that the threshold for apomorphine emesis in the dog is much lower (15-25 ug/kg i.v.) than the threshold for induction of stereotyped behaviour (0.4-0.8 mg/kg i.v.) is consistent with this possibility.

2. Dosage, route of administration and acute vs. chronic administration all might be of importance in determining behavioral outcome. Chronic orally administered l-DOPA, for example, has clear CNS stimulant effects in humans. Dunkley et al (28), however, have shown depressant effects after acute i.p. administration to dogs of 30-40 mg/kg, while at the same time Willner et al. (94) in the same laboratory have shown stimulant effects and stereotypy in dogs after acute i.p. administration of 60 mg/kg. Similarly, a case reported by Strian et al (88) suggests that apomorphine can be psychotogenic under conditions of chronic oral administration, although Cotzias (24) has reported two cases that suggest that apomorphine is less likely to cause psychosis than l-DOPA.

3. Finally, and we believe, most likely, the effects of drugs such as amphetamine and l-DOPA on the one hand and apomorphine and ET-495 on the other may be intrinsically different qualitatively and mediated by different mechanisms. The sedation seen after i.v. apomorphine and ET-495 particularly, contrasts with the stimulant effects of amphetamine and l-DOPA. We were curious as to the possibility that stimulant or psychotogenic effects might be seen after larger dose apomorphine administration, but none were noted in the experiment in which 24 mg were given intravenously.

More specific evidence for intrinsic differences in the mechanisms of action between l-DOPA and apomorphine is derived from observations by Duby et al (27) and Cotzias (24). Both described antagonism between these two drugs (surprisingly, even in their capacity to cause emesis) and not additive effects, as one would anticipate if both drugs acted via identical mechanisms. "The respective side effects were not additive; the 'awakening effect' and involuntary movements and nausea induced by levodopa were antagonized by apomorphine, whereas the sedative effects and the nausea of apomorphine were antagonized by levodopa." (27). In view of this observed antagonism it is significant that Goldberg (41) has shown that apomorphine has both "agonist and antagonist properties" on dopamine receptors in renal vasculature.

Similarly, important differences in mechanisms of action between l-DOPA and ET-495 are suggested by Chase and Shoulson's (18)
observations that ET-495 caused improvement in tardive dyskinesia
while l-DOPA causes exacerbation of this condition. These investigators also suggest ET-495 to be "a partial dopamine receptor
agonist".

Further evidence suggesting that apomorphine and ET-495 act
via mechanisms different from those of presynaptic agonists comes
from studies of dopaminergic neurons using extracellular single
unit recording techniques (Walters et al [93]). These investigators
showed development of tolerance to the effects of apomorphine and
ET-495, that one induced cross tolerance to the effects of the other,
and that once established this tolerance extended to blockade the
effects of presynaptic agonists.

Our findings with regard to induction of psychosis or worsening of schizophrenic pathology are consistent with the hypothesis
that postsynpatic agonist stimulation activates an inhibitory feedback loop to the presynaptic neuron and this causes self-limiting
clinical effects. Presynaptic agonists, on the other hand, apparently
either do not activate this negative feedback or are capable of
overcoming it and thus are more potently psychotogenic.

MAOI

These agents may act as behavioral activating agents through
effects on the neurotransmitter amines. They can precipitate manic
episodes and produce exacerbations of psychotic symptomatology in
some schizophrenic patients (14,46,74). They appear to potentiate
the psychotomimetic effects of some amino acids, including
l-Methionine and possibly l-DOPA (12,72,89).

IMIPRAMINE

The administration of tricyclic compounds may also precipitate
a manic episode in bipolar manic depressive patients (16).

A review of the literature makes it appear fairly clear that
the production of a manic episode is highly associated with a history of manic-depressive disorder. The mechanism by which imipramine
might act as a trigger for mania in some cases is not clear. It is
possible that there is some commonality in the underlying biochemical effects produced by both the tricyclic anti-depressants
and l-DOPA in their interactions with manic-depressive and schizophrenic substrates, albeit, the incidence of such activation effects
in both diagnostic categories seems higher, more predictable, and
consistent with l-DOPA than with the tricyclics.

It has been reported that imipramine hydrochloride activates
the psychotic process in schizophrenic patients (32,56,57,71).

Therefore, it seemed plausible that imipramine might be used
as a pharmacologic tool to reveal differences among diagnostic
processes (38). Three different diagnostic groups were studied -
(a) 15 schizophrenic patients (six chronic with deterioration -
apathetic, withdrawn, anergic, inactive; seven responsive and still
showing some evidence of active schizophrenic processes; and two
whose diagnosis was not unanimous); (b) seven non-schizophrenic
patients (two chronic brain syndromes with syphilis, two chronic
brain syndromes with alcoholism, one epileptic, and two uncertain)
with psychotic reaction; and (c) eight nonschizophrenic nonpsychotic
(five sociopaths and three alcoholics).

Psychiatric Observation

Imipramine was given in a dose of 3 mg/kg body weight. The
six chronic deteriorated patients did not show any specific change
in their clinical condition, whereas the other nine schizophrenics
showed some degree of activation of their psychotic state with
either appearance or increase in delusions, hallucinations, and
disturbed behavior. Psychotic material was produced freely and
there was an increase in general activity; in some subjects there
was evidence of hostility. The response was particularly interesting
in those cases (two) in whom the diagnosis was uncertain. An overt
psychotic picture, with freely produced delusions and ideas of
reference, aggresiveness, hostility, and unco-operativeness emerged.

The seven psychotic nonschizophrenic subjects showed increased
psychotic activity, with the exception of an epileptic on Dilantin
and phenobarbital, who became more drowsy. The remainder of the
group in varying degrees became more aggressive, hostile, abusive,
overactive, and generally more difficult to manage. Hallucinatory
phenomena became clearly apparent in two subjects in whom it could
previously be deduced only from their behavior. One subject began
to write voluminous notes and incessantly replied to his hallucinations almost to the point of breathlessness.

The eight nonpsychotic subjects showed no striking changes nor
did they exhibit any psychotic features (38).

There have been no reports of imipramine-induced psychotic
manifestations in character disorders (43) or neurotics (55,60).
Klein and Fink noted that 19% of their schizophrenic group developed a pattern of "agitated disorganization" and a "manic" pattern
in 6% of the schizophrenics, whereas in 20% of manic depressive
patients a manic episode occurred. Pilkington reported on the effect
of imipramine in mental defectives; in his group with schizophrenic

traits 72% developed florid schizophrenic symptoms (70).

THE LITHIUM ION

Therapeutic specificity intimately depends on diagnostic
accuracy. In order to appreciate the specific therapeutic effects
of lithium, it should be prescribed for patients showing a clear
diagnostic indication for this drug. The manic phase of manic-
depressive illness is the prime indication for lithium treatment.
The ambiguities surrounding the diagnosis of manic illness, and
especially that shadowy interface between manic phase, manic-
depressive disorder and schizophrenia, schizoaffective type,
excited phase, present a diagnostic dilemma in that both illnesses
share large components of both affective as well as behavioral
disturbance. The resolution of this problem of differential diagnosis is critical, however, because several studies have indicated
that patients do not do as well on lithium when the manic picture
is clouded with "atypical" features (80,35,50). This "atypical"
group includes subjects with schizophrenic symptoms, and the significance of such differential drug responsiveness has been underlined
in several recent studies (52,70,82). In discussing their trial of
lithium, Arnoff and Epstein (70) noted that some of their schizoaffective cases, which they acknowledged might well have been
designated "atypical manic-depressive illness" by others, showed
only moderate response or symptom aggravation under lithium treatment. It is on this sort of explicitness about diagnostic amgi-
guities that progress in delineating the therapeutic usefulness
of lithium depends. The studies by Johnson et al (52) and Shopsin
et al (82) underscore the specificity of action of lithium; both
investigations indicate strongly that lithium has no apparent
sedative or neuroleptic properties and that it can, in fact, precipitate or contribute to further decompensation of schizophrenic
symptomatology.

Central to the issue of lithium specificity, our group (83)
reported toxic-confusional states as well as activating effects in
a considerable number of schizophrenic patients (11 of 17) receiving
lithium carbonate. Significant features in these cases are a general
worsening of previously manifest psychoses with the appearance of
bizarre affect and behavior patterns, inconsistent changes in
psychomotor activity, aggravation of delusional thought, and florid
hallucinatory phenomena. The frequently concomitant appearance of
reduced comprehension, clouding of sensorium with confusion, memory
impairment, and disorientation indicate organic brain dysfunction
in these patients.

Blood lithium levels were quite modest in all instances (mean
0.750 mEq/liter) and, paradoxically, the common lithium effects or
toxic manifestations were not consistently present. The most con-

sistent laboratory abnormalities consisted of EEG changes including alterations in the alpha activity, diffuse slowing, accentuation of previous focal abnormalities, or the appearance of previously absent focal changes or both. The occurrence of neurotoxicity corresponds, therefore, to the presence and severity of EEG changes.

Previous reports of psychotogenic effects and confusion during lithium treatment have appeared in the literature (11,40,47,58,64, 79,84,87).

Several studies have offered convincing evidence of changes in electrical activity of the brain during lithium treatment, relating these changes to electrolyte effects or shifts (9,65,69) Johnson et al (53) noted that the most significant changes in EEG during chronic lithium administration were seen in individuals showing base-line abnormalities. Underlining the possible relevance of premorbid conditions to such changes, Rochford et al (75) indicated that neurologic abnormalities were found in nearly 40% of young adult psychiatric patients, significantly more than in controls (5%). The incidence of neurologic impairment did not differ significantly from one diagnostic group to another, except for those patients with affective disorders. It is interesting that no neurologic abnormality was found among subjects in this latter diagnostic category. One would anticipate from such findings that neurotoxicity following lithium administration would be highest in patients with other than primary affective disorders, that is, in subjects not diagnosed as having manic-depressive illness. This is supported by the findings in two double-blind studies using lithium or chlorpromazine in schizophrenic patients (52,82). Indications are that such patients, whether by differential handling (excretion), differences in electrolyte or endocrine substrate, or "abnormal" base-line neuropathy, exhibit a decreased threshold tolerance or sensitivity for the lithium ion, which exposes them to CNS toxicity at moderate to low levels of serum lithium.

ACETYLCHOLINE

Diisopropyl fluorophosphonate(DFP) is an anticholinesterase with 30 times the potency of physostigmine. It is an irreversible inhibitor of acetylcholinesterase. It produces in animals and man effects similar to the muscarinic and nicotinic actions of acetyl-choline. Grob et al (49), after acute administration of DFP, have described EEG changes in man and mental symptoms such as tremulous-ness, insomnia, nightmares, and confusion. Rountree et al (77) examined the effects of this agent given chronically (13 mg i.m. over 7 days) to schizophrenic and manic-depressive patients and to a group of controls.

Changes in blood pressure were significantly different in the two psychotic groups. In all the manic-depressive patients (nine, except for the two in a euthymic phase), there was a gradual fall of blood pressure from the beginning of the injection period until approximately 7 days after the withdrawal of the drug.

In the schizophrenic patients (19), however, there was a tendency for the blood pressure to rise. No schizophrenic patient showed a progressive fall in blood pressure, and no manic-depressive patient showed a progressive rise.

Although the schizophrenic and manic-depressive patients received the same total dosage of DFP and showed comparable cholinesterase inhibition, both the incidence and severity of the muscarinic effects were considerably less in the schizophrenic group. The remarkable tolerance to the drug exhibited by certain schizophrenic patients is exemplified by one patient who received a total dosage of 63 mg of DFP over 35 days without showing any characteristic effects of the drug. The few schizophrenics who showed a response to DFP comparable with that of the manic-depressive group were of the paranoid type.

In general, the EEG changes were much more marked in the manic-depressive than in the schizophrenic patients, particularly in the appearance of slow activity.

Mental Changes

In six of the 17 schizophrenic patients, a most pronounced mental effect was observed. This consisted of an "activation" of the psychosis or of the reappearance in chronic cases of the florid symptoms that had characterized the onset of the illness - bizaare behavior, thought disorder, ideas of reference, and auditory hallucinations - without impairment of consciousness. These changes persisted for a number of months after withdrawal of DFP.

Of the manic-depressive group, the two euthymic cases showed only slight mental changes. Sleeplessness and increased dreaming occurred, and slight depression in one. Two of the six hypomanic cases were unaffected by the drug. In the remainder (four hypomanic and one depressed), significant mental changes occurred, with the appearance of a marked depressant effect.

In the normal subjects, a very characteristic picture of clinical depression, irritability, lassitude, and apathy appeared. They looked dejected and felt unhappy. They were retarded and talked little and despondently.

After this report, in 1961, Gershon and Shaw (39) reported the results of an accidental series of chronic exposures to organophosphorus insecticides. Sixteen cases were reported - three were scientists studying the efficacy of sprays, eight worked in these test greenhouses, and five were farm workers. Of the 16 cases, seven were depressive and five schizophrenic; in one, a fugue state was the presenting symptom.

The fact that only two forms of psychiatric illness were induced - depressive and schizophrenic reactions - suggests that perhaps some interaction with a specific substrate produces a particular psychiatric response pattern. Follow-up of our cases showed that the effects persisted for about 6 months after the exposure ceased.

Discussion

In attempting to synthesize the effects of this array of drugs on the various diagnostic entities and disease substrates, we find that certain limited conclusions may be offered - that some drugs have an apparent specific interaction with different diagnostic and disease substrates. When the organophosphorus insecticides interact with manic-depressive disorder, a change is produced in the direction of depression, and when given to schizophrenic states an activation of psychopathology is induced. Then, when administered to normal individuals, two distinct diagnostic patterns emerge - schizophrenia and depression. This example would tend to support the view that a continuum does not exist across diagnoses, but that there is a continuum in those predisposed individuals from normal through to manifest illness.

We have one class of agents - l-DOPA, the amphetamines and related agents, and imipramine - which may be considered together.

l-DOPA, in its interaction with three diagnostic types - schizophrenics, manic-depressives, and nonpsychotic subjects - seems to induce a threshold response pattern. That is, in schizophrenics, an activation of psychosis is seen in most subjects at about one-half the dose given to nonpsychotics and in whom only a very low incidence of psychosis appears, which exibits the form of a schizophrenic reaction when it appears. In a manic-depressive population, the reaction pattern is of a manic type.

Imipramine essentially follows this reaction pattern, i.e. in manic-depressives, the pathologic reaction is that of mania; in schizophrenics, about 20 to 30% show an activation of their psychosis. The nonpsychotics, given the same dose and duration of administration, showed no pathologic reaction patterns.

The amphetamines and related agents in schizophrenic and non-schizophrenic groups demonstrate responses similar to those seen

with l-DOPA. That is, these agents demonstrate a lower threshold
of psychotogenicity in the schizophrenic substrate than in the
nonschizophrenics, but there exist a continuity of the reaction
across both groups that is somewhat dose- and time- dependent.

These data might support a concept of disease and diagnosis
specificity; the drugs emplyed here produce reaction patterns
based on the specificity of the substrate.

The therapeutic responses with lithium in manic, schizophrenic
and schizoaffective patients suggest a degree of specificity also.

The cholinergic activation data again seemed to suggest a
specific drug interaction with diagnosis, but no simple biochemical
explanations can be made.

I would like to draw some other conclusions from this
material.

We have described our ability to induce psychotic states de
novo or activate the endogenous psychosis in several conditions;
viz. schizophrenia and manic-depressive disorder. We have done
this by affecting quite different central neurotransmitter systems
and still producing the same psychopathological end point. For
example, we can induce or activate a schizophrenic-like state by
activating cholinergic systems and can produce the same end point
by activating dopaminergic systems. A similar situation exists in
regard to manic-depressive illness.

These findings tend to suggest rather strongly that we cannot implicate a unitary concept of neurotransmitter involvement.
It seems clear that if we manipulate one in a massive or significant fashion, it is exceedingly probable that others are affected
secondarily.

REFERENCES

1.   ANDEN, N.D., CORRODI, H., FUXE, K.: Turnover studies using
        synthesis inhibition. In: Metabolism of amines in the
        brain, G. Hopper, ed. Macmillan, New York, pp. 38-47,
        1969.

2.   ANGRIST, B.M., GERSHON, S.: The phenomenology of experimen-
        tally-induced amphetamine psychosis: Preliminary
        Observations. Biol. Psychiat. 2. pp. 95-107, 1970.

3.   ANGRIST, B., SATHANANTHAN, G., and GERSHON, S.: Behavioral
        effects of l-DOPA in schizophrenic patients. Psycho-
        pharmacologia 31: 1-2, 1973.

4. ANGRIST, B.M., SATHANANTHAN, G., WILK, S., and GERSHON, S.:
        Behavioral and biochemical effects of 1-DOPA in psychi-
        atric patients. In: Frontiers in Catecholamine Research
        ed. by E. Usdin and S. Snyder, Pergamon, Oxford,
        pp.991-994.,1973.

5. ANGRIST, B.M., and GERSHON, S.: The phenomenology of experi-
        mentally-induced amphetamine psychosis. Preliminary
        Observations. Biol. Psychiat. 2:95-107, 1970.

6. ANGRIST, B., GERSHON, S.: Dopamine and psychotic states:
        Preliminary remarks, In: Advances in Biochemical
        Psychopharmacology, Vol. 12, edited by E. Usdin,
        Raven Press, New York. pp. 211-219, 1974.

7. ANGRIST, B.M., SHOPSIN, B., and GERSHON, S.: The comparative
        psychotomimetic effects of stereoisomers of amphetamine.
        Nature, 234: 152-153, 1971.

8. ANGRIST, B.M., THOMPSON, H., SHOPSIN, B., and GERSHON, S.:
        Clinical studies with dopamine receptor stimulants.
        Psychopharmacologia (Berl.) 44:273-280, 1975.

9. ARAKI, I., ITO, M., KOSTYUK, P., OSCARSSON, O., and OSHIMA, I.:
        The effects of alkaline cations on the responses of cat
        spinal neurons and their removal from the cell. Proc.
        R. Soc. Lond. (Biol.), 162:319, 1965.

10. ARONOFF, M.S., and EPSTEIN, R.S.: Lithium failure in mania:
        A clinical study. Annual Mtg. of American Psychiatric
        Association, Bal Harbor, Florida. 1969.

11. BALDESSARINI, R.J., and STEPHENS, J.H.: Lithium carbonate for
        affective disorders. Arch. Gen. Psychiatry, 22:72,
        1970.

12. BERLET, H.H., MATSUMOTO, K., PSCHEIDT, G.R., SPAIDE, J.,
        BULL, C., and HIMWICH, H.E.: Biochemical correlates
        of behavior in schizophrenic patients. Arch. Gen.
        Psychiatry, 13: 521-531, 1970.

13. BROGDEN, R.N., SPIEGHT, T.M., and AVERY, G.S.: Levodopa:
        A review of pharmacological properties and therapeutic
        uses with particular reference to Parkinson's disease.
        Drugs. 2:257-408, 1971.

14. BRUNE, G.G., PSCHEIDT, G.R., and HIMWICH, H.E.: Different
        responses of urinary tryptamine and of total catechol-
        amines during treatment with reserpine and iscarboxazid
        in schizophrenic patients. Int. J. Neuropharmacol.
        2:17-23, 1963.

15.   BUCHSBAUM, M., GOODWIN, F., MURPHY, D.L., and BORGE, G.:
       Average evoked response in affective disorders.
       Am. J. Psychiatr., 128 (1): 19-25, 1971.

16.   BUNNEY, W.E., Jr., MURPHY, D.L., GOODWIN, F.K. and BORGE, G.:
       The switch process from depression to mania: Relation-
       ship to drugs which alter brain amines. Lancet, 1:
       1022-1027, 1970.

17.   CHASE, T.N.: Clinical studies of dopaminergic mechanisms. In:
       Neuropsychopharmacology of monoamines and their
       regulatory enzymes, E. Usdin, ed. Raven Press, New
       York, pp. 427-434. 1974.

18.   CHASE, T.N., SHOULSON, I.: Dopaminergic mechanisms in patients
       with extrapyramidal disease. In: Advances in neurology,
       Vol. 9, D.B. Calne, T.N. Chase and A. Barbeau, eds.
       Raven Press, New York, pp. 359-366. 1975.

19.   CONNELL, P.H.: Amphetamine Psychosis. Maudsley Monographs No.5
       Oxford Univ. Press, London. 1958.

20.   COOPER, J.E., KENDALL, R.E., GURLAND, B.J., SARTORIUS, N.,
       and FARKAS, T.: Cross national study of diagnoses of
       mental disorders. Am. J. Psychiatry, 125: 21-29,1969.

21.   CORRODI, H., FUXE, K., UNGERSTEDT, U.: Evidence for a new type
       of dopamine receptor stimulating agent. J. Pharm.
       Pharmacol. 23:989-991, 1971.

22.   COSTALL, B., NAYLOR, R.J.: On the mode of action of apomorphine,
       Europ. J. Pharmacol. 21: 350-361, 1973b.

23.   COSTALL, B., NAYLOR, R.J.: Is there a relationship between
       the involvement of extrapyramidal and mesolimbic brain
       areas with the cataleptic action of neuroleptic agents
       and their clinical effect? Psychopharmacologia (Berl.)
       32:161-170. 1973a.

24.   COTZIAS, G.C.: Levodopa, manganese and degenerations of the
       brain, harvey society lectures. Delivered 1972 under
       the auspices of the Harvey Society Series 68, pp. 115-
       147, New York, Academic Press. 1974.

25.   CREESE, I.: Behavioral evidence of dopamine receptor stimula-
       tion by piribedil (ET-495) and its metabolite S 584.
       Europ. J. Pharmacol. 28: 55-58, 1974.

26.   DAVIS, J.M. and JANOWSKY,D.S.: Amphetamine and methylphenidate
        psychosis. In: Frontiers in Catecholamine Research
        Pergamon, Oxford, pp. 977-981, 1973.

27.   DUBY,S.E., COTZIAS, G.C., PAPAVASILIOU, P.S., LAWRENCE, W.H.:
        Injected apomorphine and orally administered levodopa
        in Parkinsonism. Arch. Neurol. (Chic). 27:474-480.
        1972.

28.   DUNKLEY, B., SANGHVI. I., FRIEDMAN, E., GERSHON, S.: Comparison
        of behavioral and cardiovascular effects of l-DOPA
        and 5-HTP in conscious dogs. Psychopharmacologia (Berl.)
        26:161-172, 1972.

29.   ELLINWOOD, E.H., Jr., SUDILOWSKY, A., NELSON, L.: Behavioral
        analysis of chronic amphetamine intoxication. Biol.
        Psychiat. 4:215-230, 1972.

30.   ERNST, A.M.: Mode of action of apomorphine and dexamphetamine
        on gnawing compulsion in rats. Psychopharmacologia
        (Berl.) 10:316-323, 1967.

31.   EVERETT, G.M., BORCHERDING, J.W.: l-DOPA: Effect on concentra-
        tion of dopamine, norepinephrine, and serotonin in
        brains of mice. Science, 168: 849-850, 1970.

32.   FELDMAN, P.E.: The treatment of anergic schizophrenia with
        imipramine. J. Clin. Exp. Psychopath., 20:235, 1959.

33.   FRAM, D.H., MURPHY, D.L., GOODWIN, F.K., KEITH, H., BRODIE, H.,
        BUNNEY, W.E., Jr. and SNYDER, F.: l-DOPA and sleep in
        depressed patients. Psychophysiology 7:316-317, 1970.

34.   FRIEDMAN, E., GERSHON, S.: l-DOPA: Centrally mediated emission
        of seminal fluid in male rats. Life Sci., 11:435-440,
        1972.

35.   FRIES, H.: Experience with lithium carbonate treatment at a
        psychiatric department in the period 1964-1967. Acta
        Psychiatr. Scand. (Suppl), 207:41, 1969.

36.   FUXE, K., AGNATE, L.F., CORRODI, H., EVERITT, B.J., HOKFELT, T..
        LOFSTROM, J., UNGERSTEDT, U.: Action of dopamine recep-
        tor agonists in forebrain and hypothalamus: Rotational
        behavior, ovulation and dopamine turnover. In: Advances
        in neurology, Vol. 9, D.B. Calne, T.N. Chase, and
        A. Barbeau, eds., Raven Press, New York, pp. 223-242,
        1975.

37.   GARRATINI, S., BARREGGI, S., MARC, V., CALDERINI, G.,
          MARSELLA, P.L.: Effects of pirobedil on noradrenaline
          and MOPEGSO$_4$ levels in the rat brain. Europ. J.
          Pharmacol. 28:214-216,

38.   GERSHON, S., HOLMBERG, G., MATTSON, E., and MATTSON, N.:
          Imipramine hydrochloride. Arch. Gen. Psychiatry.
          6: 96-101. 1962.

39.   GERSHON, S., and SHAW, F.H.: Psychiatric sequelae of chronic
          exposure to organophosphorus insecticides. Lancet,
          1:1371-1374, 1961.

40.   GLESSINGER, B.: Evaluation of lithium in treatment of psychotic
          excitement. Med. J. Aust. 41:277, 1954.

41.   GOLDBERG, L.I.: Comparison of putative dopamine receptors in
          blood vessels and the central nervous system. In:
          Advances in neurology, Vol. 9, D.B. Calne, T.N. Chase,
          and A. Barbeau, Eds. Raven Press, New York, pp. 53-56.
          1975.

42.   GOLDSTEIN, M., BATTISTA, A.F., OHMOTO, T., ANAGNOSTE, B.,
          FUXE, K.: Tremor and involuntary movements in monkeys:
          Effects of l-DOPA and of a dopamine receptor stimulating
          agent. Science, 179:816-817, 1973.

43.   GOLDNER, R.D.: Control of minor sexual compulsions with imi-
          pramine and amine oxidase regulators. Third World
          Congr. Psychiatry, 2:1155, 1961.

44.   GOODWIN, F.K.: Behavioral effects of l-DOPA in man. In:
          Psychiatric Complications of Medical Drugs, Ed. by
          R.I. Shader, Raven Press, New York, pp. 149-174, 1972.

45.   GOODWIN, F.K., MURPHY, D.L., BRODIE, H.K.H. and BUNNEY, W.E.,
          Jr.: l-DOPA, catecholamines and behavior: A clinical
          and biochemical study in depressed patients. Biol.
          Psychiatry. 2:341-366, 1970.

46.   GREENBLATT, M., GROSSER, G.H., and WECHSLER, H.: A comparative
          study of selected antidepressant medications and EST.
          Am. J. Psychiatry , 119:144-153, 1962.

47.   GREENFIELD, I., ZUGER, M., BLEAK, R.M., and BAKAL, S.F.:
          Lithium chloride intoxication. New York State J. Med.
          50:549, 1950.

48.   GRIFFITH, J.J., CAVANAUGH, J.H., and OATES, J.A.: Psychosis
          induced by the administration of d-amphetamine to
          human volunteers. In: Psychotomimetic Drugs, edited
          by D.H.Efron, Raven Press, New York, p. 28, 1970.

49.   GROB, D., HARVEY, A.M., LANGWORTHY, O.R., and LILIENTHAL, J.R.,
          Jr.: The administration of di-isopropyl fluorophosphate
          (DFP) to man. III. Effect on the central nervous
          system with special reference to the electrical
          activity of the brain. Johns Hopkins Med. J., 81:217,
          1947.

50.   HARTIGAN, G.P.: The use of lithium salts in affective disorders.
          Br. J. Psychiatry, 109:810, 1963.

51.   JANOWSKY, D.S., DAVIS, J.M.: Dopamine, psychomotor stimulants
          and schizophrenia: Effects of methylphenidate and the
          stereoisomers of amphetamine in schizophrenics. In:
          Neuropsychopharmacology of monoamines and their
          regulatory enzymes, E. Usdin, ed. Raven Press, New York,
          pp. 317-323, 1974.

52.   JOHNSON, G., GERSHON, S., and HEKIMIAN, L.J.: Controlled eva-
          luation of lithium and chlorpromazine in the treatment
          of manic states: An interim report. Compr. Psychiatry,
          9:563, 1968.

53.   JOHNSON, G., HEKIMIAN, L., and GERSHON, S.: Differential drug
          responsiveness in psychiatric subjects. 8th Annual
          ACNP Mtg., San Diego, California. 1970.

54.   KAROBATH, M., DIAZ, J.L., HUTTUNEN, M.O.: The effect of 1-DOPA
          on the concentrations of tryptophan, tyrosine, and
          serotonin in rat brain. Europ. J. Pharmacol. 4:393-396.
          1971.

55.   KLEIN, D.F.: Delineation of two drug-responsive anxiety syn-
          dromes. Psychopharmacologia, 5:397, 1964.

56.   KUHN, R.: Uber die Behandlung depressiver Zustande mit einem
          Iminobenzyldervat. Schweiz. Med. Wochenschr. 87:1135,
          1957.

57.   KUHN, R.: The treatment of depressive states with G-22355.
          Am. J. Psychiatry, 115-459, 1958.

58.   LEHMANN, H.E., and BAN, T.A.: Clinical use of other antipsy-
          chotic agents. In: Principles of Psychopharmacology,
          edited by W.G. Clark and J.del Giudice, Academic Press,
          New York, p. 621. 1970.

59.   LEIBERMAN, A., LE BRUN, Y., DINKAR, B., ZOLFAGHARI, M.: The
          use of dopaminergic receptor stimulating agent
          (Piribedil, ET-495) in Parkinson's disease. In:
          Neuropsychopharmacology of monoamines and their regu-
          latory enzymes, E. Usdin ed. Raven Press, New York,
          pp. 415-425,

60.   LEYBERG, J.T., and DENMARK, J.C.: The treatment of depressive
          states with imipramine hydrochloride. Br. J. Psychiat.
          105:1123, 1959.

61.   LEWANDER, T: Effect of chronic-treatment with central stimu-
          lants on brain monoamines and some behavioral and
          physiological functions in rats, guinea pigs and
          rabbits. In: Advances in Biochemical Psychopharmacology
          Vol. 12 edited by E. Usdin, Raven Press, New York,
          pp. 221-239, 1974.

62.   LEWANDER, T.: Effect of chronic-treatment with central stimu-
          lants on brain monoamines and some behavioral and
          physiological functions in rats, guinea pigs and
          rabbits. In: Neuropsychopharmacology of monoamines
          and their regulatory enzymes, E. Usdin, ed., Raven
          Press, New York, pp. 221-239, 1974.

63.   MAJ., J., PAWLOWSKI, L: The hypothermic effect of l-DOPA in the
          rat. Life Sci. 13:141-149,1973.

64.   MAYFIELD, D., and BROWN, R.G.: The clinical laboratory and
          electroencephalographic effects of lithium. J. Psychiat.
          Res. 4:207, 1966.

65.   MORACCI, E.: AZ ione di alcuni sali applicati direttamente
          sui centri corticali sensitivo-Motori del cane. Arch.
          Fisiol., 29:487, 1931.

66.   MURPHY, D.L., BRODIE, H.K.H., GOODWIN, F.K., and BUNNEY, W.E.
          Jr.: l-DOPA: Regular induction of hypomania in bipolar
          manic-depressive patients. Nature. 229:135-136, 1971.

67.   NYMARK, M.: Apomorphine provoked stereotypy in the dog.
          Psychopharmacologia (Berl.) 26: 361-368, 1972.

68. PAUL, M.I., CRAMER, H., and BUNNEY, W.E. Jr.: Urinary cyclic
     AMP in the switch process from depression to mania.
     Science, 171:300-313., 1971.

69. PFEIFFER, C.Z., SINGH, M., and GOLDSTEIN, L.: Single dose-
     effect relationship of lithium on the electrical
     activity of cerebral cortex and of the heart.
     J. Clin. Pharmacol., 9:298, 1969.

70. PILKINGTON, T.L.: A report on "Tofranil" in mental deficiency.
     Am. J. Ment. Defic., 66:729, 1962.

71. POLLACK, B.: Clinical findings in the use of Tofranil in
     depressive and other psychiatric states. Am. J.
     Psychiatry, 116:312, 1959.

72. POLLIN, W., CORDON, P.V. and KETY, S.S.: Effects of amino acid
     feedings in schizophrenic patients treated with ipro-
     niazid. Science, 133: 104-105, 1961.

73. RANDRUP. A., MUNKVAD, I.: Stereotyped activities produced by
     amphetamine in several animal species and man.
     Psychopharmacologia (Berl.) 11, 300-310, 1967.

74. REES, L., and BENAIM, S.: An evaluation of iproniazid in the
     treatment of depression. Br. J. Psychiatry, 106:193-
     202, 1960.

75. ROCHFORD, J.M., DETRE, T., TUCKER, G.J., and HARROW, M.:
     Neuropsychological impairments in functional psychia-
     tric disease. Arch. Gen. Psychiatry, 22:114, 1970.

76. ROTROSEN, J., WALLACH, M.B., ANGRIST, B., GERSHON, S.:
     Antagonism of apomorphine induced stereotypy and emesis
     in dogs by thioridazine, haloperidol, and pimozide.
     Psychopharmacologia (Berl.) 26:185-194, 1972.

77. ROUNTREE, D.W., NEVIN, S., and WILSON, A.: The effects of
     diisoprophylfluorophosphonate in schizophrenia and
     manic depressive psychosis. J. Neurol. Neurosurg.
     Psychiatry. 13:47-62, 1950.

78. SATHANANTHAN, G., ANGRIST, B.M., and GERSHON, S.: Response
     threshold to 1-DOPA in psychiatric patients. Biol.
     Psychiatry, 7:139-149, 1973.

79. SCHOU, M.: Lithium in psychiatric therapy. Psychopharmacologia,
     1:65, 1959.

80.   SCHOU, M., JUEL-NIELSON, N., STROMGREN, E., and BOLDBY, H.:
        The treatment of manic psychoses by the administration
        of lithium salts. J. Neurol. Neurosurg, Psychiatry.
        17:250, 1954.

81.   SCHWAB, R.S., AMADOR, L.V., LETTVIN, J.Y.: Apomorphine in
        Parkinson's disease. Trans. Amer. Neurol. Ass.
        76:251-263, 1951.

82.   SHOPSIN, B., KIM, S.S. and GERSHON, S.: A controlled study
        of lithium vs. chlorpromazine in acute schizophrenics.
        Brit. J. Psychiatry, 119:435-440, 1971.

83.   SHOPSIN, B., JOHNSON, G., and GERSHON, S.: Neurotoxicity with
        lithium: differential drug responsiveness. Int. Pharma-
        copsychiatry. 1970.

84.   SIVADON, P., and CHANOIT, P: Clinical experience with lithium
        treatment of psychomotor excitation. Ann. Medicopsychol.
        113:790, 1955.

85.   SNYDER, S.H.: Amphetamine psychosis: a "model" schizophrenia
        mediated by catecholamines. Am. J. Psychiatry, 130:
        61-67, 1973.

86.   SPENSLEY, J. and ROCKWELL, D.A.: Psychosis during methylpheni-
        date abuse. New Engl. J. Med. 286:880-881, 1972.

87.   SPRING, G.K., SCHWEID, D., GRAY, C., STEINBERG, J. and HARWITZ,
        M.: A double blind comparison of lithium and chlor-
        promazine in the treatment of manic states. Am. J.
        Psychiatry, 126:1306, 1970.

88.   STRIAN, F., MICHLER, E., BENKERT, P.: Tremor inhibition in
        Parkinson syndrome after apomorphine administration
        under 1-DOPA and decarboxylase inhibitor basic therapy.
        Pharmakopsychiat.5:198-205, 1972.

89.   TURNER, W. and MERLIS, S.:A clinical trial of pargyline and
        and 1-DOPA in psychotic subjects. Dis. Nerv. Syst.
        24:538-541, 1964.

90.   UNGERSTEDT, U.: Postsynaptic supersensitivity after 6-hydroxy-
        dopamine-induced degeneration of the nigrotriatal
        dopamine system. Acta. Physiol. Scand., Suppl. 367:
        69-93, 1971.

91.   VAN BEEK, M.C., TIMMERMAN, H.: Some benzhydryl derivatives as
        central dopamine receptor stimulating agents.
        J. Pharm. Pharmacol. 26:57-58, 1974.

92.   WALLACH, M.B.: Drug-induced stereotyped behaviour: similarities
          and differences. In: Advances in Biochemical Psycho-
          pharmacology, Vol. 12, edited by E. Usdin, Raven Press,
          New York, pp. 241-260, 1974.

93.   WALTERS, J., BUNNEY, B.S., ROTH, R.H.: Piribedil and apomor-
          phine: Pre- and postsynaptic effects on dopamine
          synthesis and neuronal activity. In: Advances in
          neurology, Vol. 9, D.B. Calne, T.N. Chase and A. Barbeau
          eds., Raven Press, New York, pp. 273-284, 1975.

94.   WILLNER, J.H., SAMACH, M., ANGRIST, B.M., WALLACH, M.B.,
          GERSHON, S.: Drug-induced stereotyped behavior and
          its antagonism in dogs. Commun. Behav. Biol. 5:135-141.
          1970.

95.   WYATT, R.J., CHASE, T.N. and ENGLEMEN, K.: Effect of 1-DOPA
          on the sleep of man. Nature, 228:999-1001, 1970.

THE MEASUREMENT OF BIOGENIC AMINE TURNOVER USING OXYGEN-18

David Samuel

Isotope Department, Weizmann Institute of Science

Rehovot, Israel

Although the precise relationship between the level and turnover of biogenic amines in brain and mental disorders is not known, there is almost general agreement that these neurotransmitters play a central role in Parkinsonism, manic-depression and schizophrenia.

The evidence for this, most of it indirect, has been discussed extensively, but until recently, experimental difficulties prevented a proper study of biogenic amine turnover in man. These difficulties stem from the inaccessibility of the human brain to direct chemical and pharmacological analysis, thereby necessitating the isolation, identification and measurement of low concentrations of these amines and their major metabolites (both acids and alcohols) in blood, urine and to a more limited extent in the cerebrospinal fluid (CSF) extracted by lumbar puncture.

The origin and time course of the formation of all these metabolites has not yet been entirely elucidated (1), but it appears that practically all of the homovanillic acid (HVA) in CSF, at least, originates from dopamine (DA) in the brain. The evidence for the origin of methoxyhydroxy-phenylethylene glycol (MOPEG or MHPG), the major metabolite of norepinephrine (NE) is less certain, and it has been suggested that most of the 5-hydroxyindole acetic acid (5-HIAA), the major metabolite in blood and urine is from serotonin (5-HT) in the periphery (2). Much of this type of neurochemical research has been done on experimental animals - the rat, the cat and the monkey. Various analytical methods have been used, with some success, to study _in vivo_ rate of the turnover and transport of biogenic amines in the central nervous system of these animals, including the use of inhibitors of amine biosythesis, various precursors labelled with radioactive isotopes and extensive

95

studies on the effect of various psychoactive drugs.

The application of the techniques used in research in animals
to study mental and neurological disorders in man is limited by
the restrictions on the use of enzyme inhibitors and of precursors
labelled with radioactive isotopes in human subjects. It has, however been suggested that precursors labelled with stable isotopes
(of hydrogen, carbon, nitrogen or oxygen) could be used. The large
amounts of these materials required, to enable a measureable amount
to penetrate the blood-brain barrier, causes changes in the dyna-
mics of the system by altering relative pool sizes and by over-
loading various active transport systems. The recent application
of semi-automated gas-chromatographic-mass spectrometry (GC/MS)
methods for the quantitative analysis of nanogram quantities of
biogenic amines and their metabolites extracted from tissues and
body fluids, has been very successful in many areas of biomedical
and psycho-pharmacological research. Using these methods, a great
deal of information has been obtained in human patients and volunteers, which has provided further evidence of the involvement of
biogenic amines in psychiatric and neurological disorders. Various
techiques have been used to increase both the reliability and the
sensitivity of these GC/MS techniques, such as the use of probenecid, a drug which can block the transport of the acid metabolites
(HVA, VMA and 5-HIAA) from CSF to blood and urine, thus enabling
the rate of turnover and of the effect of psycho-active drugs to
be determined. However, in many instances it is difficult to obtain
consistent values for the blockade of transport; particularly when
the results for different individuals are compared.

The development of mass fragmentography (MF) (3,4) in which
the mass spectrometer is used for the detection and determination
of complex mixtures of volatile organic compounds separated by gas
chromatography, has been a great step forward. By using various
electronic devices, most of the biogenic amines and their metabolites can be measured in a single small sample using deuterated
standards i.e. identical synthetic compounds containing one or more
deuterium atoms. These deutero-compounds are introduced into the
sample at an early stage in the processing, and behave chemically
almost identically to the materials to be analysed, throughout all
phases of the MF analysis. However, they appear in the final mass-
spectrometric stage as peaks displaced by an integral number of
mass units (depending on the number of deuterium atoms in the standard) on the mass spectrometer chart.

The peak heights of the standard and original material can
then be compared, and a measure of the relative amount of each
determined, from which the concentration of the biogenic amines
or their metabolites in blood, urine or CSF can be calculated.

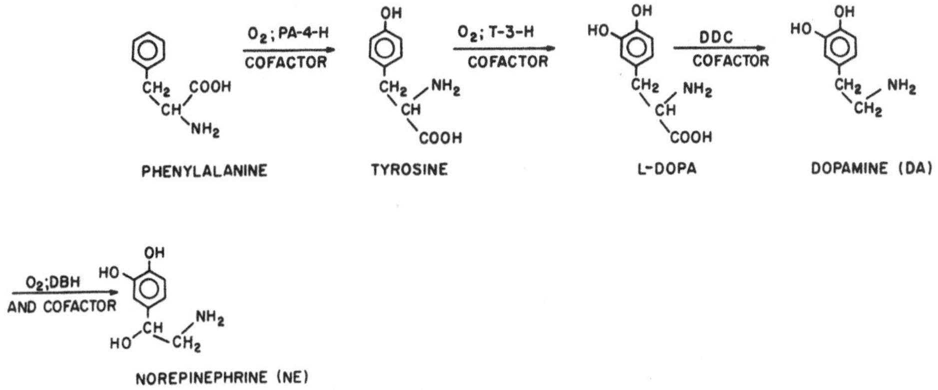

Fig. 1.   Biosynthesis of Dopamine (DA) and
           Norepinephrine (NE).

An important and fortunate fact in the biochemistry of all
three amines (DA, NE and 5-HT) is that they are synthesised in
brain from amino acid precursors (4,5) by enzymes which use <u>molecular</u>
<u>oxygen</u> and appropriate cofactors to hydroxylate the substrate
(Fig. 1 and 2). Since oxygen is readily transported to all parts of
the brain by cerebral blood flow, this presents a most useful method
for the <u>in vivo</u> labelling of the amines in both animals and man, by
using one of the two stable isotopes of oxygen (^{17}O or ^{18}O). Oxygen
-17 and oxygen-18 are present at low concentrations in all oxygen
containing materials and can be concentrated by fractional distil-
lation of water or thermal diffusion of oxygen gas, so that materials
containing over 90% ^{17}O or of ^{18}O are now available (6).

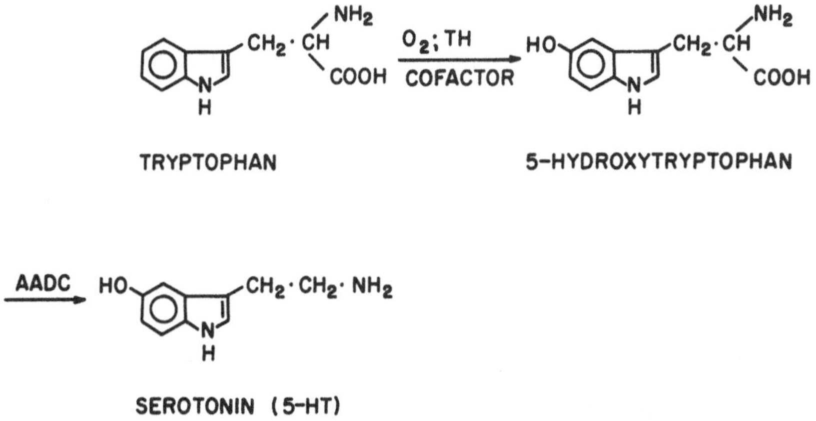

Fig. 2.   Biosynthesis of Serotonin (5-HT).

In the first series of experiments rats were caused to breathe air in a specially designed apparatus (7) (Fig. 3) in which the circulating oxygen is gradually replaced over a period of an hour or more by highly enriched oxygen-18, thereby introducing a label into the system, which is transported to the brain and incorporated into the amines, in a rate determining step. Very few, if any, other materials in the brain are labelled in this way.

Fairly extensive experiments (8) have shown that mice at least can breathe this oxygen-18 enriched atmosphere (which has the overall composition of ordinary air, i.e. 20% oxygen and 80% nitrogen) for long periods of time - up to 60 days - without apparent ill effects to their health. Since high concentrations of deuterium are known to be toxic, specific experiments are now being carried out on various experimental animals in order to insure that repeated ^{18}O treatments have no ill effects.

The ^{18}O label introduced into the meta-hydroxyl group of dopamine and norepinephrine and the 5-hydroxy group of serotonin is an extremely stable one and like all phenolic substances, does not undergo isotopic exchange with water (9), or other oxygen-containing materials in the brain or body. The label (containing up to 20% ^{18}O) is retained throughout all the catabolic processes which produce the metabolites HVA, VMA MOPEG, DOPAC and 5-HIAA. Compounds, such as steroids, which are also labelled in vivo by oxygenases are formed on an entirely different time scale, are readily separated during the chemical processing and present no problem in MF analyses. It should be noted however, that following an exposure to $^{18}O_2$, all "body water" and many substances that undergo isotopic exchange such as sugars, phosphates, etc. also contain oxygen-18 at low concentration (less than 1%) which do not affect the results in any way.

Our first experiments, which have already been published (10, 11, 12), using the technique described above, indicated that ^{18}O-labelled dopamine, HVA and other metabolites could be quantitatively determined in whole brain homogenates of the rat. We were able to measure the rate of turnover of dopamine in the corpus striatum and show that an i.p. injection of chlorpromazine (CPZ) (10 mg/kg) causes a threefold increase in the rate of incorporation of ^{18}O into HVA. This is what is to be expected, since CPZ is thought to increase the rate of conversion of dopamine to HVA, by increasing the rate of release of the amine neurotransmitter from its stores. Having established the basic applicability of this technique, we have now extended these studies further and examined the effect of α-methyl-p-tyrosine (AMPT), which blocks dopamine and NE biosynthesis and p-chlorophenylalanine (PCPA) which blocks 5HT biosynthesis, and reserpine, which by blocking biogenic amine storage has been used to produce an animal model of "depression". It must,

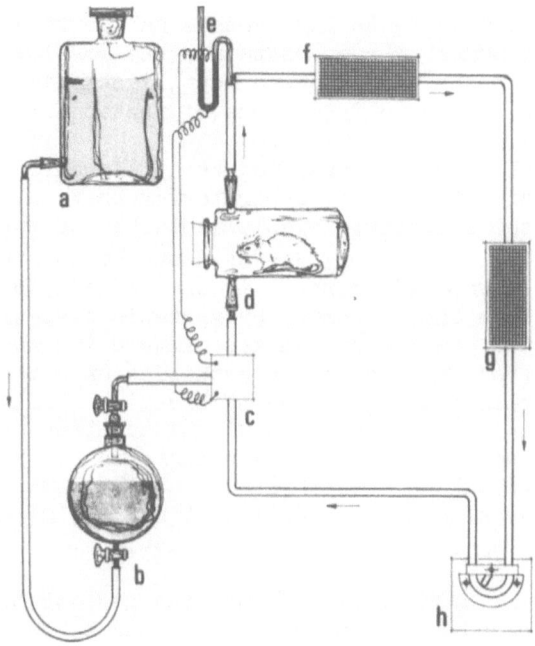

Fig. 3.   Apparatus for exposure of rats to $^{18}O_2$
          enriched atmosphere.
          a. Water pressure head.
          b. Vessel containing highly enriched $^{18}O_2$.
          c. Magnetic valve.
          d. Vessel containing rats.
          e. Manometer of CO_2 absorber.
          f. CO_2 absorber.
          g. Drying tube.
          h. Peristaltic pump.

however, be admitted that the value of animal models of psychoses
is very restricted and more revelant information of clinical and
pharmacological interest can only be obtained in man.

    In order to examine the feasibility of using this technique
with human patients, we have conducted an extensive series of
^{18}O-labelling experiments in non-human primates. A colony of young
male olive baboons (Papio anubis) which have been used at the
Weizmann Institute for various behavioural studies (13) were used
for this purpose. Each monkey (weighing 18-20 kg) was first anesthetised by an intramuscular injection of Ketalar (Ketamine; 2 mg/kg),

and a tracheal tube and a urinary catheter inserted into the throat
and bladder respectively. An intravenous saline infusion (4 ml/kg/hr)
was also made in order to compensate for the loss of fluids during
the experiment and the animals were kept lightly anesthetised for
up to 12 hours by periodic injections of pentobarbitol (5-10 mg/kg).

The tracheal tube was connected by a T-junction through a CO_2-
absorber and drying tube to a respiratory rubber balloon and to a
large glass vessel containing highly isotopically enriched oxygen
gas (over 90% ^{18}O). As the oxygen was consumed and the carbon
dioxide and water vapour absorbed, it was replaced by enriched $^{18}O_2$
gas introduced into the system by hydrostatic pressure. At regular
intervals, the ^{18}O content of the gas mixture was sampled in order
to monitor it. The effect of the anesthetics on amine and metabolite
turnover and levels was determined by baseline studies using first
ordinary oxygen and then $^{18}O_2$ without further treatment. Samples
of blood and urine from each monkey were taken every hour and in
later experiments CSF samples (0.5 to 1 ml) by lumbar puncture.
Rectal temperatures were measured from time to time and the animals
temperature kept at 35-36°C by warming pads.

The oxygen-18 content of the respired gas and of the water
distilled from blood and urine was determined by mass spectrometry
[using the CO_2 equilibration method (6)] at Rehovot. The ^{18}O analyses of serotonin and the catecholamines in CSF, blood and urine
were determined in samples which were frozen, packed in dry ice
and flown to Stockholm for MF (3) at the Karolinska Institute. The
biogenic amines, DA, NE, 5HT and their main metabolites (HVA, MOPEG,
DOPAC & 5-HIAA) (see Fig. 4) were converted to volatile derivatives,
appropriate deutero-standards added and the mixture analysed by MF.
The results indicate that in each case, one ^{18}O atom is incorporated
into the aromatic ring in the rate-determining hydroxylation. A
second labelled oxygen atom is also present, at a very low concentration (barely above background) in HVA indicating that some ^{18}O
is incorporated into tyrosine, during the hydroxylation of phenylalanine, probably in the periphery.

The time course of the rise and fall of the ^{18}O content of HVA
and DOPAC and 5-HIAA in the urine of a baboon (Tinton; No. 9) is
shown in Fig. 5. The ^{18}O concentration reaches a maximum in between
one to two hours after the start of the experiment. DOPAC and HVA
seem to reach a maximum at about the same time, whereas the 5-HIAA
maximum occurs somewhat later. The incorporation returns to baseline levels on a somewhat different time scale, the 5-HIAA, the
metabolite of serotonin in 3 hours, whereas the two catechoamine
metabolites only after 5 or 6 hours. Preliminary figures have also
been obtained for HVA and MOPEG in the CSF, obtained by lumbar
puncture from the same baboon (No. 9). Here, an extremely different
time course is seen for the two metabolites. In MOPEG a second
labelled oxygen is also found at a low concentration, which may be

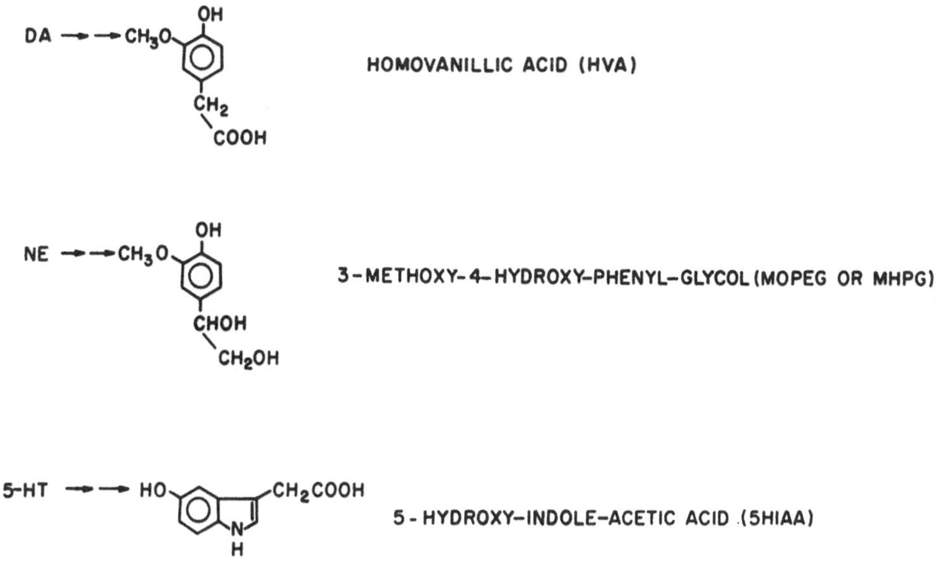

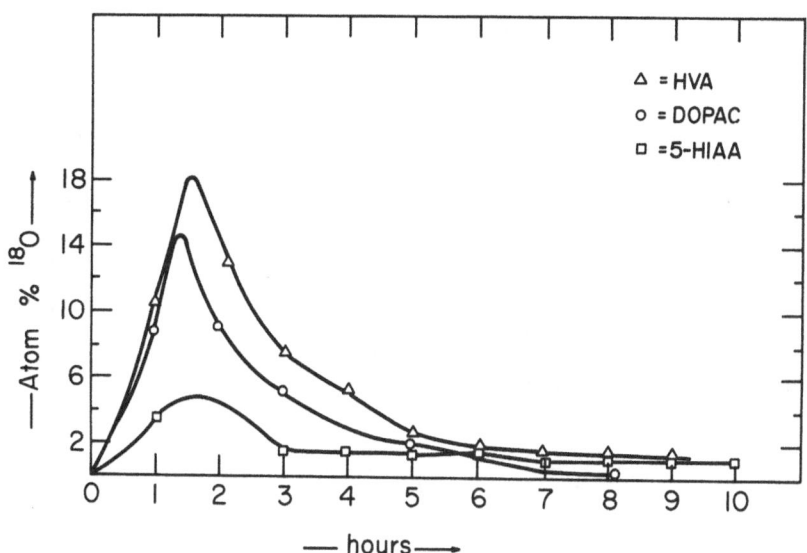

DA
OH
CH_3O
CH_2
COOH
HOMOVANILLIC ACID (HVA)
NE
OH
CH_3O
CHOH
CH_2OH
3-METHOXY-4-HYDROXY-PHENYL-GLYCOL (MOPEG OR MHPG)
5-HT
HO
CH_2COOH
N
H
5-HYDROXY-INDOLE-ACETIC ACID (5HIAA)

Fig. 4. Main metabolites of principal biogenic amines.

△ = HVA
○ = DOPAC
□ = 5-HIAA
—Atom % 18O—
18
14
10
6
2
0
1
2
3
4
5
6
7
8
9
10
— hours —

Fig. 5. Time course of ^{18}O incorporation into metabolites in urine of baboon (No. 9).

that introduced in the oxidation of DA by dopamine-β-hydroxylase (DBH).

The effect of CPZ (1.5 mg/kg given in two doses) in the monkey, is as expected from the rat experiments. The rate of incorporation of ^{18}O into HVA is faster than that in controls indicating a probable interference with DA metabolism (see ref. 14). Similar studies using clozapine and chlorimipramine are underway.

Repeated experiments on the same baboon have so far not shown any ill effects on their health or behaviour, which indicates that ^{18}O can be breathed without risk. It is hoped, before long, to use this technique in clinical studies in man. The intention is to study the involvement of biogenic amines in various neuropsychiatric disorders. This technique will also be useful in the elucidation of the mode of action, and evaluation of many of the drugs used in the alleviation and treatment of Parkinsonism, manic-depression and schizophrenia.

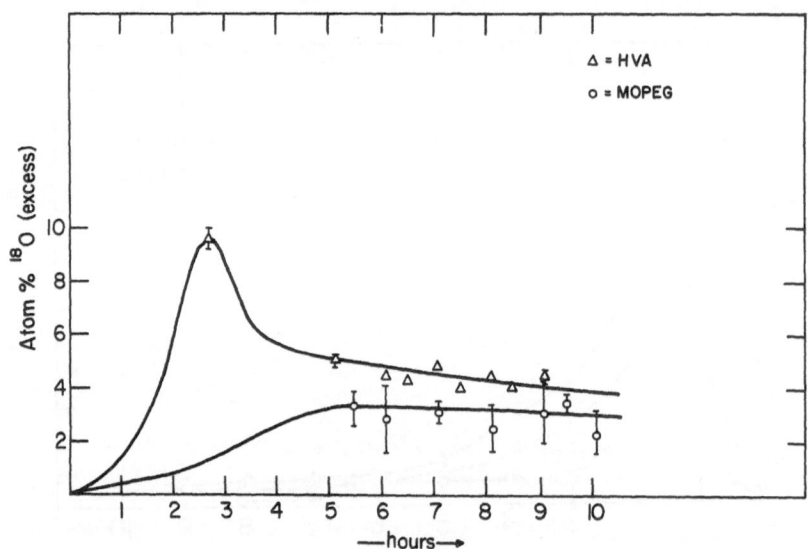

Fig. 6. Time course of ^{18}O-incorporation into
metabolites in CSF of baboon (No. 9).

ACKNOWLEDGEMENTS

This research is part of a collaborative project involving
G. Sedvall and coworkers of the Division of Neuropsychopharmacology
in the Department of Pharmacology of the Karolinska Institute,
Stockholm; E. Geller of the Department of Neurology and Anesthesiology, Ichilov Hospital, Tel-Aviv; and V.E. Grimm, E.Benhar and
I.Wasserman of the Isotope Department, Weizmann Institute, Rehovot.
It was supported by grants from Israel Center for Psychobiology,
the Swedish Medical Research Council and the National Institute
of Mental Health.

REFERENCES

1. SCHILDKRAUT, J., Am. J. Psych. 22:509, 1965.

2. PAPESCHI, R., SOURKES, T.L., POIRER, L.J. and BOUCHER, R.:
   Brain Res. 28:527, 1971.

3. SWAHN, C.G., and SEDVALL, G., Psychopharmacologia (in press).

4. NAGATSU, T., LEVITT, M., and UDENFREIND, S., J. Biol. Chem.
   239:2910 (1964).

5. SHIMAN, R., AKINO, M., and KAUFMAN, S.J., Biol. Chem. 246:1330,
   1971.

6. SAMUEL, D. In: Oxygenases ed. O. Hayaishi, Academic Press, 1962.

7. MAYEVSKY, A. and SAMUEL, D., Physiology and Behaviour 12:679,
   1974.

8. SAMUEL, D., WOLF, D., MESHORER, A. and WASSERMAN, I., Proc.
   Int. Conf. Stable Isotopes in Chem. Biol. and Med., USAEC,
   1973.

9. SAMUEL, D. and SILVER, B.L., Adv. Phys. Org. Chem. 3:123, 1965.

10. MAYEVSKY, A., SJOQUIST, B., FRI, C.G., SAMUEL, D. and SEDVALL, G.
    Biochem. Biophys. Res. Commun. 51;746, 1973.

11. SEDVALL, G., MAYEVSKY, A., SAMUEL, D. and FRI, C.G., In: Frontiers in Catecholamine Research eds. E. Usdin and S. Snyder,
    Pergamon Press, 1973.

12.   SEDVALL, G., MAYEVSKY, A., FRI, C.G., SJOQUIST, B., and SAMUEL,
      D., In: Adv. Biochem. Psychopharmacol. eds. E. Costa and
      B. Holmstedt, Raven Press, 1973.

13.   BENHAR, E., and SAMUEL, D., J. Med. Primatol. 2:11, 1973.

14.   SEDVALL, G., BECK, O., BENHAR, E., GELLER, E., GRIMM, V.,
      SAMUEL, D. and WASSERMAN, I., In: Chemical Tools in Catechol-
      amine Research Eds. O. Alingren, A. Carlsson and J. Engel.
      North Holland Publ. Co., p.17, 1975.

ANTIBODY LEVELS TO VIRUSES IN PSYCHIATRIC ILLNESS

Ranan Rimon* and Pekka Halonen**

* Jerusalem Mental Health Center, Jerusalem, Israel

** Department of Virology, University of Turku, Finland

It has long been known that certain viruses are neurotropic and that they can cause encephalitis and post-encephalitic syndromes which can be confused with psychotic disorders (1,2). It has, however, only recently been shown that viruses may have incubation periods of twenty years or more before signs of central nervous system (CNS) disease appear. Such viral infections are referred to as slow or latent to indicate the time lag between the introduction of the virus into the host and the production of the clinical symptoms.

Kuru was the first slow-virus disease in man to be successfully transmitted to primates and proven to be of viral origin (3). Kuru is a progressive, subacute and ultimately fatal degenerative disease of the CNS which has been transmitted by cannibalism among natives in certain parts of New Guinea. In addition to kuru, the Creutzfeld-Jacob disease, a presenile progressive brain atrophy, is also presumed to be caused by a slow-acting persistent viral agent. Like kuru, it may be transmitted to monkeys by intracerebral inoculation of highly diluted suspensions of brain tissues from patients with this disease (4). The perhaps most convincing evidence of slow-virus etiology in neurological disorders originates from the studies on subacute sclerosing panencephalitis (SSPE). Patients with this relatively rare disease have shown to have high measles antibody titres in their cerebrospinal fluid (CSF), and measles viruses have been cultured from their brains (5,6). Presently research continues on other human neurological diseases suspected of being caused by slow-viral infections, including multiple sclerosis (MS), Alzheimer's and Pick's presenile dementias, amyotrophic lateral sclerosis, and progressive multifocal leucoencephalopathy (7,8).

In contrast to the great interest now being taken in the search for viral agents in many neurological diseases of unknown etiology, much less attention has been paid to a possible relationship between slow virus infections in the CNS and psychiatric disorders. After Lycke and Roos (9) and Lycke et al (10) were able to demonstrate a clear correlation between dysfunction of monoamine metabolism and abnormal behavior in mice infected intracerebrally with herpes simplex virus, our group initiated a series of studies to elucidate the possible role of viral agents in the etiology and pathogenesis of psychiatric disorders.

Table 1 summarizes the results of two studies focusing on herpes simplex complement-fixing (CF) antibody in psychiatric patients (11,12).

The incidence of the positive specimens in the group of psychotic depression is significantly greater (p < 0.001) than in the control group consisting of non-depressed psychiatric patients (N = 185) and healthy medical personnel (N = 46). Furthermore, the incidence of high CF antibody titres (> 64) is also significantly greater (p < 0.05) in patients with depressive illness than in the controls.

TABLE 1. Herpes simplex complement-fixing antibody in 100 patients with psychotic depression and 231 non-depressive subjects

Group		< 4	4	8	16	32	64	≥128	Positive Ratio
Psychotic depression	No.	6	3	8	16	25	19	23	94/100
	(%)	(6)	(3)	(8)	(16)	(25)	(19)	(23)	(94)*
Controls	No.	53	10	13	16	73	45	21	178/231
	(%)	(23)	(4)	(6)	(7)	(32)	(19)	(9)	(77)*

* p < 0.001

Following these preliminary studies serum specimens were collected from three psychiatric hospitals in Southern and Eastern Finland (13). Altogether 318 specimens were from psychiatric patients and 32 from healthy medical personnel of the same hospitals. The diagnoses of the patients were made by concensus among at least three staff psychiatrists who placed emphasis upon phenomenological and behavioral criteria. All patients in the various diagnostic subgroups were either short-admission or medium-stay in-patients. The medical personnel from whom specimens were collected lived in the hospital areas or in the communities nearby.

Rubella haemagglutination test was performed on 348 specimens, measles haemagglutination test on 349 specimens and herpes simplex type 1 neutralization test was assayed on 174 serum specimens.

The mean titres of the rubella haemagglutination inhibition test were not significantly different in the psychiatric groups compared with the controls, as shown in Table 2.

Similar results were obtained with measles haemagglutination inhibition test (Table 3), but the mean titres were slightly lower in each psychiatric group than in the medical personnel, the difference being statistically significant only in the group of personality disorders (p $<$ 0.05).

The k-values of herpes simplex type 1 antibody were higher in each of the psychiatric groups than in the medical personnel (Table 4). This difference was highly significant (p $<$ 0.001) in patients with psychotic depression but also significant in the schizophrenic group (p $<$ 0.01), and in the group of other psychiatric diseases (p $<$ 0.05). In addition to the high median k-values, many serum specimens in the depression group had unusually high k-values and 15/56 (27 percent) were higher than 2.4, which was the highest k-value in the controls. The highest k-values in the schizophrenic group were not as high as in the depressed patients but there were, however, 13/54 (24 percent) specimens with higher values than the highest in the control series.

After the publication of these studies several research groups have shown interest in serum antibodies to viruses in psychiatric syndromes. Cleobury et al (14) compared 13 aggressive psychopaths with 27 other psychiatric or general hospital patients. They found an unusually high mean kinetic neutralization constant against type 1 herpes simplex virus but not against type 2 in patients with aggressive personality deviation. Carranza-Acevedo (15) corroborated our findings by demonstrating significant differences in neutralizing antibodies to herpes simplex virus between depressed patients and patients with other psychiatric illness. Additional confirming evidence to our results comes from the study of Lycke et al (16) who in a large series of psychiatric patients (N = 539) demonstrated

TABLE 2. Rubella haemagglutination inhibition antibody titres in
          348 serum specimens of psychiatric patients and medical
          personnel

Group	Number of subjects	Geometric mean titer	SEM log	p compared to medical personnel
Psychotic depression	88	39 (+ 101, -29)*	0.05986	N.S.
Schizophrenia	75	31 (+ 94, -21)	0.06865	N.S.
Neurotic syndromes	80	36 (+ 102, -27)	0.06539	N.S.
Personality disorders	74	28 (+ 55, -18)	0.05472	N.S.
Medical personnel	31	36 (+ 87, -26)	0.09681	----

  * Asymmetry due to standard deviation being calculated on
    logarithmic titer values.

TABLE 3. Measles haemagglutination inhibition titres in 349 serum
          specimens of psychiatric patients and medical personnel

Group	Number of subjects	Geometric mean titer	SEM log	p compared to medical personnel
Psychotic depression	88	123 (+545, -105)*	0.07820	N.S.
Schizophrenia	75	160 (+531, -123)	0.07340	N.S.
Neurotic syndromes	81	143 (+525, -112)	0.07431	N.S.
Personality disorders	74	104 (+319, - 78)	0.07087	< 0.05
Medical personnel	31	191 (+513, -139)	0.10160	----

  * Asymmetry due to standard deviation being calculated on
    logarithmic titer values.

higher prevalence of CF antibodies to herpes group viruses in patients with depressive psychosis (herpes simplex, cytomegalo, varicella-zoster) and in patients with dementia (herpes simplex, cytomegalo) than in the controls. In their study also the mean titres against herpes simplex were significantly higher in the group of depressed and demented patients.

The results of the above mentioned studies indicate that a considerable number of patients with psychotic depression have unusually high antibody levels to herpes simplex virus. As a rational explanation it would be tempting to maintain that there is an etiological relationship between the unusually high herpes simplex antibody pattern and psychotic depression in some of the patients. We have, however, no direct evidence to support such a hypothesis, but before other interpretations are available the etiological possibilities must be considered. The fact that neither measles nor rubella antibody titres are increased in psychotic depression rules out a general change in circulating antibody in these patients and thus enlarges the importance of the findings with herpes simplex virus and probably other herpes viruses. The increased level of neutralizing herpes simplex antibody in schizophrenia and some other psychiatric diseases, although less marked than in the depression group, must be further studied before its significance can be assessed. This could imply that there may be a general herpes-induced vulnerability to a wide range of psychiatric disorders, although this possibility must be further elucidated before a conclusion of this kind can be drawn. In addition, the effects of psychopharmacological drugs used in the treatment of most patients in our series must be investigated. Although at present time in relation to herpes viruses there are no reports of false positive immune responses caused by psycholeptic drugs, this possibility cannot be discarded.

In our opinion a similar etiological relationship as between slow virus infections and neurological diseases should be systematically searched for in psychiatric disorders. In this search, all known viruses isolated from the CNS must be included and even new viruses should be sought with primate inoculation and by other means. Approaching this problem with serological techniques, several tests measuring different antibodies to the same virus should be used. The usefulness of this has been demonstrated in our studies where schizophrenic patients had high neutralizing antibody to herpes simplex whereas the level of the CF antibody to the same virus did not differ from that of the controls. Great individual variations in measles antibody pattern of patients with SSPE and MS were found when serum and CSF specimens were tested with neutralization, haemagglutination inhibition, haemolysis-inhibition, complement fixation and immunodiffusion techniques, each measuring more or less different antibodies to the same virus (17). These findings indicate that the etiological agent in slow virus infections of the CNS may be in an incomplete form in which no mature virus can

TABLE 4. Herpes simplex type 1 k-values of kinetic neutralization test in 174 serum specimens of psychiatric patients and medical personnel

Group	Number of subjects	Median	Maximum	U	Z	P
				compared to medical personnel		
Psychotic depression	56	1.1	7.8	546	3.05	<0.001
Schizophrenia	54	1.2	5.7	573	2.63	<0.01
Other psychiatric diseases (neurotic syndromes, personality disorders)	32	0.89	3.6	365	1.99	<0.05
Medical personnel	32	0.29	2.4			

Titer distribution was analysed statistically according to the one-tailed Mann–Whitney U-test (Siegel, 1956). U is the statistic of the test. Z is the difference of the mean of the sampling distribution of U and the computed U in standard deviations. The sampling distribution of U is approximately the normal distribution.

be found. In such an unusual type of infection, especially if it
is not as fulminating as SSPE, the immunological response may not
be typical for this virus in regular infection, and this unusual
infection may cause difficulties in serological studies even with
well-known viruses.

REFERENCES

1. SHEARER, M.L. and FINCH, S.M.: Periodic organic psychosis
   associated with recurrent herpes simplex. New Engl.
   J. Med. 271, 494-497, 1964.

2. RASKIN, D.E. and FRANK, S.W.: Herpes encephalitis with cata-
   tonic stupor. Arch. Gen. Psychiat. 31, 544-546, 1974.

3. GAJDUSEK, D.S. and GIBBS, C.J. Jr.: Transmission of two sub-
   acute spongiform encephalopathies of man (kuru and
   Creutzfeld-Jacob disease) to New World monkeys.
   Nature (Lond.), 230, 588-591., 1971.

4. GAJDUSEK, D.C.: Kuru and Creutzfeld-Jacob disease. Experimental
   models of noninflammatory degenerative slow virus disease
   of the central nervous system. Ann. Clin. Res. 5, 254-261,
   1973.

5. HORTA-BABOSA, L., FUCCILLO, D.A., SEVER, J.L. and ZEMAN, W.:
   Subacute sclerosing panencephalitis: Isolations of
   measles virus from a brain biopsy. Nature (Lond.) 221,
   974-976, 1969.

6. SALMI, A.A., NORRBY, E. and PANELIUS, M.: Identification of
   different measles virus-specific antibodies in the serum
   and cerebrospinal fluid from patients with subacute
   sclerosing panencephalitis and multiple sclerosis.
   Inf. Immun. 6, 248-254, 1972.

7. PANELIUS, M., JA HALONEN, P.: Koskushermoston hitaat virus-
   infektiot. Duodecim, 87, 1465-1480, 1971.

8. TORREY, E.F. and PETERSON, M.R.: Slow and latent viruses in
   schizophrenia. Lancet, II, 22-24, 1973.

9. LYCKE, E. and ROOS, B.E.: Effect on the monoamine-metabolism
   of the mouse brain by experimental herpes simplex
   infection. Experientia, 24, 687-690, 1968.

10.   LYCKE, E., MODIGH, K. and ROOS, B.E.: Aggression in mice
      associated with changes in the monoamine-metabolism
      of the brain. Experientia, 25, 951-953, 1969.

11.   RIMON, R. and HALONEN, P.: Herpes simplex virus infection
      and depressive illness. Dis. Nerv. Syst. 30, 338-340,
      1969.

12.   RIMON, R., HALONEN, P., ANTTINEN, E. and EVOLA, K.:
      Complement fixing antibody to herpes simplex virus in
      patients with psychotic depression. Dis. Nerv. Syst.
      32, 822-824, 1971.

13.   HALONEN, P.E., RIMON, R., AROHONKA, K. and JÄNTTI, V.:
      Antibody levels to herpes simplex type I, measles and
      rubella viruses in psychiatric patients. Brit. J.
      Psychiat. 125, 461-465, 1974.

14.   CLEOBURY, J.F., SKINNER, G.R.B., THOULESS, M.E. and WILDY, P.:
      Association between psychopathic disorder and serum
      antibody to herpes simplex virus (Type I). Brit. Med. J.
      i, 438-439, 1971.

15.   CARRANZA-ACEVEDO, J.: Virus induced resistant depressions.
      Pharmacopsychiat. 7, 164-168, 1974.

16.   LYCKE, E., NORRBY, E. and ROOS, B.E.: Serological study of
      mentally-ill patients with particular reference to the
      prevalence of herpes virus infections. Brit. J. Psychiat.
      124, 273-279, 1974.

17.   PANELIUS, M., SALMI, A.A., HALONEN, P. and PENTTINEN, K.:
      Measles antibodies detected with various techniques
      in sera of patients with multiple sclerosis. Acta
      Neurol. Scand. 47, 315-330, 1971.

A TISSUE-BINDING FACTOR IN THE SERUM OF SCHIZOPHRENIC PATIENTS

I.P. Witz[*], R. Anavi[*] and H. Weisenbeck[**]

[*] Department of Microbiology, Tel-Aviv University, Israel

[**] Gehah Psychiatric Hospital, Tel-Aviv, Israel

SUMMARY

Studies using an indirect radioimmunofixation assay, have revealed the presence of a serum factor (or factors) in schizophrenic patients with the capacity to bind to human brain tissue, as well as to other human and mouse tissues.

The tissue binding property is detected in the serum of 50%-60% of schizophrenic patients, and in the serum of about 10% or less of blood-bank donors.

The serum factor precipitates with 33% saturated ammonium sulfate but does not seem to be IgG.

It is unknown whether or not this tissue-binding property of schizophrenic serum is an immunological reaction.

INTRODUCTION

The possibility that schizophrenic patients have autoantibodies reactive with components of human brain has been repeatedly raised by some investigators (1-4) but disputed by others (5-7).

Possibly related to some of these findings, were reports on alterations in the concentration or function of some serum constituents, including immunoglobulins, of schizophrenic patients (8-12).

The aim of the present study was to obtain additional information on circulating brain-fixing factors in the serum of schizophrenic patients. This was done by utilizing a radioimmunofixation assay.

MATERIALS AND METHODS

Human Brain Tissue Sections

The septal region of 2 postmortem human brains was obtained 10 hours, at most, following death. The first brain (a) was of a 36 year-old schizophrenic male who committed suicide by kerosene ingestion. The second (b) was of a 56 year-old male deceased as a result of a myocardial infarction. The tissue was sliced into blocks of approximately 1cm^3 and immediately frozen in dry ice and kept at -70°C until the time of experimentation. Four to six μ thick tissue slices were prepared in a cryostatic microtome. The sections were mounted on cover glasses and fixed with 95% ethanol for 30 min. The slices were kept dry, at 4°C until used.

Human Liver Tissue Sections

Liver tissue was obtained from case (a) (see above). The tissue and the sectioning was handled as described above.

Mouse Tissue Sections

Brain, liver and thymus were obtained from C57BL mice. The tissues and the sectioning was handled as described above.

Blood From Schizophrenic Patients

Blood (ca 20ml) was drawn from male patients aged 15-40.

All patients were initially diagnosed as schizophrenics, and the diagnosis was confirmed later on, in about 80% of the cases.

No differentiation between the various forms of schizophrenia was attempted in the frame of this study and blood was drawn from both acutely and chronically-ill patients. Most patients were treated with phenothiazines at the time of the study.

The blood was allowed to clot at room temperature for 2-3 hours, and the serum was separated by centrifugation. In order to prevent thawing the serum was distributed in small (ca 0.5 ml) aliquotes and kept frozen, until used, at -20°C.

Blood from Blood-Bank Donors

Blood samples from 15-40 years old male donors were obtained from the Marcus Memorial Blood Institute, Magen David Adom in Israel, Jaffa. The blood was treated as described above.

Human Globulin

The globulin fraction of human serum was prepared by salting out with ammonium sulfate at 33% saturation. The dissolved precipitate was dialyzed against pH 8.0 borate buffered saline, distributed in small aliquotes and kept frozen, until used, at -20°C.

Human IgG

Globulin fractions from blood-bank donors or schizophrenic patients were dialyzed against a pH 6.8, 0.017M phosphate buffer and applied to DEAE cellulose columns equilibrated with the same buffer. The IgG that eluted with this buffer was concentrated and dialyzed against borate-buffered saline.

Antisera

1) Anti sera directed against globulin from schizophrenic patients, were prepared in rabbits. Rabbits were injected subcutaneously and intracutaneously at several sites with 1 mg pooled globulin, derived from several schizophrenic patients, in complete Freund's adjuvant. Three to 4 weeks later an additional dose of 1 mg pooled "schizophrenic" globulin was administered, this time in incomplete Freund's adjuvant. The rabbits were bled 10 days following the second immunizing dose. Additional bleedings of the same animals were performed 10 days following a booster dose of 1 mg of globulin.

2) Anti sera directed against bovine serum albumin (BSA) were also produced in rabbits using the same immunizing technique described above. Purified antibodies from such antisera (see below) served as control reagents in some of the experiments.

Globulin From Immunized or Normal Rabbits

In the experiments described below we used iodinated globulin from rabbits immunized with human globulin as test reagents and globulin from normal rabbits, as control reagents. The globulin from the normal or immunized rabbits was prepared by salting out with ammonium sulfate at 33% saturation. The dissolved precipitate was dialyzed against pH 8.0 borate buffered saline.

Purification of Antibodies by Affinity Chromatography

In some assays specifically purified antibody reagents (purified reagents) rather than the globulin fraction of antisera (non-
purified reagents), have been utilized. Antibodies were purified
by affinity chromatography (13) on antigen-conjugated sepharose
(Pharmacia, Uppsala, Sweden) columns. As test reagents we used
antibodies that had been reacted with and eluted from sepharose
columns conjugated either with human globulin or with human IgG.
Purified antibodies directed against BSA had been used as control
reagents. Unfractionated antisera were applied onto sepharose columns conjugated with the appropriate antigen. Only the corresponding
antibodies are retained on such columns, while the other constituents
of the antiserum pass without retention. The antibodies were eluted
from the antigen-conjugated columns by means of a pH 2.5 glycine-
HCl buffer. The eluted antibodies were concentrated and dialyzed
against a pH 8.0 borate buffered saline.

Iodination Procedure

Rabbit globulin, human IgG or purified antibodies were radio-
iodinated with ^{125}I (The Radiochemical Centre, Amersham, England)
or with ^{131}I (Nuclear Research Centre, Negev, Israel) using the
chloramine T method (14), as described earlier (15). Pair-labeled
mixtures (PLM) were prepared by mixing an ^{125}I or ^{131}I labeled test
reagent (i.e. the globulin fraction from a rabbit immunized against
human globulin or purified antibodies directed against human globulin or IgG) with an ^{131}I or ^{125}I, respectively, labeled control
reagent (i.e. the globulin fraction of an unimmunized rabbit or
purified anti BSA antibodies).

In the direct radioimmunofixation experiments we used pair-
labeled mixtures composed of ^{125}I or ^{131}I IgG from schizophrenic
patients paired with ^{131}I or ^{125}I, labeled IgG, respectively, from
blood bank donors.

The Indirect Radioimmunofixation Assay (RIFA)

1)   The assay   Brain sections were incubated at 37°C for 30 min,
either with undiluted normal serum or with undiluted serum from
schizophrenic patients. The washed (x6) sections were then incubated
at 37°C for 30 min with a pair-labeled mixture (PLM) containing an
^{125}I labeled globulin from rabbit antisera directed against globulin
isolated from schizophrenic patients and a ^{131}I labeled control
globulin (either the globulin fraction of an unimmunized rabbit or
antibodies directed against a non-cross reactive antigen - see
above). The slices were washed again 6 times, and the radioactivity
retained on the brain slices was measured in a Packard, double-

channel, autogamma analyzer. The labels could be reversed with equal success.

The uptake of the control globulin would measure the non-specific or background fixation of the rabbit reagent while the uptake of the anti-globulin reagent measures globulin retained on the brain slice from the previous incubation.

2) The calculation: The ratio between the anti-globulin radio-activity (cpm) retained on the tissue section and the control radio-activity retained on the same section was calculated. This ratio was termed standard ratio (SR), if the brain section was incubated with a known normal human serum prior to its exposure to the PLM. The test ratio (TR) was the ratio between the antiglobulin radio-activity and the control radio-activity retained on tissue sections preincubated with the unknown, tested schizophrenic sera. We pre-ferred to compare such ratios rather than to compare the amount of antiglobulin reagent fixed onto brain sections preincubated with these 2 types of human sera in view of the varying sizes of the brain-tissue-sections. Normalized ratios were obtained by dividing each of the individual TRs or SRs by the mean SR. The value of the normalized ratio of the non-schizophrenic population approached thus 1.00.

Any TR value higher than the mean SR value ($\overline{m}$SR) + 2 standard deviations (SD) calculated for the standard sera tested on this particular day, was considered significantly higher than the $\overline{m}$SR and hence the serum was marked as having affinity to brain tissue. The $\overline{m}$SR had to be calculated for each different experiment since those values depend on the degree of labeling of the reagent in the PLM.

RESULTS

The use of the indirect fixation assay, in contrast to a direct one, enables the screening of numerous sera by the utilization of a single or, as in the present assay, a pair of radiolabeled reagents.

A. The Detection of Brain-Fixing Factors in the Serum of
    Schizophrenic Patients

Table 1 summarizes the results of 12 fixation experiments using 106 normal sera and 171 sera from schizophrenic patients. It was found that in 5 experiments the $\overline{m}$TR (i.e. the average ratio of anti-globulin radioactivity over control radioactivity retained on brain sections preincubated with sera) was higher than with the $\overline{m}$SR.

These values as well as others were normalized and the $\overline{m}$TR of all assays was significantly higher than the $\overline{m}$SR (Table 2).

TABLE 1.   Radioimmunofixation assays employing sera from
            Schizophrenic patients and from normal blood bank donors

Experiment	$\overline{m}$SR + SD (normals)	No. of Sera	$\overline{m}$TR + SD (patients)	No. of Sera	P
1	0.16 + 0.02	8	0.16 + 0.07	24	NS
2	7.90 ∓ 1.39	8	9.64 ∓ 1.78	24	0.02
3	0.94 ∓ 0.25	7	0.99 ∓ 0.39	21	NS
4	0.75 ∓ 0.11	8	0.72 ∓ 0.19	24	NS
5	1.60 ∓ 0.79	5	2.00 ∓ 0.81	5	NS
6	0.48 ∓ 0.09	6	0.67 ∓ 0.09	5	0.01
7	0.82 ∓ 0.15	13	1.04 ∓ 0.38	14	NS
8	1.60 ∓ 0.24	6	2.55 ∓ 0.82	6	0.05
9	3.39 ∓ 0.82	6	4.10 ∓ 1.77	6	NS
10	1.32 ∓ 0.30	19	1.61 + 0.35	22	0.01
11	1.83 ∓ 0.48	10	2.40 ∓ 1.31	10	NS
12	1.73 + 0.24	10	2.83 ∓ 0.81	10	0.01

TABLE 2.   Over all results[a] of radioimmunofixation assays

Reagents	Schizo ($\overline{m}$ ± SD)	Normal ($\overline{m}$ ± SD)	P
Non-purified	1.33 ± 0.46 (78)	1.01 ± 0.24 (75)	<0.01
Purified[b]	1.29 ± 0.59 (203)	1.00 ± 0.24 (71)	<0.01

[a] The values are normalized. Normalization was achieved by
     dividing each individual SR or TR by $\overline{m}$SR obtained in the
     corresponding experiment.

[b] Antibody reagents were purified by affinity chromatography.

The use of purified reagents (see Materials and Methods) was not advantageous over the use of unpurified reagents (Table 2). The results in Table 2 also indicated the heterogeneity of the schizophrenic serum population in terms of fixation properties, compared to the normal serum population. The standard deviation of the schizophrenic group being higher than the standard deviation of the normal group. This suggested to us that the sera of schizophrenic patients could be subdivided into 2 subgroups, those with brain-fixing components and those which do not show this property. The necessity thus arose to identify positive sera, i.e. sera which express brain-fixing properties. Arbitrarily, we defined as positive any serum giving a TR higher, by 2 standard deviations, than the $\overline{m}$SR.

Analysing the results obtained with 128 sera of schizophrenic individuals and 113 normal sera we found that 59% of the former (76/128) and 7% of the latter (9/113) sera to be positive. The difference between the two groups was statistically significant (P $<$ 0.01).

B. Reproducibility of Results

It was frequently observed that sera giving a high TR in a particular test, gave in a subsequent test TR values that were not significantly higher than the $\overline{m}$SR, and vice versa. The necessity arose, therefore, to perform multiple assays of the same sera.

Table 3 shows that 11/12 sera of schizophrenic patients tested 13 times or more, could be identified as positive whereas only 1/10 normal sera were positive. A serum was considered positive if it gave a TR value higher than the $\overline{m}$SR in at least one of the test repetitions. The average frequency of the times a given schizophrenic serum showed a positive fixation out of the total number of times it was assayed was 1/4. The results also show that in general, normal sera do not manifest fixation properties in spite of multiple assays. Only one of the normal sera in this particular serum group was identified as positive. This serum reacted positively only once out of 23 times it was assayed.

The fact that some sera were positive in a certain test while other known positive sera were negative in the same test indicates the heterogeneity of the brain components that fix the active schizophrenic serum factor and/or the heterogeneity in the activity spectrum of these serum factors.

C. The Specificity of the Components Involved in the Fixation of Serum Factors from Schizophrenic Patients by Brain Tissue

If the interaction of schizophrenic serum factors and human brain tissue is of an immunological nature, it is expected that the

TABLE 3.   Analysis of radioimmunofixation assays of sera
            assayed multiple times[a]

Individual results

Schizo[b]   4/13; 5/13; 2/13; 0/13; 3/14
                 3/16; 5/16; 3/16; 5/16; 3/17; 3/20; 8/22

Normals[b]   0/13; 0/15; 0/17; 0/17; 0/20
                 0/21; 0/21; 0/23; 0/23; 1/23

Summary of results

Serum Group	No. positive[c] per no. assayed	% Positive	P
Schizo	11/12	91	< 0.01
Normals	1/10	10	

---

[a] Sera were assayed 13 times or more.

[b] The frequency of positive tests (number of positive per
     number of total tests performed) of individual sera.

[c] A serum was considered positive if it showed a positive
     fixation reactivity in at least one of the tests.

serum factor be an immunoglobulin, and that the tissue component
has a definite and reproducible pattern of distribution.

Two types of experiments were performed in trying to answer
the question whether the brain-fixing factor from schizophrenic
serum can be characterized as IgG. i) Direct pair-label assay
employing IgG fractions isolated from normal and schizophrenic
serum. ii) Comparison of results obtained in the RIFA using purified
antibodies directed against either human globulin (fraction preci-
pitating at 33% saturation of ammonium sulfate) or isolated human
IgG. The former fraction contains in addition to IgG, also other
serum proteins.

IgG was purified from sera of schizophrenic patients and blood
bank donors. Individual IgG preparations were labeled either with
^{125}I or with ^{131}I. Pair-labeled mixtures (PIMs) were prepared by
pairing, at random, an ^{125}I or ^{131}I labeled IgG preparation from a
schizophrenic patient with an ^{131}I or an ^{125}I labeled IgG preparation from a normal individual. Brain slices were incubated with
such pair-labeled IgG mixtures and the uptake of the two IgG preparations was calculated.

A total of 157 PLMs were studied. These were made up by 28 IgG
preparations of schizophrenic patients (SIgG) and by 23 IgG preparations of blood-bank donors (NIgG). Some PLMs were tested on sections
from 2 different brains and some IgG preparations were tested twice.
Once the SIgG was labeled with ^{125}I and paired with an ^{131}I labeled
NIgG preparation and the second time vice versa.

The results of these experiments permitted the tentative conclusion that the schizophrenic serum factor having affinity to brain
tissue is not IgG.

Antiserum directed against schizophrenic serum globulin under-
went affinity chromatography on sepharose columns conjugated with
either human globulin or human IgG. The resulting purified antibodies were directed against whole globulin and IgG respectively.
The purified antibodies were radiolabeled and paired with radiolabeled purified antibodies directed agaist BSA (see above). Results
of assays using these purified antibodies were compared. The results
indicated that antibodies directed against the less homogeneous
globulin fraction detected schizophrenic sera having brain-fixing
components while purified antibodies directed against IgG failed
to do so. Although the number of experiments using this approach
was relatively small, the results of these experiments confirm
those reported above that the component with affinity to human
brain in patients diagnosed for schizophrenia is not IgG. The
question whether this component belongs to another immunoglobulin
class remains open.

As indicated above, a clear pattern of specificity (or cross reactivity) is one of the requisits in order to be able to define the fixation of schizophrenic serum factors by human brain tissue as an immune reaction.

Twenty-four schizophrenic and 8 normal sera were assayed three times each for their capacity to fix to human brain as well as to mouse brain, liver and thymus. These mouse tissues were tested in view of a recent paper on antibodies to mouse thymus cells in schizophrenic patients (16). A serum was considered positive if a TR higher than the $\overline{m}SR + 2SD$ was determined in at least one of the 3 test repetitions.

The results indicated that tissue fixation reactivity of schizophrenic sera was considerably more frequent than that of normal sera. Although the data are yet insufficient to draw meaningful conclusions the pattern of tissue distribution points to a wide cross-reactivity. It is, also, possible to suggest that mouse tissues are at least as suitable-targets for the tissue fixing serum components as is human brain, if not better.

DISCUSSION

In this study we have shown that a certain proportion of schizophrenic patients have in their serum a factor (or factors) exhibiting tissue binding capacity in vitro.

This serum factor was detected by the aid of an antiserum reagent directed against the globulin fraction of serum from schizophrenic patients. The use of reagents directed against schizophrenic globulin allowed the detection of tissue fixing serum components in schizophrenic patients which are antigenically different from similar components in normal serum. Moreover, by using such reagents we could detect the presence of tissue fixing components in schizophrenic serum which may not have been present in normal serum. The question whether or not the tissue-fixing components can be detected also with antiserum-reagents directed against normal globulin remains unanswered at this time.

The tissue-binding factor does not seem to be IgG and the tissue components that bind it seem to be widely distributed: they are present in tissues of both mice and men. In view of the results of this paper we cannot conclude that the tissue binding capapcity of these serum factors is of an immunological nature, neither can we exclude the possibility that it is an immune reaction.

ACKNOWLEDGEMENTS

The authors wish to thank Dr. S. Bar-Shany from the Marcus
Memorial Blood Institute, Magen David Adom in Israel, Jaffa, for
help in collecting the blood samples from blood bank donors.

Our thanks to Dr. M. Steiner, Dr. L. Feuerman, Dr. A. Elizur
and Dr. S. Tyano from Gehah Psychiatric Hospital, Beilinson Medical
Center, Faculty of Medicine, Tel-Aviv University and the William
S. Schwartz Institute for Psychiatric Treatment and Research, for
their assistance and advice. We also wish to express gratitude to
Dr. M. Baron and Dr, M. Stern from the Shalvata Psychiatric Hospital
for blood samples of schizophrenic patients. We thak Mr. Yacob
Shlomo-David for his valuable technical assistance.

The study was supported by the Benevolent Foundation of
Scottish Rite Freemasonry, Northern Jurisdiction, U.S.A.

REFERENCES

1.   HEATH, R.G., KRUPP, I.M.: Schizophrenia as an immunologic
         disorder. I. Demonstration of antibrain globulins by
         fluorescent antibody techniques. Arch. Gen. Psychiatry
         16:1, 1967.

2.   CERF, G.A.: Donness recents en immuno-neurologie; effects
         electro-physiologiques anticorps dirgees contre le
         systeme nerveux. Actual Neurophys. 8:315, 1968.

3.   SEMENOV, S.F.: The study of autoimmune processes in a psychia-
         tric clinic. Int. Rev. Neurobiol. 11:291, 1968.

4.   HEATH, R.G.: An antibrain globulin in schizophrenia. In:
         Hinwich H.W. (ed): Biochemistry; Schizophrenia and
         affective illness. Williams & Wilkins Co. Baltimore,
         pp. 171-197, 1970.

5.   WHITTINGHAM, S.,MACKAY I.R., JONES, I.H., DAVIS, H.: Absence
         of brain antibodies in patients with schizophrenia.
         Brit. Med. J. 1:347, 1968.

6.   LOGAN, D.G., DEODHAR, S.D.: Schizophrenia, an immunological
         disorder? JAMA 212:1703, 1970.

7.   BOEHME, D.H., COTTRELL, J.C., DOHAN, F.C., HILLEGASS, L.M.:
         Fluorescent antibody studies of immunoglobulin binding
         by brain tissues. Arch. Gen. Psychiatry 28:202, 1973.

8.   FROHMAN, C.E., HARRISON, C.R., ARTHUR, R.E., GOTTLIEB, J.S.:
          Confirmation of a unique plasma protein in schizophrenia.
          Biol. Psychiatry, 3:113, 1971.

9.   GOTTLIEB, J.S., FROHMAN, C.E., HARRISON, C.R.: Schizophrenia:
          New concepts. South Med. J. 64:743, 1971.

10.   FESSEL, W.J.: Blood proteins in functional psychoses. Arch.
          Gen. Psychiatry. 6:134, 1962.

11.   SOLOMON, G.F., ALLANSMITH, M., McCLELLAN, B., AMKRAUT, A.:
          Immunoglobulin in psychiatric patients. Arch. Gen.
          Psychiatry, 20:272, 1969.

12.   AMKRAUT, A., SOLOMON, G.F., ALLANSMITH, M., McCLELLAN, B.:
          Immunoglobulins and improvement in acute schizophrenic
          reactions. Arch. Gen. Psychiatry: 28:673, 1973.

13.   CUATRECASES, P.: Protein purification by affinity chromato-
          graphy. Derivatization of agarose and polyacrylamide
          beads. J. Biol. Chem. 245:3059, 1970.

14.   GREENWOOD, F.C., HUNTER, W.M., GLOVER, J.S.: The preparation
          of ^{131}I-labeled human growth hormone of high specific
          radioactivity. Biochem. J. 89:114, 1963.

15.   WITZ, I.P., YAGI, Y., PRESSMAN, D.: A normal component in
          rabbit IgG with affinity for mouse tissues. Immunology
          15:765, 1968.

16.   LURIA, E.A., DOMASHNEVA, I.V.: Antibodies to thymocytes in
          sera of patients with schizophrenia. Proc. Nat. Acad.
          Sci. U.S.A. 71:235, 1974.

FACTORS INFLUENCING THE DEAMINATION AND FUNCTIONAL ACTIVITY OF

BIOGENIC MONOAMINES IN THE CENTRAL NERVOUS SYSTEM

M.B.H. Youdim

University Department of Clinical Pharmacology

Radcliffe Infirmary, Oxford

INTRODUCTION

In 1861 Griesinger was one of the first to point out that disturbed function of the brain may be the underlying cause of mental disease. In his text book he stated that all mental disease must "necessarily and invariably" be due to an improper functioning of the brain cells (1861). Yet it is only comparatively recently that the challenge of the possible pathological and biochemical lesions in mental disease have been taken up by neurobiologists. However, in most cases no such lesion has been discovered. This does not mean that they do not exist, but merely indicates that we need further methodological techniques and knowledge to discover them. However, there has been a greater success in discovering drugs for use in the chemotherapy of affective disorders. It is of interest to note that some of the important psychoactive drugs used in the treatment of psychiatric disturbance were not discovered for their use in mental disease but were the result of accidents. To mention one, the first and still important anti-psychotic drug, chlorpromazine, was not envisaged as potentially valuable in the treatment of psychiatric disturbance (Courvoisier et al, 1953). Indeed, chlorpromazine was first used in psychiatric patients (Delay et al, 1952) only because it seemed to have a powerful effect on the central nervous system. Another example is the important class of antidepressant agents, the monoamine oxidase (MAO) inhibitors (also sometimes called psychic energizers). Iproniazid (a potent and irreversible hydrazine inhibitor of mono-amine oxidase) was originally used as an antituberculosis agent until it was discovered to have central psycho-energizing action in patients receiving it. Zeller (1952) discovered its MAO inhibitory properties and it was not until 1957 that this drug was

introduced into clinical use as an antidepressant. It is true to
say that monoamine oxidase inhibitors together with reserpine are
among the most important pharmacological drug tools yet discovered.
Much of what we know about the synthesis, catabolism and release
of biogenic monoamine neurotransmitters in the central nervous
system is due to the results obtained using these two drugs. Both
compounds have had their place in chemotherapy of affective disorders. However, they fell into disrepute largely because of their
unwanted side effects (for review see Youdim, 1975a).

In the present paper I would like to discuss some of the new
information about monoamine metabolsim and functional activity
that has accumulated recently using "selective" monoamine oxidase
inhibitors.

MONOAMINE OXIDASE (MAO) PHYSIOLOGY

It is well recognised that monoamine oxidase (MAO) plays an
important role in the catabolism of biologically active monoamines
in the central nervous system and peripheral tissues (Youdim, 1975b).
The biogenic amines are stored in an inactive form in the sub-
cellular particles (amine storage granules) of the nervous system.
Such amines can be released into the circulation either by nerve
stimulation or by pharmacological agents and could cause pharmacological effects which might be drastic if the excess is not degraded. Possibly it is for this reason that an enzyme such as MAO
capable of catabolising the amines is provided. Thus the activity
of this enzyme may be very important in regulating the amine content of the central nervous system (Davis et al, 1975). The enzyme
is present both in the extraneuronal as well as in the intraneuronal tissue. Although re-uptake mechanism is now thought to be
acting as a primary system for non-chemical inactivation of biogenic monoamines released at the receptor site (Iversen, 1967),the
function of intra-neuronal MAO may, therefore, be to metabolise
released neurotransmitter monoamines before or after re-uptake. The
process itself may depend on the state of MAO activity present
in the nerve terminal and appears to be governed by the relative
concentration of free intra and extra-neuronal amines (Trendelenberg
et al, 1972). The result suggests that MAO activity is essential
for keeping cytoplasmic levels of noradrenaline (Trendelenberg
et al, 1972) and 5-hydroxytryptamine (Green and Grahame-Smith, 1975)
in the neuron low. Under conditions when MAO is fully inhibited,
the amine storage capacity of granules, which is limited, becomes
gradually exhausted with time and the level of neuronal amines
rises and spills over into the "functional pool" to produce functional activity resulting in neurotransmission. Further support
for the physiological importance of neuronal MAO comes from recent
observations that MAO exists in multiple forms _in vitro_ as well as

<u>in vivo</u> (Youdim and Collins, 1975) having different substrate
specificities and inhibitor sensitivities (Houslay et al, 1976).

MULTIPLE FORMS OF MAO, THEIR INHIBITION AND 5-HYDROXYTRYPTAMINE
                        FUNCTIONAL ACTIVITY

     When rats are given L-dopa (L-3,4, dihydroxyphenylalanine)
Everett et al, 1963) or L-tryptophan (Grahame-Smith, 1971)
following an intraperitoneal injection of an irreversible MAO
inhibitor (pargyline or tranylcypramine) they display characteristic behavioural changes including hyperactivity. Since these
changes are only seen in animals in which MAO has been inhibited
it has been concluded that this demonstrates the ability of intraneuronal MAO to metabolize the increased dopamine (DA) or 5-hydroxy-
tryptamine (5-HT) being formed. When the enzyme is inhibited the
increased amine synthesis results in the transmitters being released
into the symaptic cleft, stimulating the receptor and producing the
behavioural changes. Using these behavioural models together with
biochemical measurements we have made an investigation into the
action of various "selective" MAO inhibitors and the functional
importance of different forms of MAO.

     It is now accepted that MAO exists in multiple forms having
different substrate specificities and inhibitor sensitivities
(Youdim and Collins, 1975), however, the controversy still exists
as to whether they are a function of a single protein or derived
from different protein molecules (see Houslay et al, 1976).

     With the selective MAO inhibitors clorgyline and deprenil two
forms of MAO can be distinguished; MAO "type A" which is "selectively" inhibited by clorgyline and oxidatively deaminates 5-HT,
noradrenaline and octopamine and MAO "type B" which deaminates
phenylethylamine, benzylamine, kynuramine and tryptamine, but is
resistant to inhibition by clorgyline and is "selectively" inhibited
by deprenil. Dopamine and tyramine are substrates for both enzyme
species (see Houslay et al, 1976).

     To answer the question as to whether either "type A" or "type
B" enzyme is responsible for the hyperactivity syndrome we used
these selective MAO inhibitors to alter functional activity of rat
brain 5-HT and possible interactions with other monoamines (Green
and Youdim, 1975). We found that tryptophan administration (100mg/
kg intraperitoneally) to rats pretreated with tranylcypramine at
doses above 2.5 mg/kg intraperitoneally resulted in the hyperactivity syndrome and total inhibition of both "type A" and "type
B" MAO. Brain 5-HT concentrations were greater than 1 μg/g wet
weight brain 90 min after L-tryptophan administration. A dose of
1 mg/kg did not result in hyperactivity and inhibition of MAO

activity was below 85%. Nor did the brain 5-HT levels reach 1 μg/g 90 min after L-tryptophan. In contrast neither clorgyline or deprenil even at doses as high as 10 mg/kg produce the hyperactivity syndrome after intraperitoneal injection of tryptophan (100 mg/kg) nor did they inhibit both "type A" and "type B" MAO. Administration of either drug did not produce a brain 5-HT increase as large as that seen after tranylcypramine (2.5 mg/kg). However when clorgyline and deprenil were given together at doses of 25 mg/kg or more prior to tryptophan administration the animals became hyperactive. Bio- chemical investigation showed that both forms of the enzyme were inhibited above 85% and brain 5-HT accumulation was similar to values seen when tranylcypromine (2.5 mg/kg or more) was the inhibitor (Green and Youdim, 1975).

Several points emerge from these experiments regarding the brain 5-HT, MAO inhibition and hyperactivity syndrome. Our results suggest that while in vivo deamination of 5-HT is normally the function of MAO "type A" nevertheless when this form of the enzyme is inhibited by clorgyline the increased 5-HT can spill over on "type B" MAO which will continue to metabolise this amine. When deprenil is also given with the clorgyline, the "type B" enzyme is now also inhibited and the hyperactivity is seen and the brain 5-HT increases as occurs when a non-specific inhibitor such as tranyl- cypramine is given.

Valuable information has been obtained from the study of selective MAO inhibitors and their specificities in vitro.It must be remembered that conditions in vivo may be very different. Our present findings support the view (Youdim , 1973) that in vivo multiple forms of MAO may act as an integrated enzyme system having properties different from the individual enzyme forms examined in vitro. This view is reflected in the results which are obtained with regard to 5-HT and hyperactivity. It seems that although MAO "type A" may be responsible for deamination of 5-HT, only when both forms of enzyme are inhibited above 85% does the phenomenon of hyperactivity occur and the rate of 5-HT synthesis reaches a value above 0.40 μg/h.

These findings suggest that 85% of MAO activity present in the brain is grossly in excess of normal physiological requirements; but it seems that the pharmacological and behavioural changes are seen only when the remaining 15% "functionally active MAO" is inhibited. At present it is not known whether this MAO activity is located intraneuronally or not, and whether it is part of the same or another form of the enzyme. Of great interest is the finding of Robinson et al (1975) that therapeutic responses of MAO inhibitors as antidepressants depend on the inhibition of "total MAO" by more than 85%. If true, this may be one reason why successful therapy of depressive states by MAO inhibitors has been difficult to achieve.

Previous studies of human brains obtained at autopsy from patients
treated with therapeutic doses of inhibitors have indicated that
MAO activity is not inhibited above 75% when dopamine was used as
the substrate (Youdim et al, 1972).

We have confirmed that in the rat brain like that of human
brain (Collins et al, 1970) dopamine is metabolised by MAO "type
A" and "type B" (Green and Youdim, 1975). Recent observation
suggests that the steady state level of brain dopamine is important
for the hyperactivity syndrome observed after an irreversible non-
selective MAO inhibitor and tryptophan (Green and Grahame-Smith,
1974; Green et al, 1976; Youdim et al, 1976a). The fact that neither
clorgyline or deprenil is able to produce the tryptophan hyperactivity syndrome would also suggest that when MAO activity is
blocked with either of these two inhibitors dopamine can be
deaminated by either of the two enzyme species.

MONOAMINE OXIDASE ACTIVITY AND CLINICAL SITUATIONS

The present knowledge of the physiology of MAO and the intraneuronal regulation of its activity is very limited. However
Youdim and Holzbauer (1973, 1976) have shown that the activity of
the enzyme can be influenced by a number of biological factors
e.g. oestrous cycle, growth and as well as by drugs (naturally
occurring steroids).

Dietary components such as iron can also influence the enzyme.
Because of the apparent importance of iron in determining monoamine
oxidase activity (Symes et al, 1969; Symes et al 1971) we have
studied platelet MAO activity in patients with iron deficiency.
The activity of MAO when assayed with four substrates was significantly lowered in the platelets from the blood of patients with
iron-deficiency anaemia and treatment with oral iron restored MAO
activity (Youdim et al, 1975). Platelet MAO activity has been
determined in patients with psychiatric diseases with the implications that it may reflect brain MAO activity (Murphy and Wyatt,
1972; Meltzer and Stahl, 1974) and thus it is important to determine factors such as iron states, which may influence MAO activity
in the platelet.

There is little doubt that this enzyme plays an important
role in the catabolism of biogenic monoamines which are transmitter
substances. The behavioural studies reported in the present paper
support this conclusion (Green and Youdim, 1975). Any disturbance
in its function such as either an increase or a decrease in the
brain may thus lead to a change in the functional activity of
neuro-transmitters. Disturbances of its activity can occur for
many reasons and have been reported in a number of clinical
situations such as schizophrenia and unipolar depression (see

Sandler et al, 1975). This must be kept in mind in the quest for
a causal link between MAO function and any psychiatric disorder.
Clinical research in this field is in addition limited to studies
on MAO activity in blood platelets and measurements of deaminated
monoamine metabolites in the urine and cerebrospinal fluid (CSF).

Human platelet MAO is "type B" with regard to substrate specificities and inhibitor sensitivities (Youdim et al, 1976b), whereas the brain possesses both "type A" and "type B". Much more
evidence is needed to decide whether changes in the MAO activity
in the blood platelet can be used as an indication of similar
changes in the brain MAO activity and monoamine deamination.

When measuring in vitro activities of enzymes in tissue homogenates or isolated cells the question arises whether such measurements can be used as an indication for the events occurring in vivo.
Animal experiment studies have shown that at least in the rat the
development of the monoamine oxidase activity towards dopamine
in vitro follows a similar change as the tissue concentrations of
homovanillic acid and dihydroxyphenylacetic acid, the two acid
metabolites of dopamine formed by the action of MAO (Davis et al,
1975). Further studies are needed to correlate MAO activity with
appearance of other monoamine neurotransmitter metabolites.

Animal experiments have also provided evidence that the concentration of 5-hydroxyindole-3yl-acetic acid in the CSF can reflect the 5-hydroxytryptamine metabolism in the central nervous
system (Moir et al, 1970; Bulat and Zivkovic, 1971).

There is evidence that the beneficial effects achieved in
certain mental conditions by drugs which inhibit MAO in vitro
can be attributed to the inhibition of the enzyme in vivo and thus
to a slower rate of catabolism of biogenic monoamines in the brain.
The crucial question whether changes in the normal rate of amine
metabolism can lead to mental disturbance is still far from settled.
The response of some patients treated with MAO inhibitors to the
ingestion of certain dietary amines (tyramine in particular) with
a large rise in blood pressure suggests that MAO plays an essential
role in the disposition of these compounds (Youdim 1976a). However,
deprenil, a potent irreversible MAO inhibitor, may avoid this problem if the results from animal studies are relevant. Indeed, there
is one report that deprenil antagonises the pressor effect of
tyramine (Knoll and Magyar, 1972).

The lack of potentiation of the tyramine effect by deprenil
may be explained by the fact that tyramine is a substrate for both
"type A" and "type B" enzymes. When "type B" enzyme is inhibited
by deprenil tyramine can still be catabolised by "type A" MAO.
Another important property of this inhibitor is the relative lack
of inhibition of intestinal MAO, compared to that seen after other

MAO inhibitors. Intestinal MAO is for the most part "type A" and
thus patients treated with this inhibitor may be able to ingest
oral tyramine with impunity (Youdim, 1976a).

Because of its pharmacological and biochemical properties it
seems that deprenil is the most promising drug among the selective
inhibitors from the therapeutic point of view. The use of selective
inhibitors has been suggested as a possible treatment for depression
(Youdim et al, 1970) and Parkinsonism (Yang and Neff, 1974), since
such drugs would be expected to cause an elevation of 5-HT or dopamine levels without affecting the concentrations of the other transmitter amines. Recently we have demonstrated that deprenil is
indeed very effective in potentiating the anti-akinetic effect in
Parkinsonian patients with or without previous L-dopa (L-dihydroxy-
phenylalanine) therapy. The clinical result is an excellent kinetic
effect not only when starting L-dopa therapy or in "responders" to
L-dopa therapy but also in cases of off-effects. The drug is able
to block this effect when given before the time that off-phases set
in (Birkmayer et al, 1975).

Clinical evaluation of this drug as an antidepressant either
alone or in combination with lithium is awaited with great interest
in the light of the effectiveness of lithium and MAO inhibitors in
the treatment of certain types of depression resistant to other
forms of therapy (Zall, 1971; Himmelhoch et al, 1972). As Grahame-
Smith and Green (1974) have shown and pointed out it is more than
coincidence that tryptophan plus a MAO inhibitor and lithium plus
a MAO inhibitor both produce the same hyperactivity syndrome in
the rat through effects on brain 5-HT function.

THE USE OF RADIOLABELLED IRREVERSIBLE INHIBITORS TO STUDY
MITOCHONDRIAL MONOAMINE OXIDASE ACTIVE SITE

Membrane bound mitochondrial monoamine oxidase, an enzyme
containing 1 mol of covalently bound FAD (Youdim, 1975b; Salach
et al, 1976) has been the subject of inhibitor studies since 1952.
Fortunately, many of the drugs that inhibit the enzyme act irreversibly, presumably by binding to an active site. However, little is
known about the mechanism of the action of these inhibitors.

In order to understand how MAO and drugs that inhibit it
irreversibly function in vivo, knowledge about its cofactor requirements and the nature of its active site are required.

Phenylethylhydrazine (phenelzine), a hydrazine, and pargyline,
an acetylenic amine, have been more extensively investigated than
other inhibitors. The former has been widely used as an antidepressant in the treatment of depression. Recently it has been

shown that the inhibition of MAO by phenylethylhydrazine, pargyline
and 3-dimethylamino-1-propyne is irreversible, but the enzyme can
be protected from inhibition by benzylamine and kynuramine (Chuang
et al, 1974; Collins and Youdim, 1975; Maycock et al, 1976). When
the enzyme is fully inhibited the drugs combine with the oxidized
form of the enzyme with the formation of a 1:1 covalent adduct.

The cofactor FAD isolated from purified liver MAO is associated
with a penta peptide having the following amino acid sequence:
Ser-Gly-Gly-Cys-Tyr, the flavin being attached via the 8α-carbon
of riboflavin in a thio-ether linkage with the cysteine (Walker
et al 1971). Chuang et al (1974) and Oreland et al (1973) reported
that the inhibition of purified kidney and liver MAO by pargyline
is accompanied by the disappearance of the 450-500 nm band of
flavoquinine and the appearance of a peak at 410 nm. This fact
taken together with the observation that ^{14}C-pargyline is recovered
in the flavin penta-peptide fraction after proteolytic digestion
of the enzyme provide evidence that the covalent adduct involves
the FAD moiety together with the inhibitor. These studies led us
to examine the action of the anti-depressant deprenil (another
acetylenic amine) on MAO and its possible attachment to the cofactor FAD at the active site.

Deprenil (phenyl-isopropylmethylpropinylamine hydrochloride)
is a selective inhbitor of MAO "type B". It irreversibly inacti-
vates rat brain and liver mitochodrial MAO. The inactivation of
the purified liver enzyme results in the loss of absorption in
the 450-500 nm region of flavin spectrum and a concomitant increase
in absorbance at 410 nm. The inhibition is prevented by monoamine
substrates, is time dependent, and is the function of the amount
of ^{14}C-inhibitor bound to the enzyme. The inhibition is accompanied
by the formation of 1:1 covalent adduct between the enzyme and the
inhibitor (Youdim, 1976b).

Since the studies of Chuang et al (1974) and others (Oreland
et al, 1973; Collins and Youdim 1975; Maycock et al, 1976) had
provided evidence for involvement of covalent link between MAO
inhibitors and FAD at the active center of the enzyme, an examination was made of the flavin peptide adduct isolated from ^{14}C-deprenil
treated purified rat liver MAO. The ^{14}C-deprenil could not be
resolved from the FAD-penta peptide adduct. More than 90% of the
original ^{14}C-deprenil bound to the enzyme could be recovered after
proteolytic digestion of MAO in association with the FAD. Thus 1
mol of (^{14}C)-deprenil is bound to 1 mol of flavin/1 mol of enzyme.
Maycock et al (1976) using the the simple acetylenic inhibitor
3-dimethylamino-1-propyne have elegantly determined its binding
site on liver FAD penta-peptide. From their chemical analysis (and
spectral properties of the FAD-inhibitor penta-peptide adduct,
which is identical to those observed for pargyline and deprenil)
it was concluded that the flavin-inhibitor adduct is an N-5 sub-

substituted dihydroflavine and its structure has been determined. More recently we have shown that for the most part brain MAO also contains covalently bound FAD as cofactor and the isolated FAD penta-peptide has the same structure as that isolated from the liver enzyme (Salach et al., 1976) (see Fig. 1). Thus it has been concluded that deprenil binds to brain MAO active site in a similar fachion, as indicated in Fig. 1.

TITRATION OF MAO BY RADIOLABELLED INHIBITORS

The mol to mol binding of (^{14}C)-inhibitors (pargyline, deprenil and phenylethylhydrazine) to MAO allows the investigator to titrate enzyme concentration. Since the inactivation of MAO by these inhibitors gave a linear stoichiometric inhibition, the titration end-point can be related directly to enzyme concentration (Chuang et al, 1974; Youdim, 1976b). The platelet MAO has been used as a peripheral marker for the brain enzyme and it has been reported that its activity is lower in schizophrenia (Murphy and Wyatt, 1972; Meltzer and Stahl, 1974). However, these results have not been confirmed in platelets obtained from untreated patients (Crow et al, 1976). The method of enzyme titration could be used to resolve whether there is a lowered amount of enzyme or that other factors are involved. One situation where this problem has been examined is in iron deficiency anaemia; treatment with oral ferrous sulfate restores the MAO activity (Youdim et al, 1975). Using (^{14}C) -deprenil to titrate the enzyme our studies have shown that the amount of active enzyme is lowered in iron-deficiency anaemia (Youdim et al, 1976).

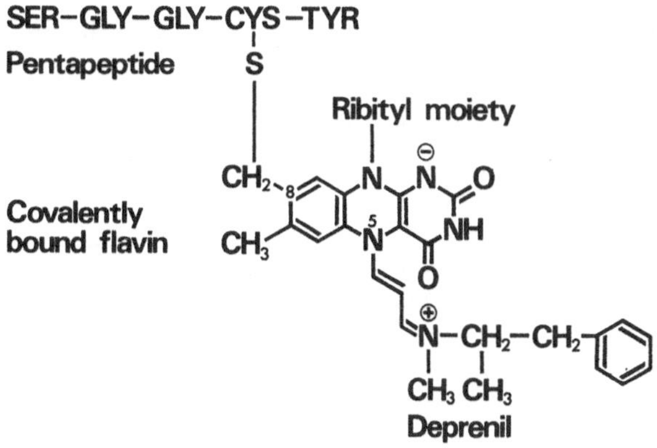

Fig. 1.   Brain monoamine oxidase active site

REFERENCES

1. BIRKMAYER, W., RIEDERER, P., YOUDIM, M.B.H. AND LINAUER, W.:
    J. Neurol. Trans. 36: 303-326, 1975.

2. BULAT, M. AND ZIVKOVIC, B.: Science, 173, 738-740, 1971.

3. CHUANG, H-Y.K., PATEK, D.R. AND HELLERMAN, L.: J. Biol. Chem.
    249, 2381-2386, 1974.

4. COLLINS, G.G.S. AND YOUDIM, M.B.H.: Biochem. Pharmacol.
    24, 703-706, 1975.

5. COLLINS, G.G.S., SANDLER, M., WILLIAMS, E.D. AND YOUDIM, M.B.H.:
    Nature (Lond). 225, 817-820, 1970.

6. COURVOISIER, S., FOURNEL, J., DUCROT, R., KOLSKY, M. AND
    KOETSCHET, P.: Arch. Int. Pharmacodyn. 92, 305, 1953.

7. CROW, T.J., JOHNSTONE, E.C. AND OWEN, F.R.: In: Monoamine
    Oxidase and its Inhibition (Ed. J. Knight) North Holland
    Amsterdam. (in press).

8. DAVIS, A.J., HOLZBAUER, M., SHARMAN, D.F. AND YOUDIM, M.B.H.:
    Brit. J. Pharmacol. 55, 558-560, 1975.

9. DELAY, J., DENIKER, P. AND HARL, J.M.: Ann. Medicopsychol.
    (Paris) 110, 112-121, 1952.

10. EVERETT, G.M., WIEGAND, R.G. AND RINALDI, F.U.: Ann. N.Y.
    Acad. Sci. 107, 1068-1080, 1963.

11. GRAHAME-SMITH, D.G.: J. Neurochem. 18, 1053-1066, 1971.

12. GRAHAME-SMITH, D.G. AND GREEN, A.R.: Brit. J. Pharmacol. 52,
    19-26, 1974.

13. GREEN, A.R. AND GRAHAME-SMITH, D.G.: Neuropharmacology, 13,
    949-959, 1974.

14. GREEN, A.R. AND GRAHAME-SMITH, D.G.: In: Handbook of Psycho-
    pharmacology (Eds. L.L. Iversen, S. Iversen and S. Snyder).
    Plenum Press, New York, pp. 169-245, 1975.

15. GREEN, A.R. AND YOUDIM, M.B.H.: Brit. J. Pharmacol. 55, 415-
    422, 1975.

16. GREEN, A.R., YOUDIM, M.B.H. AND GRAHAME-SMITH, D.G.: Neuro-
    pharmacology 15, 173-179, 1976.

17. GRIESINGER, W.: Die Pathologie und Therapie der psychischen
        Krankheiten für Aerzte und Studirende 2d ed. Stuttgart:
        Krabbe. 1861.

18. HIMMELHOCH, J.M., DETRE, T., KUPFER, J.D., SWARTZBURG, M.
        AND BYCK, R.: J. Nerv. Ment. Dis. 155, 216-220, 1972.

19. HOLZBAUER, M., AND YOUDIM, M.B.H.: Brit. J. Pharmacol. 44,
        600-608, 1973.

20. HOUSLAY, M.D., TIPTON, K.F. AND YOUDIM, M.B.H.: Life Sci.
        (in press). 1976.

21. IVERSEN, L.L.: Uptake and Storage of Noradrenaline in
        Sympathetic Nerve. Cambridge University Press, Cambridge
        1967.

22. KNOLL, J. AND MAGYAR, K.: Adv. Biochem. Psychopharmacol.
        5, 393-408, 1972.

23. MAYCOCK, A.L., ABELES, R.H., SALACH, J.I. AND SINGER, T.P.:
        Biochemistry, 15, 114-125, 1976.

24. MELTZER, H.Y. AND STAHL, S.M.: Res. Commun. Chem. Pathol.
        Pharmacol. 7, 419-431, 1974.

25. MOIR, A.T.B., ASHCROFT, G.W., CRAWFORD, T.B.B., ECCLESTON, D.
        AND GULDBERG, H.C.: Brain, 93, 357-368, 1970.

26. MURPHY, D.L. AND WYATT, R.J.: Nature (Lond.) 238, 225-226,
        1972.

27. NEFF, N.H. AND YANG, H.Y.T.: Life Sci. 14, 2061-2074, 1974.

28. ORELAND, L., KINEMUCHI, H. AND YOO, B.H.: Life Sci. 13, 1533-
        , 1973.

29. ROBINSON, D.S., NIES, A., RAVARIS, C.L., IVES, J.O. AND
        LAMBORN, K.R.: In: Classification and Predication of
        Outcome of Depression. (Ed. J. Angst). Angs. Symp.
        Medicum, Hoechst 8, Basel.

30. SALACH, J.I., YASUNOBU, K.T., MINAMURA, M. AND YOUDIM, M.B.H.:
        In: Flavins and Flavoproteins (Ed. T.P. Singer) Elsevier,
        Amsterdam, (in press) 1976.

31. SYMES, A.L., MISSALA, K. AND SOURKES, T.L.: Science, 174,
        153-155, 1971.

32. SYMES, A.L., SOURKES, T.L., YOUDIM, M.B.H., GREGORIADIS, G.
     AND BIRNBAUM, H.: Can. J. Biochem. 47, 999-1003,
     1969.

33. TRENDELENBERG, U., DRASKOCZY, P.R. AND GRAEFE, K.H.: Adv.
     Biochem. Psychopharmacol. 5, 371-379, 1972.

34. WALKER, W.H., KEARNEY, E.B., SENG, R.L. AND SINGER, T.P.:
     Eur. J. Biochem. 24, 328-336, 1971.

35. YOUDIM, M.B.H.: Brit. Med. Bull. 29, 120-123, 1973.

36. YOUDIM, M.B.H.: In: Modern Problems of Pharmacopsychiatry;
     Genetics and Psychopharmacology. (Ed. J. Mendlewicz).
     Karger, Basel. pp. 65-89, 1975a.

37. YOUDIM, M.B.H.: In: MTP International Review of Science;
     Physiology and Pharmacological Biochemistry. (Ed.
     H.K.F. Blaschko). Butterworths, London. pp. 169-211.
     1975b.

38. YOUDIM, M.B.H.: In: Neuroregulators and Hypothesis of
     Psychiatric Disorders. (Eds. E. Usdin, J. Barchas and
     D. Hamberg). Oxford University Press, Oxford (in press).
     1976a.

39. YOUDIM, M.B.H.: In: Flavins and Flavoproteins (Ed. T.P.
     Singer) Elsevier, Amsterdam. (in press) 1976b.

40. YOUDIM, M.B.H. AND COLLINS, G.G.S. In: Monoamine oxidase and
     its inhibition. Ciba Foundation Symposium No. 39.
     (ed. J. Knight). North Holland, Amsterdam (in press).

41. YOUDIM, M.B.H., COLLINS, G.G.S., SANDLER, M., BEVAN JONES, A.B.,
     PARE, C.M.B. AND NICHOLSON, W.J.: Nature (Lond). 236,
     225-228, 1972.

42. YOUDIM, M.B.H., GREEN, A.R. AND GRAHAME-SMITH, D.G.: In:
     Vth International Parkinson's Disease Symposium (Ed.
     W. Birkmayer). Springer-Verlag, Wein (in press).

43. YOUDIM, M.B.H., GRAHAME -SMITH, D.G. AND WOODS, H.F.: Clin.
     Sci. Mol. Med. (in press) 1976b.

44. YOUDIM, M.B.H., WOODS, H.F., MITCHELL, B., GRAHAME-SMITH, D.G.
     AND CALLENDER, S.: Clin. Sci. Mol. Med. 48, 289-295,
     1975.

45. ZALL, H.: Amer. J. Psychiat. 127, 136-139, 1971.

46. ZELLER, E.A., BARSKY, J., BERMAN, E.R. AND FOUTS, J.R.:
     J. Pharm. Exp. Ther. 106, 427-438, 1952.

HYPOTHERMIC EFFECTS OF ANTIPSYCHOTIC PHENOTHIAZINES

Shlomo Yehuda

Department of Psychology

Bar-Ilan University, Tel-Aviv, Israel

INTRODUCTION

D-Amphetamine-Induced Hypothermia

The thermal effects of d-amphetamine in rats depend upon the ambient temperature at which the animals are maintained. A dose of 5-15 mg/kg, i.p. causes marked hypothermia among rats kept at 4°C but results in hyperthermia for rats kept at 20-37°C (Yehuda and Wurtman, 1972a). The drug also interferes with normal behavioral thermoregulation. When d-amphetamine-treated rats are placed in a temperature-gradient apparatus they tend to locate themselves far away from a heat source when the ambient temperature is 4°C, and to locate themselves near a heat source when the ambient temperature was 30°C (Yehuda and Wurtman, 1974a).

The attempts to locate the site of action of d-amphetamine-produced hypothermia among rats maintained in a cold ambient temperature led to the hypothesis that the pharmacological as well as behavioral effects are mediated by the release of dopamine (DA) in the brain. The following results obtained from our pharmacological and neuroanatomical studies support this hypothesis:

a. Hypothermia was not observed when rats were injected with peripheral acting sympathomimetic drugs (e.g., tyramine or B'B-difluoroamphetamine). This indicates that the hypothermia is mediated by the CNS (Yehuda and Wurtman, 1972b).

b. Drugs that increase the availability of DA, or stimulate DA central receptors (e.g. apomorphine, clonidine, L-dopa, or ET-495) produce hypothermia, while pimozide and haloperidol failed to produce hypothermia. In addition, these drugs

137

even blocked the amphetamine-induced hypothermia (Yehuda
and Wurtaman, 1972b).
c. There is only a minimal effect of the monoamines NE
and 5-HT on d-amphetamine-produced hypothermia. Blockade
of NE receptors (e.g., by phenoxybenzamine or by propranolol) produces marked hypothermia. Neither the blockade
of 5-HT receptors (methysergide), nor the decrease in
5-HT concentration (p-chloroamphetamine) nor the destruction of 5-HT neurons in the brain (5,6,-DHT) result in a
reduction of d-amphetamine hypothermia (Yehuda and Wurtman, 1972b). Moreover, d-amphetamine-induced paradoxical
behavioral thermoregulation is enhanced by DA stimulants
(Yehuda and Wurtman, 1974b).

Supporting evidence for the involvement of central dopaminergic
neurons in hypothermia arises from studies of the hypothermic
effects of apomorphine- a direct selective DA-receptor stimulant
(Bennet et al., 1972; Glick and Marsanico, 1974; Kennedy and Burks,
1974; Reid et al., 1975).

Histochemical fluorescence studies have shown that much of
the dopamine in the brain is concentrated within the following
groups of neurons (Fuxe et al., 1970): (1) The nigro-striatal
pathway, which originate in the substantia nigra and terminates
in the striatum; (2) mesolimbic tract that originates in the central
tegmental area (A_{10}) and project mainly to the olfactory tubercule
and nucleus accubens; (3) the tubero-infundibular dopamine neurons
of the hypothalamus; (4) in the retina; and (5) in the limbic
cortex (Thierry et al., 1974; Hokfelt, et al., 1974). The origin of
those nerve terminals are still unknown.

In an attempt to localize the dopaminergic tract that mediates
the hypothermic response, we studied the effects of lesions in
various DA pathways. We found that d-amphetamine-induced hypothermia
and paradoxical thermoregulatory behavior can be blocked in rats
lesioned in the mesolimbic pathway. No blockade was observed, however, in caudate nucleus-lesioned rats (Yehuda and Wurtman, 1975).
No blockade of hypothermic response to d-amphetamine was observed
among rats lesioned either in olfactory bulb or in area postrema.
Both sites are rich in structure containing NE neurons (unpublished
data).

DA Hypothesis of Schizophrenia and Phenothiazines

Amphetamine-psychosis resembles "true" acute paranoid schizophrenia more than any other drug-induced model psychosis. Snyder
(1972a; In Kety and Matthysse, 1972; Banerjee and Snyder, 1973;
Snyder, 1973; Snyder et al., 1973; Snyder, 1974; Feinberg and
Snyder, 1975) suggested that brain dopamine is the mediator of this
phenomenon. His conclusion is based on studies of the structural

activity relationships in antipsychotic phenothiazines, which are
the drug-of-choice in many psychotic cases. Further support is
provided by Matthysse (In Kety and Matthysse, 1972; Matthysse, 1973)
who suggested, following Carlsson and Lindquist (1963), that the
antipsychotic activity of phenothiazines is correlated with their
ability to block central DA activity.

Indirect Measuring of DA Blockade

The possible correlation between the degree of blockade of
DA-receptor sites and the antipsychotic activity of a drug can be
studied indirectly by measuring the effect of various types of
phenothiazines on a phenomenon which is clearly mediated only by
central dopaminergic neurons. Several experimentally induced types
of behavior have been associated with changes in brain DA, e.g. the
stereotypic behavior or the rotational behavior seen in rats
previously subjected to unilateral destruction of parts of the
nigro-striatal pathway. Our studies (Yehuda and Wurtman, 1975)
showed that such stereotyped behavior is most probably mediated by
the mesolimbic pathway. But these conclusions are not in accord
with those of Asher and Aghajanian (1974) who interpreted their
data to indicate that stereotyped behavior is mediated by the nigro-
striatal pathway. Some methodological and technical differences
between the two studies might account for the different results.

We chose to test the effects of various types of phenothiazines
on the d-amphetamine-induced hypothermia, which is clearly mediated
by the dopaminergic mesolimbic pathway (Chiel et al., 1974; Yehuda,
1975; Yehuda and Wurtman, 1972a, b, 1974a, b. 1975). The aim of
this study was to investigate various phenothiazines classified as
antipsychotic as to their ability to block d-amphetamine-induced
hypothermia, and thus obtain an indirect index of their dopaminergic
blocking ability.

MATERIALS AND METHODS

Male Sabra rats (Hebrew University) weighing 90-120 gr were
housed six-seven per cage at an ambient temperature of 20°C-22°C.
The rats had free access to food and water. Immediately before
each experiment, rats were placed in individual cages; they were
then injected 10 mg/kg (i.p.) with one of several drugs in about
1.0 ml of medium (usually in 0.9% NaCl, or in a few cases in a
suspension of 1% methyl cellulose), and placed in an environmental
chamber set at 4°C. (Relative humidity was about 60%). Thirty
minutes later, half of the rats in each experimental group received
an intraperitoneal injection of 15 mg/kg d-amphetamine. Colonic
temperature was measured by a telathermometer (Yellow Spring Inst.,
Yellow Spring, Ohio) just prior to the first injection and at

15-minute interval thereafter. Each experimental group included
at least 10 rats. All experiments were performed between 10.00 h
and 14.00 h.

RESULTS

Contrary to our predictions, the phenothiazines used in our
study did not block d-amphetamine-induced hypothermia, but actually
appeared themselves to cause hypothermia and to potentiate that
produced by d-amphetamine.

As in our previous studies (Yehuda and Wurtman, 1972a, b),
d-amphetamine causes hypothermia of about -4.5°C among rats kept
at 4°C. Again as in our previous study, chlorpromazine causes even
more marked hypothermia (of about -12°C). However, unlike our
previous studies, control rats, which received saline (0.9% NaCl)
also exhibited slight hypothermia. In our previous studies, control
rats were able to regulate their body temperature over the duration
of the experiment. Perhaps this difference can be attributed to the
different strains used in the two sets of experiments. In this
study, we used the "Sabra" strain, while in previous studies the rats
were Sprague-Dawley. (We are in process of testing the thermal
response to various drugs of rats of other strains).

All phenothiazine-tested derivatives caused various degree of
hypothermia among rats kept at 4°C. There is a general correlation
between the degree of the hypothermia and the chemical structure
of the drug: Those drugs which belong to the piperidine subgroup,
isopropylamino or thioxanthene subgroups tend to cause a lower
degree of hypothermia than those drugs which belong to the piperazine
or to the propylamine subgroups (Table 1).

The order of the degree of the hypothermia induced by the injection of the drug together with d-amphetamine (Table 1) is similar to the order of the degree of hypothermia induced by the drug
alone.

Feinberg and Snyder (1975) presents a ranking of "relative
clinical potency" of 14 phenothiazines. Five of those drugs were
tested in this study. A comparison between the "relative clinical
potency" and the degree of the hypothermia induced by those drugs
(Table 2) reveals a very high correlation between the two phenomena:
antipsychotic activity and induced hypothermia.

Interestingly, the additional hypothermic effects of d-amphetamine to the hypothermia-induced by the drug itself, were inversely
related to the degree of hypothermia caused by the drug; as the
degree of hypothermia caused by the drug increased, the hypothermic
effect caused by adding d-amphetamine decreased (Table 1).

TABLE 1. Hypothermia – induced by drug alone, drug + d-amphetamine (120 min, after the first injection.)

Drug	Drug alone Rank	T°	Drug + d-amphetamine Rank	T°	Between drug alone and drug + d-amphetamine Rank	T°
Saline	–	-1.9	–	-4.5	–	2.6
Mepazine	1	-1.4	2	-4.0	8	2.6
7360 R.P.	2	-1.8	4	-5.4	11	3.6
Chloroprothixene	3	-1.8	3	-4.4	7	2.6
Thioproperazine	4	-2.4	1	3.5	2	1.1
Thioridazine	5	-3.9	5	-7.1	10	3.2
Promepazine	6	-4.0	6	-9.1	12	5.1
Trimepazine	7	-7.7	8	-10.2	6	2.5
Perphenazine	8	-9.0	7	9.7	1	0.7
Chlorpromazine	9	-11.1	9	-13.1	4	2.0
Carphenazine	10	-12.3	11	15.3	9	3.0
Triflupromazine	11	-12.4	10	14.8	5	2.4
Chloroimipiphenine	12	-14.7	12	16.6	3	1.9

TABLE 2. A comparison between "Relative clinical potency"
          and drug-induced hypothermia

Drug	Relative clinical potency*	Hypothermia (°C)
Triflupromazine	5	-12.4
Perphenazine	7	- 9.0
Chlorpromazine	10	-11.1
Promazine	11	- 4.0
Chlorprothixene	12	- 1.8

Rank of relative clinical potency out of 14 phenothiazines

*   (Feinberg and Snyder, 1975)

        In order to investigate the relative contribution of blockade
of dopamine receptors by chlorpromazine (CPZ) on the hypothermic
effect of the drug, groups of rats were pretreated with pimozide
(4 mg/kg) or with haloperidol (3mg/kg). Half an hour later, each
group received a dose of d-amphetamine (15 mg/kg) or CPZ (10 mg/kg).
Half·an hour later, each group received the other drug. Therefore,
each group received 3 treatments, at 30-minute intervals. The
results (Table 3) showed that (a) only pretreatment with pimozide
resulted in relative blockade of hypothermia induced by the combination of d-amphetamine + CPZ (in this order of treatment). In
all other 3 groups an increase of the hypothermia was found. (b)
that order of treatment (d-amphetamine, CPZ) is important in
pimozide-pretreatment groups but not for the haloperidol-pretreat-
ment groups. The increased output of DA which may be expected by
arousal of the neuronal feedback system can be logically initiated
by a drug which seems to block the DA receptors. On the other hand,
a drug which interferes with the production of DA or with the
interaction of DA and its receptors, but not with the receptor sites
will not lead to an increase in the feedback loop. This may explain
the blockage of hypothermia of the combined treatment of d-amphetamine and CPZ (in this order) in pimozide-treated rats, and the
increased hypothermia in the other group (additive effects).

TABLE 3. Effects of combined treatment on body temperature

Treatment	Time (min) after the first injection				
	30'	60'	90'	115'	120'
Pimozide (4) + d-Amp (15) + CPZ (10)	-0.3 ± 0.2	-2.9 ± 0.9	-5.4 ± 2.3	-7.4 ± 4.1	-9.3 ± 4.1
Halop (3) + d-Amp (15) + CPZ (10)	-1.6 ± 0.6	-5.2 ± 0.6	-12.0 ± 1.2	$-15. \pm 1.4$	More than -20
Pimozide (4) + CPZ (10) + d-Amp (15)	-0.9 ± 0.9	-5.6 ± 0.4	-12.4 ± 1.1	-15.8 ± 1.3	More than -20
Halop (3) + CPZ (10) + d-Amp (10)	-1.1 ± 0.3	-6.3 ± 1.4	-14.5 ± 2.6	-16.9 ± 1.9	More than -20

d-Amp = d-amphetamine

CPZ = chlorpromazine

Halop = haloperidol

Data expressed as Mean $\pm$ S.D.

DISCUSSION

Our hypothesis that antipsychotic phenothiazines should block d-amphetamine-induced hypothermia was not substantiated. On the contrary, phenothiazines classified as an antipsychotic themselves produced hypothermia, and the reported hallucogenic phenothiazine (R.P. 7630) was unable to produce significant hypothermia even in 400 mg/kg dose (our unpublished data).

The correlation found between the degree of hypothermia produced by the drug and the degree of antipsychotic activity is dependent upon several factors. The present study was based upon the injection of a fixed drug dose, 10 mg/kg, i.p., and d-amphetamine was added 30 minutes after the first injection. No consideration for dose-response relationship or to individual time-course was taken into account in this preliminary study. The study of dose-response and time course of selective antipsychotic phenothiazine is in progress now.

There are several possibilities to explain the apparent paradox that both dopamine receptor blockers (i.e. phenothiazines) and a DA striatal stimulant (i.e. d-amphetamine, Groves, 1974) both cause the same phenomena, that of hypothermia:
  (a) The hypothermia - induced by phenothiazines is not mediated by the action of these drugs on central DA receptors. Chlorpromazine, for an example, acts upon other brain and peripheral loci. Since chlorpromazine causes a depression in the activity of catecholamine neurons in the autonomic centers in the brain stem, this may affect thermoregulatory mechanisms. However, it seems from our results that DA does play a role in chlorpromazine-induced hypothermia, as this hypothermia is markedly attenuated by pretreatment with pimozide.

  (b) If DA neurons are involved in the hypothermic effects of antipsychotic phenothiazines, then the existence of a neuronal feedback loop within a DA system might explain the effect. Such a neural loop was proposed by Carlsson and Lindquist (1963), Snyder (1974), Bunney et al., (1973). Our present data do not contradict this hypothesis. However, it may suggest additional neural loop controlling interaction between DA pathways. New research is in progress in order to a) substantiate this hypothesis and b) to determine if the interaction between the two pathways is pre- or postsynaptic.

  (c) Our previous studies indicated that the hypothermic effect of d-amphetamine is mediated by its action on the central dopaminergic mesolimbic pathway (Yehuda and Wurtman, 1975). On the other hand, it has been suggested (Anden, 1964; Asher and Aghajanian, 1974; Burki et al., 1975; Carlsson and Lindquist, 1963; Horn and Snyder,

in the striatum are mediating psychotic behavior. The antipsychotic effects of phenothiazines may be explained by the ability of these drugs to block central striatal dopaminergic receptor sites (e.g. York, 1972).

Further research on d-amphetamine hypothermia is important because it is the only behavioral parameter that can be ascribed with certainty to the DA mesolimbic pathway.

D-amphetamine causes marked hypothermia among rats kept at 4°C. This hypothermia is due to the effect of the drug on central neurons in the dopaminergic mesolimbic pathway. However, we could not demonstrate blocking with antipsychotic phenothiazines of the d-amphetamine induced hypothermia. Indeed, our results showed that all phenothiazines tested cause hypothermia. The degree of the hypothermia is generally correlated with antipsychotic activity.

Acknowledgements

These studies were supported in part by a research grant from the Israeli Psychobiology Center, and by the Research Committee, (Bar-Ilan University). The author wishes to thank Mr. P. Frommer for his excellent technical assistance. Dr. H. Babkoff for many helpful suggestions, and Dr. H. Green, (Smith, Kline and French Co.) for d-amphetamine and chlorpromazine. Other drugs were generously provided by: Wyeth (carphenazine), Asta (chlorimipiphenine), Lederle (chlorprothixene), Warner-Lambert (mepatine), Bayer (trimprazine and promepuzine), Schering (perphazine), Sandoz (thioridazine), Rhene-Poulene (Thioproperazine and 7360 R.P.), Upjohn (Triflupromazine), and Janssen (pimozide and Haloperidol).

REFERENCES

1.   AGHAJANIAN, G.K., AND BUNNEY, B.S.: Pre- and postsynaptic feedback mechanisms in central dopaminergic neurons. In: Seeman, P. and Brown, G.M. (eds.) Frontiers in Neurology and Neuroscience Research, Uni. of Toronto Press, 4-11, 1974.

2.   ANDEN, N.E., ROSS, B.E., WERDINIUS, B.: Effects of chlorpromazine, haloperidol and reserpine on the levels of phendic acids in rabbit corpus striatum. Life Sci. 3, 149-154, 1964.

3.   ASHER, I.M. AND AGHAJANIAN, G.K.; 6-OH-DA lesions of olfactory tubercules and caudate nuclei: Effect of amphetamine-induced stereotyped behavior in rats. Brain Res.

4.   BANERJEE, U. AND LIN, G.S.: On the mechanism of central action
         of amphetamine: The role of catecholamines.
         Neuropharmacol:12, 917-931, 1973.

5.   BARNETT, A., GOLDSTEIN, J., AND TABER, H.I.: Apomorphine-
         induced hypothermia in mice: a possible dopamine effect.
         Arch. Int. Pharmacodyn. 198, 242-247, 1972.

6.   BUNNEY, B.S., WALTERS, J.H., ROTH, R.H., AND AGHAJANIAN, G.K.:
         Dopaminergic neurons: effects of antipsychotic drugs
         and amphetamine on single cell activity. J. Pharmacd.
         Expt. Therp. 185, 560-570, 1973.

7.   BUNNEY, B.S. AND AGHAJANIAN, G.K.: A comparison of the effects
         of chlorpormazine, 7-hydroxychlorpromazine and chlor-
         promazine sulfoxide on the activity of central dop-
         aminergic neurons. Life Sci. 15, 309-318, 1974.

8.   BURKI, H.R., EICHENBERGER, E., SAYERS, A.C., AND WHITE, T.G.:
         Clozapine and the dopamine hypothesis of schizophrenia.
         Pharmakopsychiat. 8, 115-121, 1975.

9.   CARLSSON, A., AND LINDQUIST, M.: Effects of chlorpromazine
         or haloperidol on formation of 3-methoxtyramine and
         normetanephrine in mouse brain. Acta Pharmacol.17,
         140-148, 1963.

10. CHIEL, H., YEHUDA, S. AND WURTMAN, R.J.: Development of
         tolerance in rats to the hypothermic effects of
         d-amphetamine and apomorphine. Life Sci. 14, 483-488,
         1974.

11. FEINBERG, A.P., AND SNYDER, S.H.: Phenothiazine drugs, struc-
         ture activity relationships explained by conformation
         that mimics dopamine. Proc. Nat. Acad. Sci. USA.
         72, 1899-1903, 1975.

12. FUXE, K., HOKFELT, T. AND UNGERSTADT, U.: Morphological and
         functional aspects of central monoamine neurons,
         Internat. Rev. Neurobiol. 13, 93-128, 1970.

13. GLICK, S.D., AND MARSANICE, R.G.: Apomorphine-induced and
         pilocarpine-induced hypothermia in mice. Br. J.
         Pharmacol. 51, 353-357, 1974.

14. GROVES, P.M., REBEC, G.V., SEGAL, D.S.: The action of d-amphet-
         amine on spontaneous caudate nucleus and reticular
         formation of the rat. Behav. Biol. 11, 33-47, 1974.

15   GUNNE, L.M., ANGGARD, E., AND JONSSON, L.E.: Clinical trials
           with amphetamine-blocking drugs. Psychiat. Neurol.
           Neurochir. 225-226, 1972.

16. HOKFELT, T., LJUNGDAHL, A., FUXE, K. AND JOHANSSON, O.: Dopamine
           nerve terminals in the rat limbic cortex, Aspects of
           dopamine hypothesis of schizophrenia. Science, 184,
           177-179, 1974.

17.   HORN, A.S. AND SNYDER, S.H.: Chlorpromazine and dopamine,
           Proc. Nat. Acad. Sci. USA. 68, 2325-2328, 1971

18.   KENNEDY, M.S., AND BURKS, T.F.: Dopamine receptors in the
           central thermoregulatory mechanism of the cat.
           Neuropharmacol. 13, 119-128, 1974.

19.   KETY, S.S., AND MATTHYSSE, S.: (Eds.) Prospects in research
           in schizophrenia. NRP Bull. 10, 371-507, 1972.

20.   KAROBATH, M.E.: Blockade of dopamine receptor. Pharmakopsych.
           8, 151-161, 1975.

21.   MATTHYSSE, S: Implication of feedback control in catecholamine
           neuronal systems; In: E. Usdin and S.H. Snyder (Eds.)
           Frontiers in Catecholamine Research. Pergamon Press,
           Oxford, 1139-1142, 1973.

22.   MATTHYSSE, S.: Schizophrenia: Relationships to dopamine trans-
           mission, motor control and feature extraction. In:
           F.O. Schmitt and F.G. Worden (Eds.) The Neurosciences
           The MIT Press, Cambridge, Mass., 733-737, 1974.

23.   REID, J.L., LEWIS, P.J., MYERS, M.G.: Role of central
           dopaminergic mechanisms in piribedil and clonodine-
           induced hypothermia in the rat. Neuropharmacology
           14, 215-220, 1975.

24.   ROSS, B.E.: Effects of certain tranquillizers on the level of
           homovanillic acid in the corpus striatum. J. Pharm.
           Pharmacol. 17, 820-823, 1965.

25.   SEEMAN, P., AND LEE, T.: Antipsychotic drugs, Science, 188,
           1217-1219, 1975.

26.   SNYDER, S.H.: Catecholamines in the brain as mediators of
           amphetamine-psychosis, Arch. Gen. Psychiat. 27,
           168-179, 1972.

27.   SNYDER, S.H.: Catecholamines as mediators of drug effects in
      schizophrenia. In: F.O. Schmitt, and F.G. Worden (Eds.)
      The Neurosciences, The MIT Press, Cambridge, MASS.
      721-732, 1974.

28.   SNYDER, S.H., AND BANERJEE, S.P.: Amines in schizophrenia,
      In: E. Usdin and Snyder, S.H. (Eds.) Frontiers in
      Catecholamine Research. Pergamon Press. Oxford, 1133-
      1138, 1973.

29.   SNYDER, S.H., TAYLOR, K.M., COYLE, J.T. AND MEYERHOFF, J.L.:
      The role of brain dopamine in behavior regulation and
      the action of psychotropic drugs. Am. J. Psychiat.
      117-124, 1970.

30.   TAYLOR, K.M. AND SNYDER, S.H.: Differential effects of d-
      and l-amphetamine on behavior and on catecholamine
      disposition in dopamine and noradrenaline containing
      neurons of rat brain. Brain Res. 28, 295-309, 1971.

31.   YEHUDA, S.: D-Amphetamine and the sensory role of a rat's tail
      in thermoregulation, or what the rat's tail tells the
      rat's brain. Beh. Biol. 19, 233-238, 1975.

32.   YEHUDA, S. AND WURTMAN, R.J.: The effects of d-amphetamine and
      related drugs on colonic temperature of rats kept at
      various ambient temperatures. Life Sciences, 11,
      851-859, 1972a.

33.   YEHUDA, S., AND WURTMAN, R.J.: Release of brain dopamine as a
      probable mechanism for the hypothermic effects of
      d-amphetamine, Nature. 240, 477-478, 1972b.

34.   YEHUDA, S. AND WURTMAN. R.J.: Paradoxical effects of d-amphet-
      amine on behavioral thermoregulation, Possible mediation
      by brain dopamine. J. Pharmacol. Expt. Ther. 190,
      118-122, 1974a.

35.   YEHUDA, S. AND WURTMAN, R.J.: Paradoxical, thermoregulatory
      behavior in rats induced by d-amphetamine. Blockade
      by alpha-noradrenergic or dopaminergic blocking agents.
      J. Pharm. Pharmacol. 26, 210-212, 1974b.

36.   YEHUDA, S. AND WURTMAN, R.J.: Dopaminergic neurons in the nigro-
      striatal and mesolimbic pathways: Mediation of specific
      effects of d-amphetamine, Eur. J. Pharmacol. 30, 154-158
      1975.

37.   YORK, D.H.: Dopamine receptor blockage - a central action of
      CPZ on striatal neurons. Brain Res. 37, 91-99, 1971.

BIOCHEMICAL AND PHARMACOLOGICAL STUDIES ON AN ANIMAL MODEL OF

HYPERACTIVITY STATES

Marta Weinstock,[1] Zipora Speiser,[1] and Ruth Ashkenazi[2]

(1) Department of Physiology and Pharmacology, Sackler
School of Medicine, Tel-Aviv, Israel
(2) Department of Physiology, Hadassah School of Medicine
Jerusalem, Israel

One of the major contributions that the research scientist can
make to psychiatry is to elucidate the mechanism of existing psychotropic drugs and to design suitable tests for the discovery of new
ones.

When normal animals are used in such behavioral tests, one
most often detects only the neurotoxic side effects of psychotropic
drugs. Experimental studies with such agents are more meaningful if
they are carried out instead on suitable analogues in animals of the
behavioral disorder in Man that one wishes to treat. By analogy,
no-one would think of testing for potential anti-arrhythmic agents
in animals with normal cardiac rhythms.

Behavioral abnormalities in animals are most commonly produced
by giving drugs, either alone or in combination. Hyperactivity for
example, may be produced by amphetamine (1), tetrabenazine with
imipramine (2), or by 5-hydroxytryptophan with a monoamine oxidase
inhibitor (3). Potential antipsychotic agents are then tested for
their ability to reduce the hyperactivity. With these techniques
one often learns more about the drugs involved than about the
behavioral disorder they are supposed to mimic. Furthermore, such
drug combinations may create other problems unrelated to their
behavioral effects (4). For example, many drugs including the phenothiazines, interfere with the metabolism of amphetamine by liver
enzymes, thereby potentiating its effects at certain dose levels,
when as tranquilizers, one would expect them to antagonise amphetamine (5).

Such disadvantages could be eliminated by using animal models
of abnormal behavior which can be produced without the use of drugs.

Some of the most easily recognised forms of abnormal behavior in animals are hyperactivity, irritability and aggression, all characteristic of hypomania in Man.

This type of behavior can readily be reproduced in mice and rats by rearing them in social isolation (6).

The present paper presents evidence for the role of central noradrenaline function in this model of abnormal behavior. It also shows that isolation induced hyperactivity can be selectively suppressed by drugs which reduce noradrenaline activity in doses which do not show general depressant effects in normal animals.

MATERIALS AND METHODS

Male Wistar Albino rats were placed individually in opaque plastic animal cages, at the age of three weeks. They were housed at a constant environmental temperature of 22°C-24°C, on a 12-hour light-dark schedule, for 6-8 weeks. Litter-mates or rats born at approximately the same time were housed in larger cages in groups of 4-6, as previously described (7).

Behavior of isolated and group housed rats in the open field was assessed by two observers who did not know what treatment the rat had received. Three parameters, ambulation, rearing and sniffing were measured for individual rats, for 10 min. after its introduction into the open field, as previously described (7).

All rats received either the drug under test or an equal volume of saline at a stated time before exposure to the open field.

To study the effect of 6-hydroxydopamine on behavior, isolated rats were anesthetised with sodium pentobarbitone and placed in a stereotaxic instrument. A 23-gauge permanent cannula was then cemented in place just above the left lateral ventricle, (0.2mm posterior to bregma, 3.8mm below skull, lateral, 1.5mm) and fitted with a stylet to prevent clogging. Rats were then injected on each of four successive days with either 25 μg 6-hydroxydopamine (6OHDA) in 10 μl artificial C.S.F. (8) containing 1.0 mg/ml ascorbic acid or with vehicle solution alone, adjusted to pH 4.5.

α Methylparatyrosine methyl ester (αmpT) was injected i.p. and open field behavior of isolated rats determined 4 hours later, and that of group housed rats, 4 and 6 hours later.

Diazepam and chlorpromazine were each injected s.c. and phenoxybenzamine, i.p., 30 min. before the rats were exposed to the open field, while dl-propranolol was given 15 min. before the experiment.

To compare the rate at which solitary and group-housed rats adapt to the novel environment, rats from each group were exposed individually to the open field for 10 min. at approximately the same time of day on each of 5 successive days, and their behavior recorded.

Immediately after exposure to the open field, rats which had received either αmpT, 6-hydroxydopamine, or their respective saline or artificial cerebrospinal fluid treated controls, were killed by decapitation, the brain rapidly dissected out, minus the pineal body, and frozen immediately on dry ice. Brains were stored at -20°C for not more than 4 days until assayed for noradrenaline, dopamine and 5-hydroxytryptamine by the method of Barchas et al. 1972 (9).

RESULTS AND DISCUSSION

Repeated Exposure of Rats to Open Field

Solitary housed rats showed considerably higher scores for all three behavioral parameters than did group-housed controls on their first exposure to the open field. Exploratory activity of group-housed rats diminished considerably on the second day and was almost absent by day 5.

Although isolated rats also showed less activity on their second exposure, it nevertheless took 5 days before their general activity was reduced to that shown by the control rats on day 1. (see Fig. 1).

This experiment shows that not only are socially isolated rats much more active than group-housed rats on their initial exposure to the open field, but they also take longer to adapt to the novel environment.

Modification of Isolation-induced Hyperactivity by αmpT and 6-OHDA

A number of theories have indicated the involvement of catecholamines in the etiology of affective illness (10,11). Hyperactivity induced by amphetamine, somewhat resembles the behavior of isolated rats, and is also believed to result from an increase in the activity of central catecholamines (12).

Isolated and control rats were therefore pretreated with αmpT to inhibit the synthesis of both dopamine and noradrenaline, and the resulting effect on their open field behavior as determined.

Four hours after an injection of αmpT 200 mg/kg i.p. to isolated rats. total brain noradrenaline was reduced by 50% and dopamine,

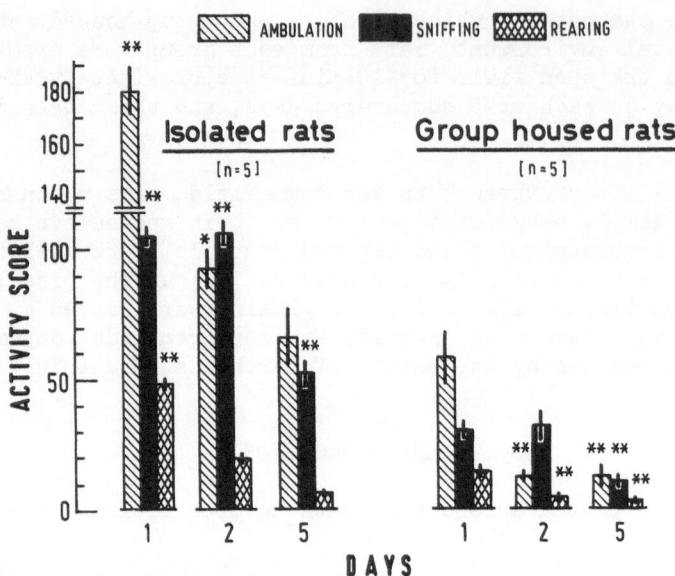

Fig. 1.   Effect on behavior of repeated daily exposure to open
           field of solitary and group-housed rats.
           Significantly different from score of group-housed rats
           on day 1.   * P < 0.05.   ** P < 0.01.

by 59%, while 5-hydroxytryptamine was not significantly altered.
This treatment reduced ambulation and rearing activity to about
the level usually seen with group-housed controls, but sniffing
was not reduced significantly. It was noticed that at the same
time αmpT treated rats were also much less irritable and aggressive
than saline treated animals. (see Fig. 2).

Treatment of group-housed control rats with 200 mg/kg αmpT
also reduced brain noradrenaline and dopamine levels by 50% and 66%
respectively. However their open field behavior did not differ significantly from that of saline pretreated controls (see Fig. 3).

These findings showed that a reduction of total brain catecholamines by 50-60% could abolish the abnormal hyperactivity while
apparently not influencing normal exploration. However, when open
field behavior of group-housed rats was assessed 6 hours after αmpT
treatment, all behavioral parameters were significantly reduced.
Brain noradrenaline and dopamine were depleted to 27% and 28% of
their control values.

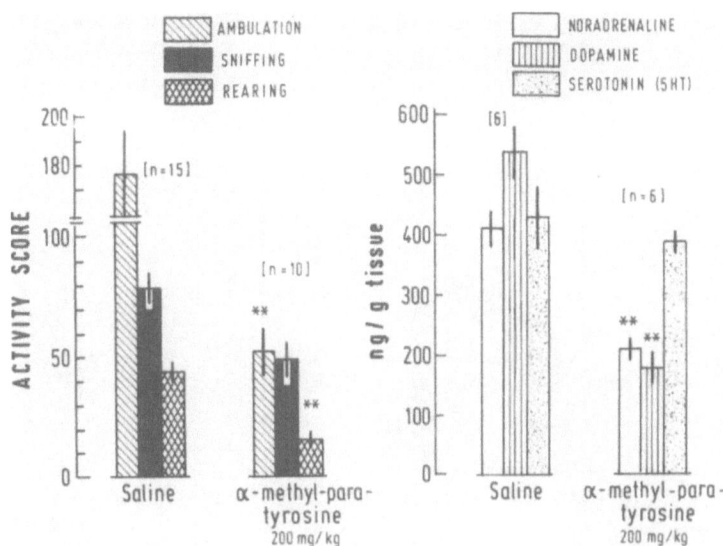

Fig. 2. The effect of αmethylparatyrosine (αmpT) on brain amine
         levels and open field behavior of socially isolated rats.
         αmpT 200 mg/kg l/P was injected 4 hours before exposure
         to open field. Significantly different from appropriate
         value of saline treated rats.
         ** P < 0.01.

It suggests that hyperactivity in the isolated rat may be
associated with the action of predominantly newly synthesised catecholamines, while normal exploratory activity can be maintained so
long as there are sufficient amounts of catecholamines in the storage
granules. Once the latter become critically depleted, normal activity
is also reduced.

In order to determine the relative importance of noradrenaline
and dopamine in the isolation-induced hyperactivity syndrome, selective lesioning of noradrenergic pathways was made with intraventri-
cular 6-hydroxydopamine. As is shown in Fig. 4, this treatment
reduced whole brain noradrenaline by 46%, while causing a slight
but non-significant rise in dopamine levels.

Although we did not determine noradrenaline levels in different
brain areas other authors (18) have shown that 6-OHDA given in several small doses results in the loss of this amine mainly from nerve
terminals, while its content in the cell bodies remains virtually
unchanged.

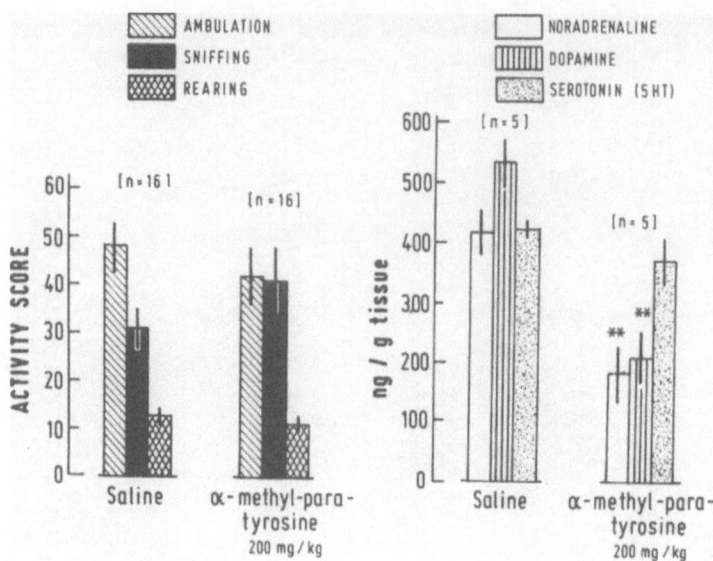

Fig. 3.   The effect of αmethylparatyrosine (αmpT) on brain amine
levels and open field behavior of group-housed rats.
αmpT 200 mg/kg i.p. was injected 4 hours before exposure
to the open field.
Significantly different from appropriate value for saline
treated rats.
** P < 0.01.

Both ambulation and rearing scores were significantly reduced
by 6-OHDA treatment, suggesting that the release of newly synthesised noradrenaline may be more important in this behavioral syndrome
than that of dopamine (See Fig. 4).

Modification of Isolation-induced Hyperactivity by Drugs.

One of the most commonly used screening tests for minor tranquilizers and anti-anxiety agents, is their ability to reduce isolation-induced fighting in male mice (14). This behavior is antago-
nised by many of the benzodiazepines as well as by phenothiazines,
butyrophenones and some tricyclic antidepressant agents. However,
a comparative study carried out by Sofia, 1969 (15) on a large number
of drugs, showed that none of these agents was apparently having a
selective effect on the aggressive behavior, since at similar or
even lower doses, they all showed general depressant activity in
normal mice in the "rotarod" test.

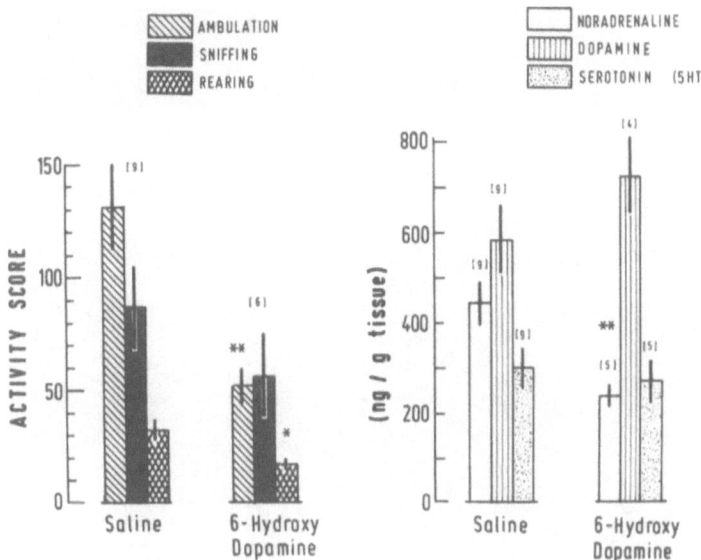

Fig. 4.   The effect of 6-hydroxydopamine (6-OHDA) on brain amine
          levels and open field behavior of socially isolated rats.
          6-OHDA - 25 μg injected on each of 4 successive days into
          left lateral ventricle. Control rats received equal volume
          of vehicle solution. Open field behavior determined 14 days
          after last injection.
          Significantly different from control rats.
          ** P < 0.01   * P < 0.02.

     The effect of various doses of diazepam and chlorpromazine were
studied on the open field behavior of socially isolated and group-
housed rats to see whether either agent could influence the abnormal
behavior preferentially. The effect of relatively low doses of diazepam is shown in Fig. 5.

     Diazepam significantly reduced the hyperactivity of isolated
rats at a dose of 1 mg/kg but this effect did not appear to be
selective as normal exploratory activity of group-housed rats was
also inhibited by the same dose.

     On the other hand, chlorpromazine did modify the abnormal
behavior at as low a dose as 0.1 mg/kg, while not significantly
reducing the activity of group-housed rats until 5-10 times the dose
was given (see Fig. 6). The inhibitory effect of chlorpromazine on
open field behavior of both types of rats was clearly dose-related,

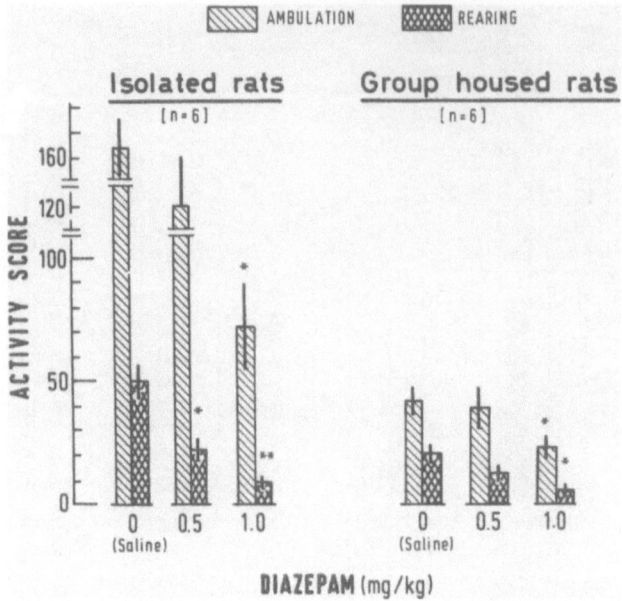

Fig. 5.   The effect of diazepam on open field behavior of socially
          isolated and group-housed rats.
          Diazepam was injected s.c. 30 min. before exposure of rats
          to the open field.
          Significantly different from the scores of rats given saline.
          * P < 0.05   ** P < 0.01.

and at 1 mg/kg, this drug almost completely abolished all activity
particularly in the socially isolated rat.

     Since it was shown that the hyperactive behavior of socially
isolated rats appeared to be related to the release of newly synthesised noradrenaline, it seemed reasonable to assume that either
α- or β-adrenoceptor blocking agents may also reduce the hyperactivity selectively. Unlike chlorpromazine, phenoxybenzamine and propranolol do not block dopamine receptors (16) but both agents have
been shown to inhibit the noradrenaline induced stimulation of adenyl
cyclase in the brain (17).

     Phenoxybenzamine, 1 mg/kg s.c. reduced the hyperactivity of iso-
lated rats to about the level of the exploratory activity of group-
housed animals. 5 mg/kg and 10 mg/kg did not further reduce the hyperactivity significantly. The same doses of phenoxybenzamine also reduced the normal exploratory activity, but unlike chlorpromazine,
did not do so in a dose related manner, neither did they suppress

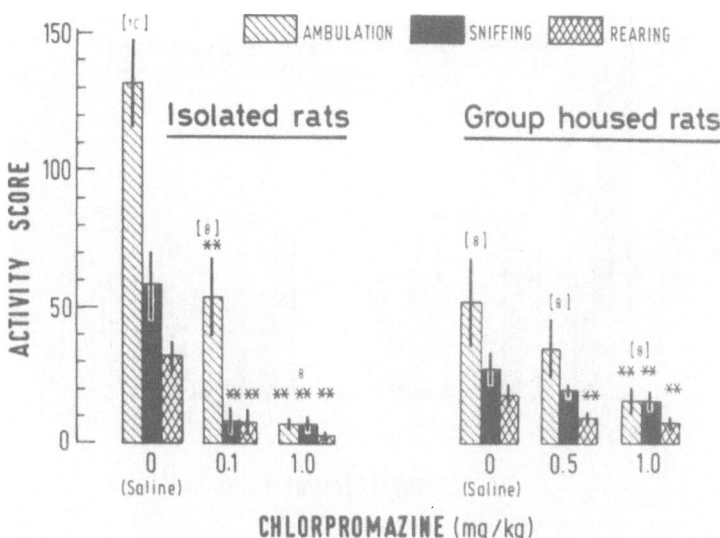

Fig. 6. The effect of chlorpromazine on open field behavior of
         socially isolated and group-housed rats.
         Chlorpromazine was injected s.c. 30 min. before exposure
         of rats to the open field.
         Significantly different from the scores of rats given
         saline.
         ** P < 0.01.

activity entirely. Thus, if phenoxybenzamine acts by blocking central
noradrenaline receptors, these findings suggest exploratory activity
may still be maintained, even if at a slightly lower level, as long
as dopamine function is unimpaired. Blockade of dopamine receptors
or selective destruction of dopamine neurones results in akinesia
(18) (see Fig. 7).

Propranolol also reduced the hyperactive behavior of isolated
rats to the level of group-housed controls. This drug was effective
at a dose of 0.2 mg/kg and doses up to and including 10 mg/kg did
not further reduce the activity (See Fig. 8). In contrast to phenoxybenzamine, propranolol had no significant effect on the open field
behavior of grouped rats, in doses below 10 mg/kg. At 20 mg/kg
general depressant effects occured unrelated to an effect on noradrenaline neurones (16) (See Fig. 8).

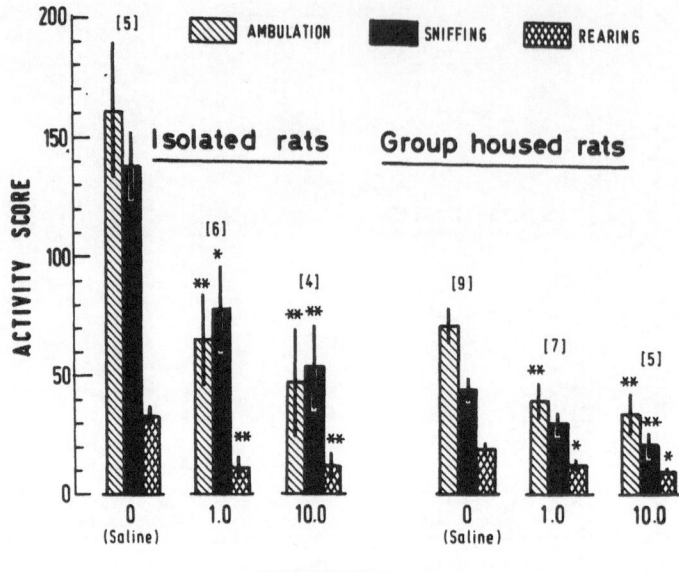

Fig. 7.   The effect of phenoxybenzamine on open field behavior of
          socially isolated and group-housed rats.
          Phenoxybenzamine was injected i.p. 3-45 min. before expo-
          sure of rats to open field.
          Significantly different from the scores of rats given
          saline.   P < 0.05.

     These experiments showed that propranolol has a highly selective
effect on abnormal hyperactivity, since 100 times the dose was required to influence the behavior of normal rats under the same conditions.

     Our findings are in agreement with the reports of the effects
of propranolol in psychotic and normal human subjects.

     In a recent study in acute schizophrenic subjects, propranolol
was found to cause a complete remission of symptoms within 3-26 days
of treatment. This drug was also effective in several patients who
had not responded to phenothiazines. Furthermore, unlike the latter
agents, propranolol caused no signs of interference with extrapyramidal function even at high doses (19) indicating that it does not
block dopamine receptors in human subjects.

     In spite of its sedative effects in psychotic patients, propra-
nolol has no significant central nervous depressant effects in normal

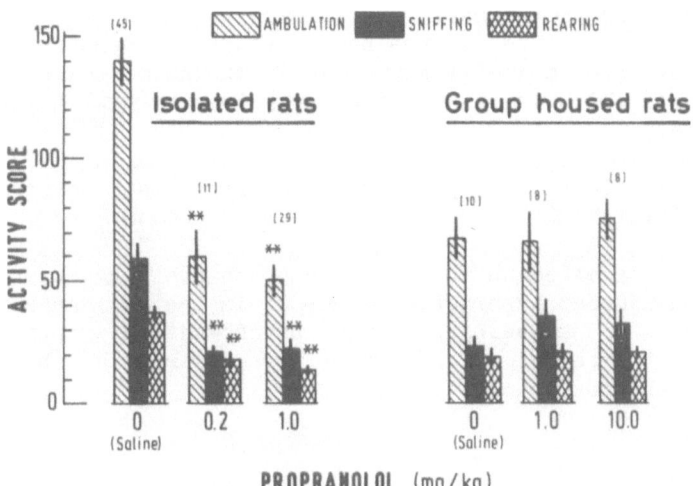

Fig. 8.   The effect of propranolol on open field behavior of
          socially isolated and group-housed rats.
          Propranolol was injected s.c. 15 min. before exposure of
          rats to open field.
          Significantly different from the scores of rats given saline.
          P ⟨ 0.01.

human subjects (20).

     As yet little is known of the mechanism of the selective action
of propranolol on abnormal hyperactivity.

     Studies in our laboratory have shown that propranolol can reduce
the release of noradrenaline from stimulated sympathetic nerves as
well as to block its effects on peripheral β-adrenoceptors (21).
This effect on noradrenaline release is shared by the d-isomer (21)
(22) which is only a very weak β receptor blocking agent, and by
practolol (23), which lacks the membrane stabilising properties of
d- and dl-propranolol (24). Both d-propranolol and practolol can
also selectively modify the open field behavior of isolated rats (7).
It is therefore possible that these agents act by inhibiting an
excessive release of noradrenaline rather than by blocking its
receptors.

This could be accomplished in one of two ways. If hyperactivity results from overstimulation of noradrenaline neurones because of a reduction of an inhibitory input to these neurones, propranolol could act selectively on this behavior by raising the level or action of the inhibitory transmitter to the normal value. Alternatively it could interfere with a specific process in the noradrenergic pathways themselves which is responsible for releasing newly synthesised noradrenaline.

Further studies are in progress to differentiate between the various possibilities.

The data presented in this paper support the suggestion that the isolation-induced hyperactive syndrome in the rat can serve as a useful model for screening potential psycho-active agents. Drugs which inhibit the release of noradrenaline appear to be able to reduce this behavior specifically.

REFERENCES

(1) RANDRUP, A. and MUNKVAD, I.: Stereotyped activities produced by amphetamine in several animal species and man. Psychopharmacologia (Berl.) II 300-310, 1967.

(2) MATUSSEK, N. and LINSMAYER, M.: The effect of lithium and amphetamine on desmethylimipramine-Ro 4-1284 induced motor hyperactivity. Life Sciences 7, 371-375, 1968.

(3) GRAHAME-SMITH, D.G.: Inhibitory effect of chlorpromazine on the syndrome of hyperactivity produced by l-tryptophan or 5-methoxy-N, N dimethyltryptamine in rats treated with a mono-amine oxidase inhibitor. Br. J. Pharmac. 43, 856-864, 1972.

(4) GARATTINI, S.: Importance of a knowledge of drug metabolism for the assessment of drug interactions. In: Importance of Fundamental Principles in Drug Evaluation. Eds. Tedeschi, D.H. and Tedeschi, R.E., 121-139, Raven Press, New York.

(5) SULSER, F. and SANDERS-BUSH, E.: Biochemical and metabolic considerations concerning the mechanism of action of amphetamine and related compounds. In: Psychotomimetic Drugs, Ed. Efron, D.H., Raven Press, New York, 83-94, 1970.

(6)   VALZELLI, L.: Drugs and aggressiveness. In: Advances in Phar-
        macology. Eds. Garattini, S. and Shore, P.A. Vol. 5,
        79-108, 1967, Academic Press, New York.

(7)   WEINSTOCK, M. and SPEISER, Z.: The effect of dl-propranolol,
        d-propranolol and practolol on the hyperactivity induced
        in rats by prolonged isolation. Psychopharmacologia,
        (Berl.) 30, 241-250, 1973.

(8)   MERLIS, J.K.: The effect of changes in calcium content of the
        cerebrospinal fluid on spinal reflex activity in the
        dog. Amer. J. Physiol. 131, 67-72, 1940.

(9)   BARCHAS, J., ERDELYI, E., and ANGWIN, P.: Simultaneous deter-
        mination of indole- and catecholamines in tissues using
        a weak cation exchange resin. Analyt. Biochem. 50, 1-17,
        1972.

(10) SCHILDKRAUT, J.J.: The catecholamine hypothesis of affective
        disorders: a review of supporting evidence. Amer. J.
        Psychiat. 122, 509-522, 1965.

(11) M.R.C. BRAIN METABOLISM UNIT: Modified amine hypothesis for
        the etiology of affective illness. Lancet II 573-577,
        1972.

(12) SULSER, F. and SANDERS-BUSH E.: Effect of drugs on amines in
        the C.N.S. Ann. Rev. Pharmacol. 11, 209-230, 1971.

(13) SORENSON, C.A. and ELLISON, G.D.: Nonlinear changes in activity
        and emotional reactivity scores following central nor-
        adrenergic lesions in rats. Psychopharmacologia (Berl.)
        32, 313-325, 1973.

(14) VALZELLI, L: The "isolation syndrome" in mice. Psychopharma-
        cologia 31, 305-320, 1973.

(15) SOFIA, R.D.: Effects of centrally active drugs on four models
        of experimentally-induced aggression in rodents. Life
        Sci. 8 Part 1. 705-716, 1969.

(16) ANDEN, N.E. and STRÖMBOM, U.: Adrenergic receptor blocking
        agents. Effects on central noradrenaline and dopamine
        receptors and on motor activity. Psychopharmacologia
        (Berl.) 38, 91-103, 1974.

(17) PALMER, G.C., SULSER, F. and ROBINSON, G.A.: Effects of
        neurohumoral and adrenergic agents on cyclic AMP levels
        in various areas of rat brain in vitro. Neuropharmacol.

(18)   ANDEN, N-E., STRÖMBOM, U. AND SVENSSON, T.H.: Dopamine and
       noradrenaline receptor stimulation: reversal of reserpine
       induced suppression of motor activity. Psychopharma-
       cologia 29, 289-298, 1973.

(19)   YORKSTON, N.J., MALIK, M.K.U., HARVARD, C.W.H., ZAKI, S.A.
       and MORRISON, R.C.: Propranolol in control of schizo-
       phrenic symptoms. Brit. Med. J. 4, 633-635, 1974.

(20)   LADER, M.H. and TYRER   : Central and peripheral effects of
       propranolol and sotalol in normal human subjects.
       Br. J. Pharmac. 45, 577-560, 1972.

(21)   ELIASH, S. and WEINSTOCK, M.: Role of adrenergic neurone
       blockade in hypotensive action of propranolol. Br. J.
       Pharmac. 43, 287-294, 1971.

(22)   MYLECHARANE, E.J. and RAPER, C.: Further studies on the
       adrenergic neuron blocking activity of some β-adreno-
       ceptor antagonists and guanethidine. J. Pharmacol.
       25, 213-218, 1973.

(23)   WEINSTOCK, M. Unpublished observations.

(24)   DUNLOP, D. and SHANKS, R.G.: Selective blockade of adreno-
       ceptive β-receptors in the heart. Br. J. Pharmac.
       32, 201-212, 1968.

DISCUSSION

<u>Dr. Belmaker</u>:   I think one of the purposes of this symposium was to
bring basic scientists and clinical scientists together. I wonder
if it would be in order if Prof. Atzmon and perhaps Prof. Sam
Gershon might be willing to say a few words on the question of the
present state of the evidence as to whether propanolol is effective
in some psychotic states.

<u>Dr. Atzmon</u>:   This is a very moot problem. Some people are of the
opinion that propanolol works in certain forms of psychosis. That
opinion is not based upon anything but clinical impressions by
psychiatrists. It is based upon uncontrolled, not double-blind,
not even single-blind clinical impressions.

     As we all know, the same clinical impressions have been made
with let's say 5,000 different drugs in all kinds of medical conditions. Nevertheless, some psychiatrists, are again convinced that
some drug, the action of which is not known, has a beneficial effect
on some forms of psychosis. They are of the opinion that it may be
beneficial to patients who have been resistant to any other form
of treatment. That is the state of the art. It certainly has nothing
to do with the state of any science, as far as propanolol and
psychosis is concerned.

     At the moment, one clinical study is underway in England, where
propanolol is being checked double-blind, against phenothiazines.
I think that within 1-2 years we will have more clearcut answers.

<u>Dr. Sam Gershon</u>: I think that Dr. Atzmon's appraisal has been
critical and cautious. The experience in the United States really
doesn't add anything. There have been single cases reported, and
then a few cases had intervening problems and all the trials
stopped. Then there was the question of puerperal psychoses which
were responsive. Then there was the statement that chronic schizophrenics would not respond to propanolol at all. So where we really
are is awaiting a properly carried out trial before this can be
resolved. The clinical data is interesting, it is provocative, and
it would be more than disastrous if proper studies are not carried
out.

SOME OLD AND NEW THEORIES IN BIOCHEMICAL PSYCHIATRY

Arnold J. Mandell

The University of California at San Diego

La Jolla, California 92093, U.S.A.

The boundary between theory and data may be clear to the outside observers of a particular field of science, particularly those who call themselves the philosophers of science, but for the practitioners, working day by day moving constructs into practice, gaining facility for translating abstract notions into operations and back again to revise their theoretical definitions, the boundary tends to dissolve. In the case of a psychiatric physician, for example, libido may start to become observable intensity, the drive behind a compulsion, attachment strength, sexual practices, characterological rigidity, or a variety of other intuitively derived clinical notions. Thousands of pages are spent untangling such confusions, and some gain in understanding results from the enterprise, but the boundary is never clarified. Perhaps the work of clarifying boundary conditions is the task indigenous to research.

The problem is less difficult with psychological theories of behavior than it is with our new, more "real" sounding biological theories. No one actually expects to find point-to-point representations in the brain of conditioned inhibition, retroflexed rage, perceptual gestalt, working through, or cognitive encoding. In addition, we in behavioral science have been warned by the Vienna school and its followers to carefully discriminate between scientific constructs that we use as orienting ideas, hypotheses, and theoretical models and their operational definitions, as when, for example, we consider extinction as a decrease in the strength of a response following its repeated practice under defined circumstances.

Lately I have noticed a trend growing from advances in biological psychiatry and psychopharmacology which suggests that this

lesson in distinguishing theory from operations, learned well with
regard to psychologically based theories, has failed to generalize
(another operationally definable term) to the area of brain and
behavior. Too many of us think we are <u>really saying something</u> when
we state about the use of tricyclics in a depressed patient that we
are "increasing the functional levels of norepinephrine at his nerve
endings" or, when reserpine is administered to a person, that we are
"depleting the norepinephrine in his catecholamine nerve endings."
We have sensed the energy level of intensity in our patient, rejected
the word <u>libido</u> as dated, and, with the pleasurable feeling of clo-
sure that accrues to those in ambiguous and responsible positions,
now declare "norepinephrine this" or "norepinephrine that." This
under-the-breath psychopharmacological litany recited while making
empirical clinical decisions is connected to the operations of the
brain no more firmly than the erstwhile <u>libido,</u> but it seems to be
so, BECAUSE IT SOUNDS BIOLOGICAL! It can be, and has been, measured
in a rat brain as well as in human urine and cerebrospinal fluid.
Can that be said about <u>libido</u>?

Before discussing our work on some of the effects of lithium
on the serotonergic system in the rat brain and its potential
implications for a model explaining lithium's symmetrical prophylactic actions against both mania and depression in some patients
with bipolar affective disease, I feel behooved to review briefly,
in oversimplified terms, the recent history of theory in biochemical
psychiatry. I hope it will become obvious that, although the
biological sophistication of the sound of the words suggests that we
know completely what we're talking about, we really don't. Not yet.
I intend also to offer a new one of those seductive biological models
which lend themselves to clinical poetry. Perhaps the brief review
is a way of warning you not to be taken in by my conclusions.

Figure 1 portrays the scene of origin of most biological
theories in psychiatry, which provokes the intuitive speculation
of therapists, using their own feelings as referents. This data
base has led to a number of erroneous concepts in biochemical
psychiatry. For example, the term <u>depletion,</u> in the case of the
action of reserpine, <u>does</u> refer to the emptying of vesicular stores
of amines, and intuitively one might think of a hypertensive patient
taking reserpine who is lethargic, depressed, and without sexual or
aggressive drive. But that image doesn't come to grips with the fact
that reserpine <u>increases</u> the synthesis of both norepinephrine
(Mueller, Thoenen, and Axelrod, 1969; Segal, Sullivan, Kuczensky and
Mandell, 1971) and serotonin (Knapp, Mandell and Geyer, 1974; Toser,
Neff, and Brodie, 1966) and increases the turnover of these neurotransmitters in intact animals (Toser et al., 1966; Neff and Costa,
1968). Given the compensatory mechanisms that I will discuss below,
such an image distorts the thinking of even some biologists into the
spurious assumption that "exhaustion" or " depletion" can occur in
an active mammalian biosynthetic system with an adequate supply of

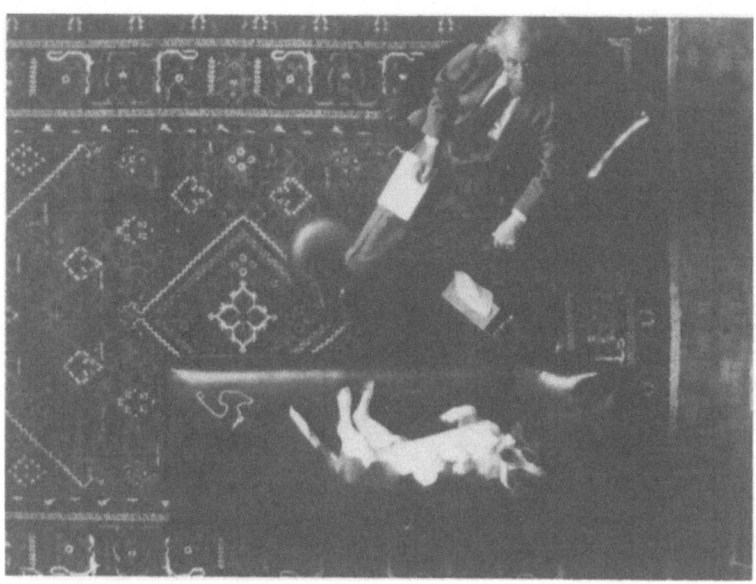

Fig. 1.   Representative seminal locus of biological theories in
          psychiatry. The therapist (top) intuitively speculates
          regarding possible biological substrates of various
          components of his patient's behavior.

substrate and cofactors. Current work suggests that, at least in
the case of neurotransmitter systems in the brain, this cannot
happen. Neurotransmitter depletion, like fatigue itself, is simply
not what it sounds like. Sleep is not the loss of wakefulness. This
is perhaps the best example of an unfortunate marriage between a
scientific-sounding term, dowered by a few pieces of animal data,
and an intuitively interpreted clinical perception. Depletion of
vesicular stores of transmitter is certainly not the major mechanism
of the behavioral result of reserpine administration. The story is
much more complex and as yet unsettled.

     Figure 2 illustrates one of the oldest biochemical theories
in psychiatry, which has surfaced from time to time over the past
few decades with reports of aberrant metabolites in the body fluids
of psychiatric patients. In the welter of well-charaterized neurometabolic genetic diseases growing up around us like wild grasses
in the spring, we in psychiatry hoped we would find one of our own:
a methylated indole, a mauve spot, a serum level of hallucinogen,
a heretofore unknown substance in the cerebrospinal fluid. The more
imaginative pursuers of this possibility speculate that the aberrant

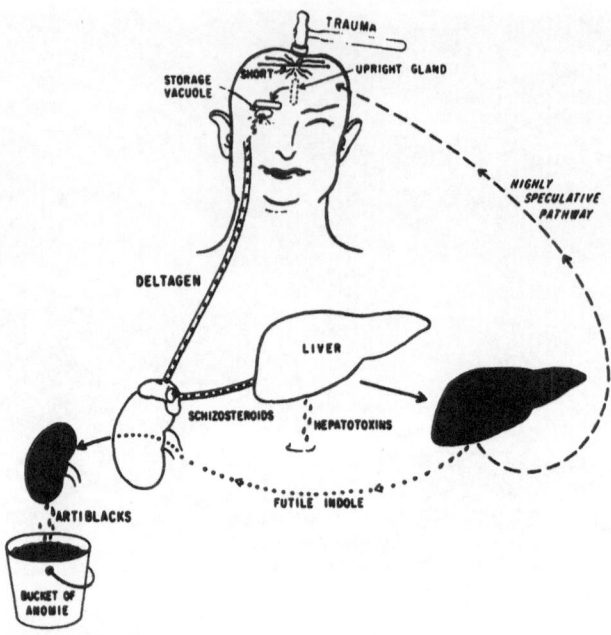

Fig. 2.   A map designed to assist the reader in conceptualizing
          the quest for aberrant metabolites and their possible
          causative roles in mental illness.

metabolite feeds back on the brain, making a bad matter worse:
the classical positive-feedback model for a decompensating or
pathological circumstance in an organism. A trauma causes a short,
the short knocks the upright gland sideways, releasing a factor
that influences peripheral glands, which then influence the liver
metabolism that leads to an aberrant metabolite, which then goes
back to the brain to cause more shorts. Again I have to say, not
yet. Moreover, we have no model disease in another organ system
that could serve as an example. The neurometabolic diseases that
manifest aberrant metabolites, do so on the basis of a shunt, a
spillover, or some other epiphenomenal manifestation of the absence
or near absence of particular enzymes. Abnormal function leads to.
manifestations of abnormal metabolites which, although they can be
diagnostic and create havoc, are secondary to a primary, demonstrable deficiency in an enzymatic step. No enzyme absence or near
absence has been reported in any classical psychiatric syndrome.
Even the statistical deviations from the norm in serum monoamine
oxidase or cerebrospinal fluid transmitter metabolites that have
been found in patients with affective disorder (Murphy and Weiss,
1972;Goodwin, Post, Dunner and Gordon, 1973) certainly reflect
nothing resembling the genetic absence of an enzyme protein such

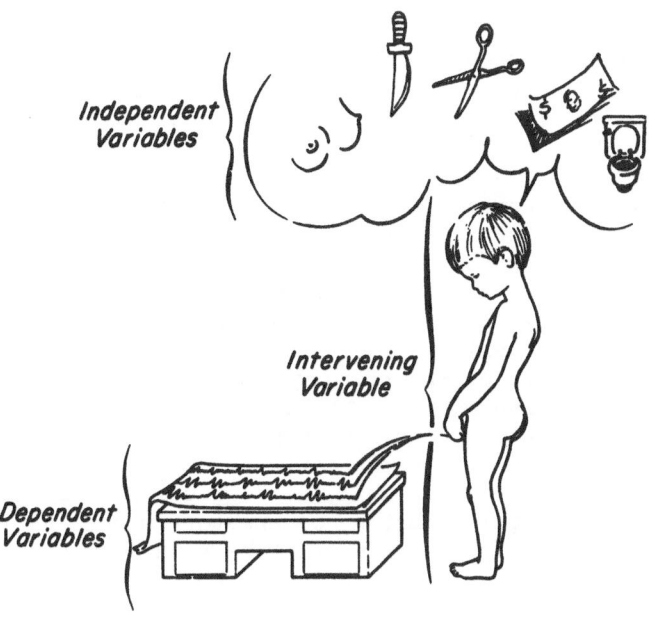

Fig. 3. Some researchers monitor known metabolites in people who
         manifest psychopathology and try to establish relationships
         on an empirical basis between body substances and symptoms.

as constitutes the core biochemical pathology in each of twenty or
so neurometabolic diseases that have been characterized (Stanbury
et al., 1972). So, although psychiatry often tries to ride in the
cloak of the terminology and operations of other, better established
pathophysiologies, I think in this instance the garb is not appropriate.

     Figure 3 represents another approach to biochemical psychiatry,
that is, monitoring normal metabolites in people with psychopathological conditions and establishing relationships on an empirical
basis. Are there relationships between psychopathological states
and deviations in peripheral hormones, neurotransmitter metabolites,
or other measures? Corticosteroid elevations in depression and
acute schizophrenia are examples of the fruits of such searches.
Ironically enough, after years of vagueness and speculation, some
workers are getting a kind of limbic, subcortical EEG out of the
blood and urine, reflecting abnormalities in the modulation by
biogenic amine transmitters of hypothalamic polypeptide control
over the pituitary in some psychopathological conditions. In this
context, which I will not review here, there is much interest in
the possibility that hyperactivity of dopamine receptors could

play a role in the expression of some psychotic states. This possibility fits some psychopharmacological work and some basic brain
chemistry, and has recently been tied a little more directly to
patients by work with pituitary hormones that depend upon dopamine
for their regulation (Snyder, 1974).

Over the past decade, biological psychiatry has been seen in
terms of a model of central synaptic function in biogenic amine
systems. We have been able to relate drug effects on man's behavior
to drug effects on a rat's biogenic amine neurons, and have used a
neuronal model to explain the drug actions (and, implicitly, as a
behavioral model as well). Drugs release, block reuptake, block
receptor impingement, or interfere with the metabolic degradation
of biogenic amine transmitters, as illustrated in figure 4. The
processes are thought of as hydrodynamic: the more transmission,
the more "up", the less transmission, the more "down". The notion
still suffers from the psychoanalytic "depletion" image described
above, with the exception that a compensatory mechanism is involved.
Apparently, the less neurotransmitter there is in the nerve ending,
the more is synthesized, depending upon the release of product-
feedback inhibition.

This "NIMH neuron" model has been dominant until very recently,
when it has been challenged increasingly by the complexity of drug
actions, the variety of compensatory mechanisms available to reverse

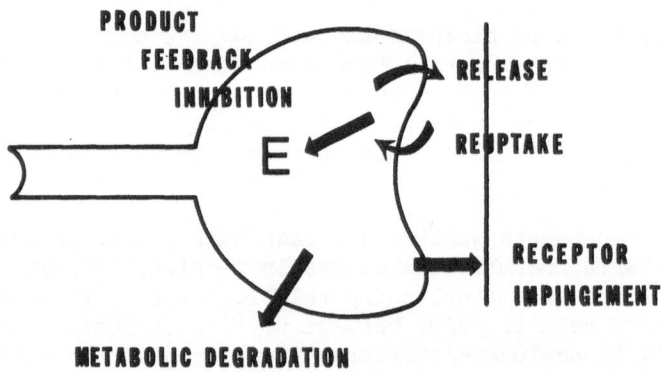

FIRST ORDER DRUG-SENSITIVE MECHANISMS

Fig. 4.   A relatively early synaptic model, the "NIMH neuron",
          showing the processes directly affected by pharmacological
          manipulation.

the effects of acute synaptic perturbation, and <u>the increasing</u>
<u>importance of transmitter synthesis over release as the determinant</u>
<u>of transmitter availability at the synapse</u>. We have begun to make
sense out of the fact that the important psychiatric drugs
(tricyclics, monoamine oxidase inhibitors, antipsychotics, and
lithium) take days, weeks, or months to work clinically, despite
the fact that they "act" acutely at the synapse in a matter of
minutes. The latency, as I will indicate, seems to depend on the
drugs triggering various complex sequences of events involving
macromolecular changes in the neurons, which reach a new steady
state of function much later. Figure 5 represents some of these
"second order" mechanisms, and I will describe them primarily in
terms of our work in the serotonergic systems in rat brain.

Tryptophan hydroxylase, called the rate-limiting enzyme in
the synthesis of serotonin, is apparently unsaturated <u>in situ</u>
with respect to its substrate, the amino acid tryptophan. Indices
of serotonin biosynthesis in brain do change in the same direction
as tryptophan levels in blood and plasma, which have been shown to
be affected by nutritional manipulation, psychotropic drugs, and
drugs affecting plasma protein binding of tryptophan hydroxylase
(Fernstrom and Wurtman, 1971; Grahame-Smith, 1971; Paoletti, Sirtori,
and Spano, 1975; Tagliamonte, Tagliamonte, Perez-Cruet, Stern and
Gessa, 1971). However, there is a dynamic barrier between whole
brain levels of substrate and the intraneuronal enzyme; a few years
ago we demonstrated that tryptophan is taken into serotonergic nerve
endings by a specific high affinity transport system, and that the
relative velocity of the uptake process is sensitive to pharmacological manipulation (Knapp and Mandell, 1972, 1973; Knapp et al.,
1974; Mandell and Knapp, 1976a).

When we assay the <u>amount</u> of soluble tryptophan hydroxylase in
the neurons, we find that both single and repeated administrations
of various psychotropic drugs can change the levels of enzyme
present in serotonergic cell bodies and nerve endings (Sanders-Bush,
Bushing, and Sulser, 1972; Knapp et al., 1974; Gal, Christiansen,
and Yunger, 1975; Knapp and Mandell, 1976). Our work suggests that
the amount of tryptophan hydroxylase available for activation in
the nerve ending (the net result of enzyme protein synthesis,
degradation, and movement down the axon) increases or decreases
<u>to compensate</u> for functional changes induced in serotonergic nerve
endings. Work is in progress in Reis's laboratories to confirm
these findings by means of immunoassays (Joh, Shikimi, Pickel,
and Reis, 1975).

We also measure the capacity of a partially enriched preparation of synaptosomes from selected brain regions to convert
radioactive tryptophan to serotonin, as an index of the integrated
function of serotonergic neurons. This measurement incorporates
the <u>amount</u> of intraneuronal enzyme, the relative velocity of the

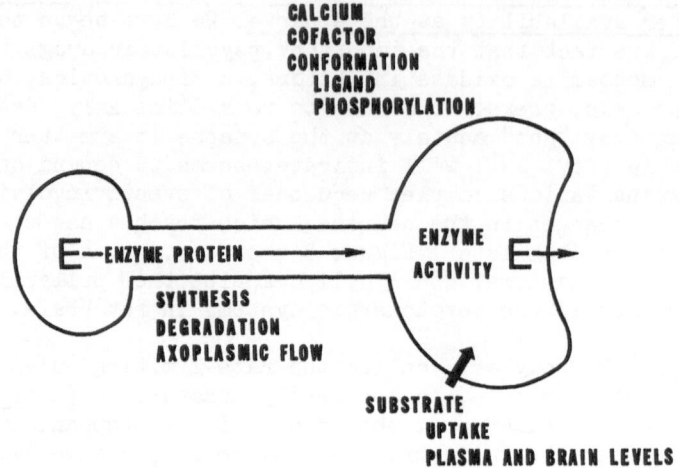

Fig. 5. Our current neuronal model, showing various parameters
thought to be involved in "second order" regulation of
synaptic function, i.e. the regulation of transmitter
synthesis.

high affinity uptake of the radioactive substrate, and another
factor, deduced from changes in conversion rate without associated
changes in either substrate uptake or soluble enzyme activity.
Changes in the conversion of tryptophan in an intact nerve ending
preparation independent of the amount of soluble enzyme present
imply that one or several intrasynaptosomal regulatory influences
may bear on the enzyme's activity state. So far only calcium has
been demonstrated to activate tryptophan hydroxylase (Knapp, Mandell,
and Bullard, 1975; Boadle-Biber, 1975), but in the case of catecholamine synthesis, conformational changes relating to model membrane
binding, cofactor levels, or phosphorylation of the enzyme protein
appear able to affect the activity of the intraneuronal mixed-
function oxidase, tyrosine hydroxylase (Kuczenski and Mandell, 1972,
1972a; Costa and Meek, 1974; Bullard and Mandell unpublished observations), so we think that comparable discoveries probably lie
ahead in the regulation of the serotonin synthesizing enzyme.

It is no accident, of course, that the drugs with which we
attempt to manipulate, and thereby elucidate, these once-obscure
mechanisms in rat brain, are substances that have observable
psychological and behavioral effects in people. The lithium ion in
particular has been a boon in our efforts to delineate these regulatory processes. In concentrations reasonably comparable to

therapeutic blood levels in man (i.e. < 1.5 meq/liter) lithium administered in vivo or added in vitro significantly increases the relative velocity of the high affinity uptake of labeled tryptophan into synaptosomally enriched preparations from rat striate cortex, and the uptake increases linearly with both time and dose (Knapp and Mandell, 1973, 1975). Because we measure the uptake in terms of the radioactivity retained in a washed pellet after incubation with the labeled substrate, we had to rule out two other possibilities. By monitoring the rate of efflux of radioactivity from samples prepared from animals treated with lithium chloride or sodium chloride, we showed that the lithium was not retarding the efflux of radioactivity (Knapp and Mandell, 1975). Also, until recently we could not be sure we were not simply labeling some intraneuronal pool via an exchange of exogenous for endogenous tryptophan. Now we have modified the techniques of Denkla and Dewey (1967) and measured endogenous tryptophan concentrations in preparations from rats treated with lithium chloride or sodium chloride. Whether we pooled the brain preparations or examined striata from individual animals, the increase in intrasynaptosomal tryptophan was significant after lithium treatment (Mandell and Knapp, 1976a).

A proportional increase in the capacity of intact synaptosomal preparations to convert labeled tryptophan to serotonin is initially associated with the stimulation of substrate uptake by lithium. Although the specific activity of the conversion measure is about two orders of magnitude lower than that of the uptake measure, the increases are invariably proportional; this is true also in studies of the alterations induced in the same parameters with other drugs and amino acid loads (Mandell and Knapp, 1976a).

With repeated daily lithium chloride injections, the activity of intraneuronal tryptophan hydroxylase decreases gradually. After three weeks of such daily injections, the substrate uptake remains elevated; the intraneuronal enzyme remains decreased; and the neuronal capacity to convert labeled substrate to transmitter has returned to control level. This last measure reflects a "buffered" steady state, achieved by the movement of two variables to their respective extremes (Knapp and Mandell, 1975; Mandell and Knapp, 1976).

By administering cocaine to rats and examining the same parameters, we have confirmed that the sequence of changes induced by lithium in the serotonergic biosynthetic system in brain is initiated by the stimulation of the high affinity substrate uptake. Cocaine inhibits this tryptophan uptake system and the conversion measure and results in a subsequent increase in tryptophan hydroxylase within the neurons (Knapp and Mandell, 1973). However, when we treat rats for three days with lithium chloride and challenge with a cocaine injection, we find that cocaine has virtually no effect on uptake, conversion, or enzyme activity; the system

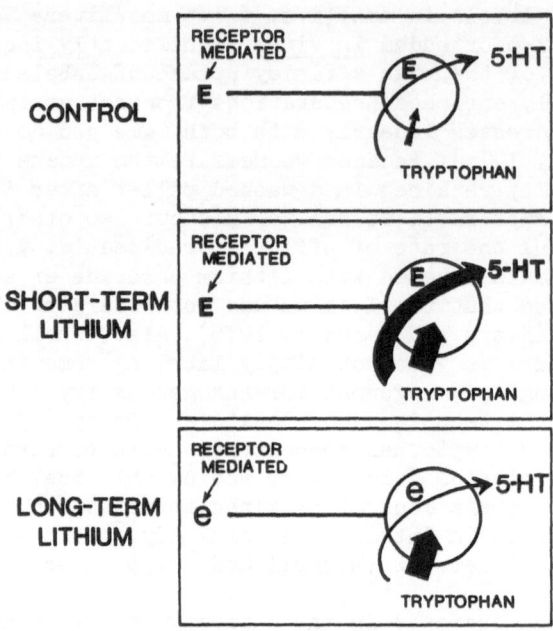

Fig. 6.   Hypothetical mechanisms in the action of lithium on
          serotonergic neurons. See the text for detailed
          explanation.

apparently has been stabilized by the lithium and rendered invul-
nerable to the cocaine challenge (Knapp and Mandell, 1976). Data
with regard to the effects of another stimulant drug, amphetamine,
on a serotonergic system that has been "buffered" with lithium are
similar (Mandell and Knapp, 1975).

     Figure 6 illustrates our model for the mechanisms in the action
of lithium. In the control neuron, tryptophan hydroxylase (E) is
optimal both in the cell body and in the nerve ending. Substrate
(tryptophan) is transported through the membrane and converted by
the enzyme to serotonin (5-HT), which is released from the nerve
terminal. After short-term lithium treatment tryptophan uptake
is augmented and consequently synthesis and release of serotonin
are increased, since intraneuronal enzyme is not saturated with
regard to substrate. After long-term lithium treatment, the
amount of enzyme has been reduced (E → e) to compensate for the
initial increase in serotonergic bombardment of the receptor.
Tryptophan uptake is still augmented, but transmitter synthesis
and release at the nerve ending have returned to control levels.

Thus, the return to control values for the synaptosomal capacity to convert tryptophan to serotonin is associated with the movement of one drug-sensitive parameter to high values (uptake), the other to low values (intrasynaptosomal enzyme). These two mechanisms resist further change (Knapp and Mandell, 1972, 1976; Knapp et al., 1974; Mandell and Knapp, 1975). Mogens Schou (1976) has suggested that a theory for the action of lithium in the affective disorders involving one neurotransmitter would require elements consonant with a symmetrical prophylactic effect (i.e. against both "ups" and "downs") and maintenance of a control level of function. We suggest that the interaction of lithium and the serotonin biosynthetic system as diagrammed in figure 6 might produce a circumstance that fulfills Schou's requirements. Several groups are currently studying indoleamine metabolites in cerebrospinal fluid during lithium treatment to see if our model is consistent with the biochemical findings in man.

ACKNOWLEDGEMENT

This work is supported by United States Public Health Service Grant DA-00265-04.

REFERENCES

BOADLE-BIBER, M: Effect of calcium on tryptophan hydroxylase from rat hind brain. Biochem. Pharmacol. 24:1455-1460, 1975.

COSTA, E. & MEEK, J.L.: Regulation of the biosynthesis of catecholamines and serotonin in the CNS. Ann. Rev. Pharmacol. 14:491-511, 1974.

DENKLA, W.D. & DEWEY, H.K.: The determination of tryptophan in plasma, liver, and urine. J. Lab. Clin. Med. 69: 160-169, 1967.

FERNSTROM, J.D. & WURTMAN, R.J.: Brain serotonin content: Physiological dependence on plasma tryptophan levels. Science (Washington) 173: 149-152, 1971.

GAL, E.M., CHRISTIANSEN, P.A. & YUNGER, L.M.: Effect of p-chloroamphetamine on cerebral tryptophan-5-hydroxylase in vivo: A re-examination. Neuropharmacology 14: 31-39, 1975.

GOODWIN, F.K., POST, R.M., DUNNER, D.L. & GORDON, E.K.: Cerebrospinal fluid amine metabolites in affective illness: The probenecid technique. Am. J. Psychiat. 130: 73-79, 1973.

GRAHAME-SMITH, D.G.: Studies in vivo on the relationship between brain tryptophan, brain 5-HT synthesis, and hyperactivity in rats treated with a monoamine oxidase inhibitor and L-tryptophan. J. Neurochem. 18: 1053-1066, 1971.

JOH, T.H., SHIKIMI, T., PICKEL, V.M. & REIS, D.J.: Brain tryptophan hydroxylase: Purification of production of antibodies to and cellular and ultrastructural localization in serotonergic neurons of rat midbrain. Proc. Nat. Acad. Sci. 72: 3575-3579, 1975.

KNAPP, S. & MANDELL, A.J.: Narcotic drugs: Effects on serotonin biosynthetic systems of the brain. Science (Washington) 177: 1209-1211, 1972.

KNAPP, S. & MANDELL, A.J.: Short- and long-term lithium administration: Effects on the brain's serotonergic biosynthetic systems. Science (Washington) 180: 645-647, 1973.

KNAPP,S. & MANDELL, A.J.: Effects of lithium chloride on parameters of biosynthetic capacity for 5-hydroxytryptamine in rat brain. J. Pharmacol. Exp. Ther. 193: 812-823, 1975.

KNAPP, S. & MANDELL, S.J.: Coincidence of blockade of synaptosomal 5-hydroxytryptamine uptake and decrease in tryptophan hydroxylase activity: Effects of fenfluramine. J. Pharmacol. Exp. Ther. 197: in press, 1976.

KNAPP, S. & MANDELL, A.J.: Cocaine and lithium: Neurobiological antagonism in the serotonin biosynthetic system in rat brain. Life Sci. 18: 679-684, 1976a.

KNAPP, S., MANDELL, A.J. & BULLARD, W.P.: Calcium activiation of brain tryptophan hydroxylase. Life Sci. 16: 1583-1594, 1975.

KNAPP, S., MANDELL, A.J. & GEYER, M.A.: Effects of amphetamines on regional tryptophan hydroxylase activity and synaptosomal conversion of tryptophan to 5-hydroxytryptamine in rat brain. J. Pharmacol. Exp. Ther. 189: 676-689, 1974.

KUCZENSKI, R.T. & MANDELL, A.J.: Allosteric activation of hypothalamic tyrosine hydroxylase by ions and sulphated mucopolysaccharides. J. Neurochem. 19: 131-137, 1972.

KUCZENSKI, R.T. & MANDELL, A.J.: Regulatory properties of soluble and particulate rat brain tyrosine hydroxylase. J. Biol. Chem. 247: 3114-3122, 1972a.

MANDELL, A.J. & KNAPP, S.: Neurobiological mechanisms in lithium
        prophylaxis of manic-depressive disease: An hypothesis.
        In: Almgren, O. et al. (eds.) Chemical Tools in Catechol-
        amine Research II, pp. 9-16 North-Holland, Amsterdam,
        1975.

MANDELL, A.J. & KNAPP, S.: A neurobiological model for the
        symmetrical prophylactic action of lithium in bipolar
        affective disorder. Pharmakopsych. (Stuttgart) 9:
        116-124, 1976.

MANDELL, A.J. & KNAPP, S.: Regulation of serotonin biosynthesis
        in brain-role of the high affinity uptake of tryptophan
        into serotonergic neurons. Fed. Proc., in press, 1976a.

MUELLER, R.A., THOENEN, H. & AXELROD, J.: Increase in tyrosine
        hydroxylase after reserpine administration. J. Pharma-
        col. Exp. Ther. 169: 74-79, 1969.

MURPHY, D.L. & WEISS, R.: Reduced monoamine oxidase activity in
        blood platelets from bipolar depressed patients.
        Am. J. Psychiat. 128: 1351-1357, 1972.

NEFF, N.H. & COSTA, E.: Application of steady-state kinetics to
        the study of catecholamine turnover after monoamine
        oxidase inhibition or reserpine administration.
        J. Pharmacol. Exp. Ther. 160: 40-47, 1968.

PAOLETTI, R. SIRTORI, C. Jr. & SPANO, P.F.: Clinical relevance
        of drugs affecting tryptophan transport. Ann. Rev.
        Pharmacol. 15: 73-81, 1975.

SANDERS-BUSH, E., BUSHING, J.A. & SULSER, F.: p-Chloroamphetamine
        inhibition of cerebral tryptophan hydroxylase. Biochem.
        Pharmacol. 21: 1501-1510, 1972.

SCHOU, M.: Clinical prophylactic effects and clinical pharmaco-
        logy of lithium. Neurosci. Research Prog. Bulletin.
        14: in press, 1976.

SEGAL, D.S., SULLIVAN, J.L. III, KUCZENSKI, R.T. & MANDELL, A.J.:
        Effects of long-term reserpine treatment on brain tyrosine
        hydroxylase and behavioral activity. Science (Washington)
        173: 847-849, 1971.

SNYDER, S.H.: Madness and the Brain, McGraw-Hill, New York, 1974.

STANBURY, J.B. et al.: The Metabolic Basis of Inherited Disease,
        McGraw-Hill, New York, 1972.

TAGLIAMONTE, A., TAGLIAMONTE, S., PEREZ-CRUET, J., STERN, S. &
        GESSA, G.L.: Effect of psychotropic drugs on tryptophan
        concentration in the rat brain. J. Pharmacol. Exp. Ther.
        177: 475-480, 1971.

TOSER, T.N., NEFF, N.H. & BRODIE, B.B.: Application of steady-
        state kinetics to the synthesis rate and turnover time
        of serotonin in the brain of normal and reserpine-
        treated rats. J. Pharmacol. Exp. Ther. 153: 177-182,
        1966.

COMBINED USE OF NEUROLEPTIC DRUGS

Amos D. Korczyn

Department of Physiology and Pharmacology

Sackler School of Medicine, Tel-Aviv University, Israel

The therapeutic approach to schizophrenia has progressed considerably during the past years. The introduction of phenothiazines, butyrophenones and newer antipsychotic drugs has resulted in shorter hospitalizations and fewer relapses. There are now several dozens different antipsychotic drugs in clinical use. These belong to only a few families and, in fact, a chemical similarity exists between all of them (1). If this similarity is related to the mechanism of action of these drugs, then all should have the same clinical indications. On the whole, controlled trials aimed at finding "the right drug for the right patient" have not been very successful (2).

A common practice among psychiatrists is the use of combined medications in a single patient, such as two phenothiazines with a butyrophenone. These combinations are reputed to achieve results superior to an increased dose of one of the drugs used separately. However, if the response to antipsychotic drugs depends upon a single activity (such as blockade of dopamine receptors), then such an assumption is unwarranted. In fact, at least one trial has demonstrated the inferiority of drug combinations when compared to a single drug in psychotic patients (3). The fact that there is a strong clinical tendency towards the use of combined medication, in spite of authoritative claims to the contrary (4), suggests that further information is needed.

There are several methods for determining the "equivalence" of antipsychotic activity in experimental animals. Surprisingly, there are hardly any reports of the responses to drug combinations in these tests. Lately, several papers have appeared suggesting a synergistic effect of neuroleptic drugs and alpha-methylpara-tyrosine (5). This may well be a promising lead for clinical psychiatry. It

should be remembered that most centrally active drugs have important interactions with other preparations used for the same indication. In the psychiatric clinical setting this is exemplified
by the combined use of tricyclic antidepressants with mono-amine-
oxidase inhibitors (6).

When two neuroleptic drugs are administered concurrently, the
interaction could theoretically take various forms. If the dose-
response curve of an antipsychotic agent for any activity follows
an S-shape, then simultaneously giving two drugs could result in
one of the following:

a) An additive effect. In this case the response when both
   drugs are given simultaneously will equal the sum of the
   responses to each drug given alone; or, when the dose-
   response curves of both drugs are adjusted to merge, the
   response will equal that resulting from a dose which is
   the sum of the two values on the abscissa.

b) Potentiation. Here the response will be bigger than in
   the additive effect. This will be the case if, for example
   two alternative parallel central pathways exist, and each
   drug relates specifically to one. An example of this type
   of interaction is that between anticonvulsants, such as
   phenytoin and phenobarbitone.

c) Occlusion. Here the response will be less than in the
   additive effect, and usually will be somewhat larger
   than the response to the more potent drug at the doses
   used in the combination. This will be the case if each
   drug acts relatively specifically on successive steps
   of a pathway. An example of this type of interaction is
   that between anti-inflammatory and narcotic analgetics.

d) Antagonism. In this case the response is smaller than to
   the more active drug given alone. This will be the case
   if both drugs act on the same receptors but with different properties. An example of this type of interaction
   is between narcotic analgetics and narcotic "antagonists"

Results demonstrating an additive effect, potentiation or
occlusion between neuroleptic drugs will have theoretical implications. Results showing occlusion or antagonism will also have
clinical importance in terms of the simultaneous use of different
anti-psychotics in psychiatric patients.

We performed experiments on the behavioral effects of various
combinations of drugs used in psychiatry aimed at evaluating the
four possible interactions described previously. Spontaneous
activity of mice was measured in a simple activity cage, in which

animals were placed in groups of fours. The hyperactivity following
amphetamine injection to the same mice was also measured. At the
time intervals used, 10-20 minutes following amphetamine (10 mg/kg),
only hyperactivity is seen without stereotyped behavior.

We first tested combinations of chlorpromazine and haloperidol.
These two potent antipsychotics are among the most widely used
agents in clinical practice, often in combination in the psychiatric setting.

The effects of chlorpromazine and haloperidol used singly and
in combination in our model are illustrated in Fig. 1. Chlorpromazine was used in the small dose of 0.3 mg/kg which only slightly
reduced the spontaneous activity and the amphetamine-induced hyperactivity. When chlorpromazine and haperidol were given together,
the response was additive. This was the result when these drugs
were given in other dosage combinations. Our interpretation from
these findings is consistent with the view that chlorpromazine and
haloperidol affect the same receptors, with a similar order of
magnitude of affinity to the receptors, at least as far as spontaneous activity and amphetamine-induced hyperactivity are involved.

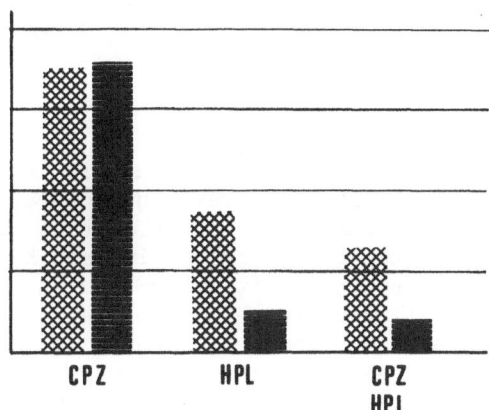

Fig. 1.   The effect of chlorpromazine (CPZ), 0.3 mg/kg s.c., and
          of haloperidol (HPL) 0.3 mg/kg s.c., given singly and
          in combination, on the spontaneous activity (hatched)
          and amphetamine-induced hyperactivity (parallel lines).
          Mice in groups of fours were injected with the neuro-
          leptics, and one hour later, d,l amphetamine (10 mg/kg)
          was added. Results are expressed in percentage of the
          performance of mice injected with saline instead of
          the neuroleptics. Top horizontal line, activity of the
          control group (100%). Note that the effect of chlor-
          promazine alone was small, and its effect when given
          with haloperidol was that expected from the additive
          model of interaction.

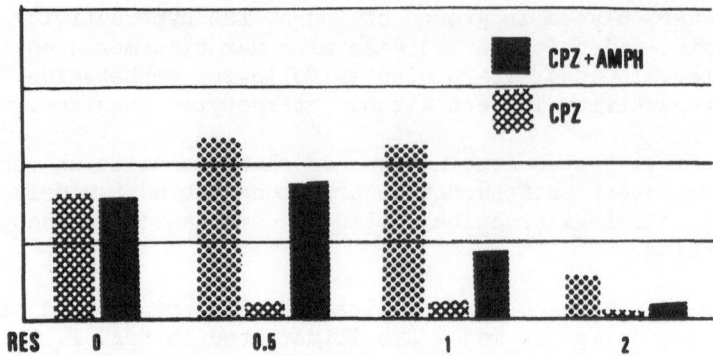

Fig. 2. The effect of reserpine (RES) pretreatment,
         given at various doses, on the spontaneous
         activity of mice. Details as in Fig. 1. Dotted
         bars, reserpine only; hatched bars, chlorpro-
         mazine (CPZ), 2.5 mg/kg; parallel line bars,
         amphetamine-induced hyperactivity in chlorpro-
         mazine treated animals. Chlorpromazine alone
         reduced spontaneous and amphetamine-induced
         activity to about 40% of control. Given after
         reserpine, the effect of chlorpromazine was
         much larger, fitting the potentiation model
         of interaction.

     Next, we tested reserpine. Although this drug is a potent
antipsychotic, it has fallen somewhat into disrepute. The reason
we have included reserpine in our study is that its mechanism of
action differs from that of chlorpromazine and haloperidol. Rather
than block dopamine receptors, it interferes in the presynaptic
terminals with the storage and release of neurotransmitter amines.
When chlorpromazine was given in the amount of 2.5 mg/kg, spontaneous activity and amphetamine-induced hyperactivity were reduced.
Pretreatment of the animals with relatively small amounts of reserpine, 0.5 and 1 mg/kg given four days previously, markedly
potentiated the chlorpormazine effect (Fig. 2). Thus, it seems
that the combination of chlorpromazine and reserpine may have
therapeutic advantages.

     The third combination which we tested was haloperidol with
promethazine. Promethazine, a phenothiazine derivative, is not
antipsychtotic; its effects in our system are small and on the
dose-response curve it is far on the right ocmpared to chlorpromazine or haloperidol. It is a sedative, however, and in high
doses can reduce spontaneous activity and later amphetamine-induced
hyperactiviity. When promethazine is given in a relatively small
dose of 25 mg/kg it has no effect on spontaneous activity, and we

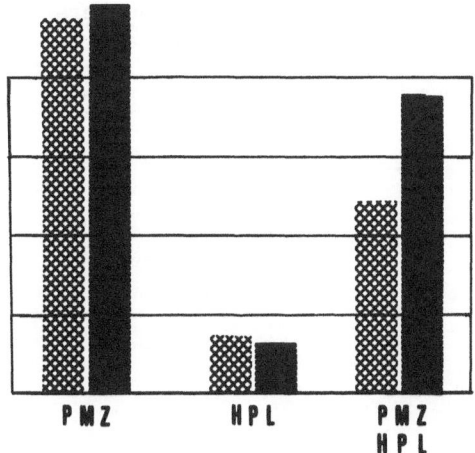

Fig. 3.   The effect of promethazine (PMZ, 25 mg/kg) and
          of haloperidol (HPL, 0.5 mg/kg) given singly and
          in combination, on spontaneous and amphetamine-
          induced hyperactivity. Details as in Fig. 1.
          Note that promethazine antagonized the effects of
          haloperidol both on spontaneous activity and on
          amphetamine-induced hyperactivity.

expected no effect on the depression of activity produced by 0.5
mg/kg haloperidol. Actually there is marked antagonism of promethazine on haloperidol-induced hypoactivity (Fig. 3).

    While our studies are still in the preliminary phase, the
results seem to indicate that the combined use of antipsychotic
drugs is not as simple as it looks, and requires considerably
more attention than it has received so far. It is suggested that
the problem can be tackled in experimental animals. Promising
combinations could be of those drugs which have different mechanisms
of actions.

REFERENCES

1.   JANSSEN, P.A. In: Neuropsychopharmacology (eds. Bente, D. and
         Bradley, P.B.) 4:151, Elsevier, Amsterdam, 1965.

2.   GARDOS, G.J.: Nerv. Ment. Dis. 159:343, 1974.

3.   MERLIS, S., SHEPPARD, C., COLLINS, L. ET AL.: Amer. J. Psychiat.
         126:1647, 1970.

4.   HOLLISTER, L.: <u>Clinical Use of Psychotherapeutic Drugs</u>.
            Charles C. Thomas, Springfield, pp. 192, 1973.

5.   AHLENIUS, S. and ENGEL, J.: <u>Eur. J. Pharmacol</u>. 15:187, 1971.

6.   SARGANT, W.: <u>Lancet</u> 2:634, 1963.

DISCUSSION

<u>Dr. Sam Cohen</u>: I have written a letter to the British Medical
Journal pleading that psychiatrists stop giving vast numbers
of different drugs to some patients.

    This is a scientific conference in a hospital and I think
it is an appropriate place to ask psychiatrists to consider more
rationally what they do. Perhaps if one drug doesn't work to give
a little bit more of the same thing instead of giving two or three.

<u>Dr. Sam Gershon</u>: I would like to second most vigorously these
previous statements. You propose a model which really doesn't
accord with the clinical data. There's very good data based on
clinical control studies that reserpine is not as effective as a
phenothiazine reference. If you do another experiment, using a
similar model to your's, and you take a phenothiazine plus a single
dose of an antidepressant, you will strongly potentiate the effect
that you see in your system, without showing increased antipsychotic
activity.

    The other clinical fact is that if you start off a patient
with three of these together and he doesn't get better, giving
them all in non-therapeutic doses, you've got no idea at all as
to which drug is the effective drug.

    I think the proposal based on your animal model is misleading.

<u>Dr. Korczyn</u>: I think perhaps the point that I made was not clear
enough. I didn't want to suggest the use of combined drugs in
psychiatry, rather the reverse, as Dr. Cohen has suggested. My
studies were based on the fact that I think too much combined
drugs are used in psychiatry and I think there is close to no
basic research on this problem. It has to be performed.

AN ANIMAL MODEL FOR THE MEASUREMENT AND MANIPULATION OF PROBLEM SOLVING ABILITY

Barry D. Berger

Department of Psychology

University of Haifa, Israel

Changes in learning, memory, attention, and other cognitive processes often accompany the mood disorders. Indeed, as in schizophrenia, disturbances of thought represent one of the central features of the disease, manifesting itself in a variety of symptoms. However, research on the etiology and treatment of these disorders has focused primarily on the mood characteristics and has more or less neglected the cognitive deficits.

One reason for this one-sided approach has been the difficulty in defining an adequate laboratory model for studying the cognitive process. The problem is a classic one in experimental psychology in that it requires a means for differentiating between performance, motivational, and associative factors. For example, a drug may indirectly influence problem solving ability by affecting sensory function, general arousal, motivation or motor coordination in addition to, or instead of, directly acting on the learning process. Thus a drugged rat may perform differently from its untreated counterpart in a maze or other learning device for a variety of reasons but it would be erroneous to presume that differences in performance were due solely or at all to the effect of the drug on the learning process (Dawson and McGaugh, 1973).

Unfortunately, with the techniques presently available it has been very difficult to separate these various factors and consequently to suggest possible therapies for dealing with specific cognitive deficits. The usual approach has been to successively use different behavioral tests to measure the various aspects of the drug effect - one to measure appetite, one for ataxia, one for general arousal and so on - and thereby to identify and perhaps

reduce the drug effect to one specifically on the learning process
(Miller, 1964). In the work to be presented here, however, we propose a different approach, one that takes the form of a single
test or battery of tests, but that makes several behavioral measures
simultaneously, thus enabling the analysis of the data into respective performance and associative categories and essentially identi-
fying whether a drug or other manipulation has an effect directly
or indirectly on cognitive function.

The apparatus consists of a rectangular Plexiglass chamber
45 cm. long, 25 cm. wide, and 36 cm. high with a stainless steel
grid floor. Mounted on one wall and serving as the response mani-
pulanda are two stainless steel panels with signal lamps above them.
A grey Plexiglass barrier separates the response panels and their
lamps and extends 29 cm. along the length of the chamber. A magazine light and liquid feeder assembly is located in the wall opposite to the response panels. The lamps, feeder and microswitches
of the response panels are connected to solid state logic circuits
for automatic programming of stimuli and recording of responses.

In the basic program, pressing either of the two response
panels triggers the 6-second feeder and magazine light cycle causing
a 0.1 cc dipper of sweetened condensed milk (two parts water to one
part milk) to be presented for 3 seconds terminating the trial. In
a variation of the basic program, only a response at the correct
panel triggers the milk reward, whereas responding at the incorrect
panel registers an error. The correction procedure is used, the
trial continuing until a correct response is made. The sequence
of occurences in which a response to the left or right panel produces reward and the presence or absence of signal lights above
the the correct and incorrect panels is also determined by the
programming circuitry.

The learning task used in the present series of experiments
consists of two sessions of 150-trials each. The problem to be
solved is a visual discrimination task, the spatial position of
the correct panel being signalled by the absence of a signal light
and the position of the incorrect panel by the presence of the
signal light.

Four behavioral measures are made on each trial: initial
errors; repetitive errors; latency; total time. An initial error
(IE) is recorded if the initial choice on any given trial is incorrect. Thus, only one initial error could be made on any given
trial with a maximum of 150 initial errors possible during any
session of 150 trials. Repetitive errors (RE) are described as all
additional incorrect responses on a given trial after an initial
error has been made. Latency is the time (in seconds) to the initial response, correct or incorrect. Total time is the time (in

seconds) to the correct response and thus to the end of the trial.

The subjects were 200-250 gram male Sprague-Dawley derived albino rats purchased from a local supplier. They were housed individually and maintained on a diet of 20 grams Purina lab chow per day with water available ad lib. Prior to the start of the experiment, the animals were handled and pretrained in the learning apparatus to press either of the panels to receive milk reward.

Under normal conditions, control rats learn the solution to the discrimination problem in the course of the two test sessions (Figure 1). The reduction of initial errors is particularly relevant since this score measures the initial choice on each trial. At the beginning of the first session, animals respond correctly only on about 46.2% of the trials (26.9 initial errors in the first block of 50-trials). However, by the end of the first session, the animals have reached 72% correct initial choices (14 incorrect choices out of 50 trials) and by the end of the second session, animals make only 4.8 initial errors out of 50 trials (90.4% correct).

Elimination of repetitive errors represents another indication of learning. In the case of this measure, animals learn not to repeat an incorrect response more than once on any given trial. In other words, animals learn to eliminate perseveration of incorrect responding and to make the correct response after obtaining feedback from an error. In the illustration of Figure 1, for example, 207 repetitive errors were made in the first 50 trials of session 1 and only 13.3 errors in the last 50 trials of session 11. However, it should be pointed out that the reduction of repetitive errors is not a perfect indicator of solving the discrimination problem. Firstly, as can be seen in the illustration, the course of improvement in eliminating initial errors does not precisely mirror the rate of decline of repetitive errors suggesting that the improvement of performance according to two measures may be by different mechanisms. Secondly and more important, improvement on the repetitive error measure is achievable even if the problem is made insolvable with respect to initial errors. This is achieved by disconnecting the signal lamps above the response panels thereby eliminating the relevant cue for making the initial correct choice. Under these circumstances, initial errors remain at chance level but repetitive errors continue to be eliminated at nearly normal rates. This observation points out the necessity for recording both types of errors and not simply relying on a measure of total errors per trial (initial and repetitive errors combined) as an indicator of problem solving.

The latency score measures performance independantly of learning rate since it is based on the first response of the trial whether or not that response is an error or a correct choice. Indeed as can be seen in the figure, the average latency at the beginning of

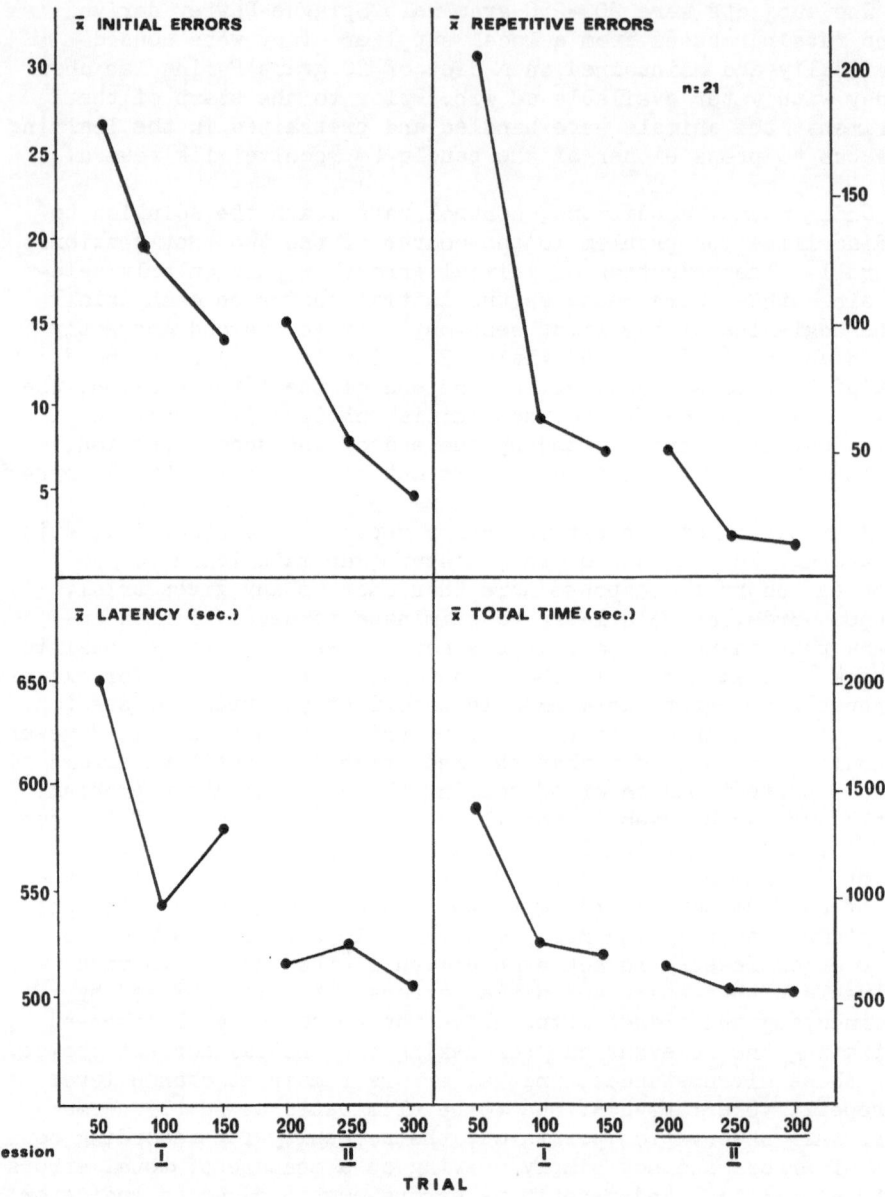

Fig. 1. Acquisition of a visual discimination problem in a
         group of 21 untreated rats. Performance measures include:
         initial errors; repetitive errors; latency; total time.

learning is about the same as the latency after the problem has been solved. This measure is not particularly sensitive to changes in learning but is very useful as an indicator of performance change. As will be shown further in this discussion, some drugs can affect response latency but have no effect, retard, or even facilitate learning.

Total time indicates the rate of making the correct response. As such, it may be considered as a measure of learning. Indeed, total time generally decreases as learning increases (Figure 1). However, since some manipulation may affect running speed, motivation, or motor coordination, but not learning ability, it is important to consider the total time measure together with the initial error score. As in the case of latency, and since the total time measure includes the latency score, it is entirely conceivable to observe an animal that performs slowly but accurately.

Thus, it should be possible to identify and separate performance from associative factors in the learning task by evaluating the overall pattern of the data that is based on the four behavioral measures. By means of illustration, Figure 2 describes the combined results of two experiments on the effects on learning of parachlorophenylalanine (PCPA), an inhibitor of the synthesis of serotonin in the brain (Tenen, 1967). PCPA (300 mg/kg) was injected intraperitoneally 48-hours (replication 1) or 72-hours (replication 2) prior to the first of the two daily training sessions. Control animals were injected with the vehicle, 1% Tween - 80.

As can be seen from Figure 2, PCPA facilitated the acquisition of the learning task by a specific effect on the elimination of initial errors. This was particularly apparent by the last 50 trials of the first training session at which time the PCPA group had an average of only 9.6 initial errors whereas the control group an average of 15.2 initial errors (t = 1.87; df = 27; p < .05). No significant differences between the two groups were observed using the other behavioral indicators although there was a tendency for the overall average number of repetitive errors in the PCPA group (281.3) to be less than that of the control group (354.8). The general direction for the latency and total time measures was for the PCPA group to respond more slowly than controls, but this difference did not approach statistical significance. On the basis of this overall picture, it would seem that PCPA may exert a specific facilitative effect on the rate of problem solving in a discrimination task and that this effect is independant of effects of the drug on response rate.

In other experiments now being conducted in our laboratory, we are testing a variety of brain manipulations including drugs in this learning paradigm. One goal of this work is to develop a

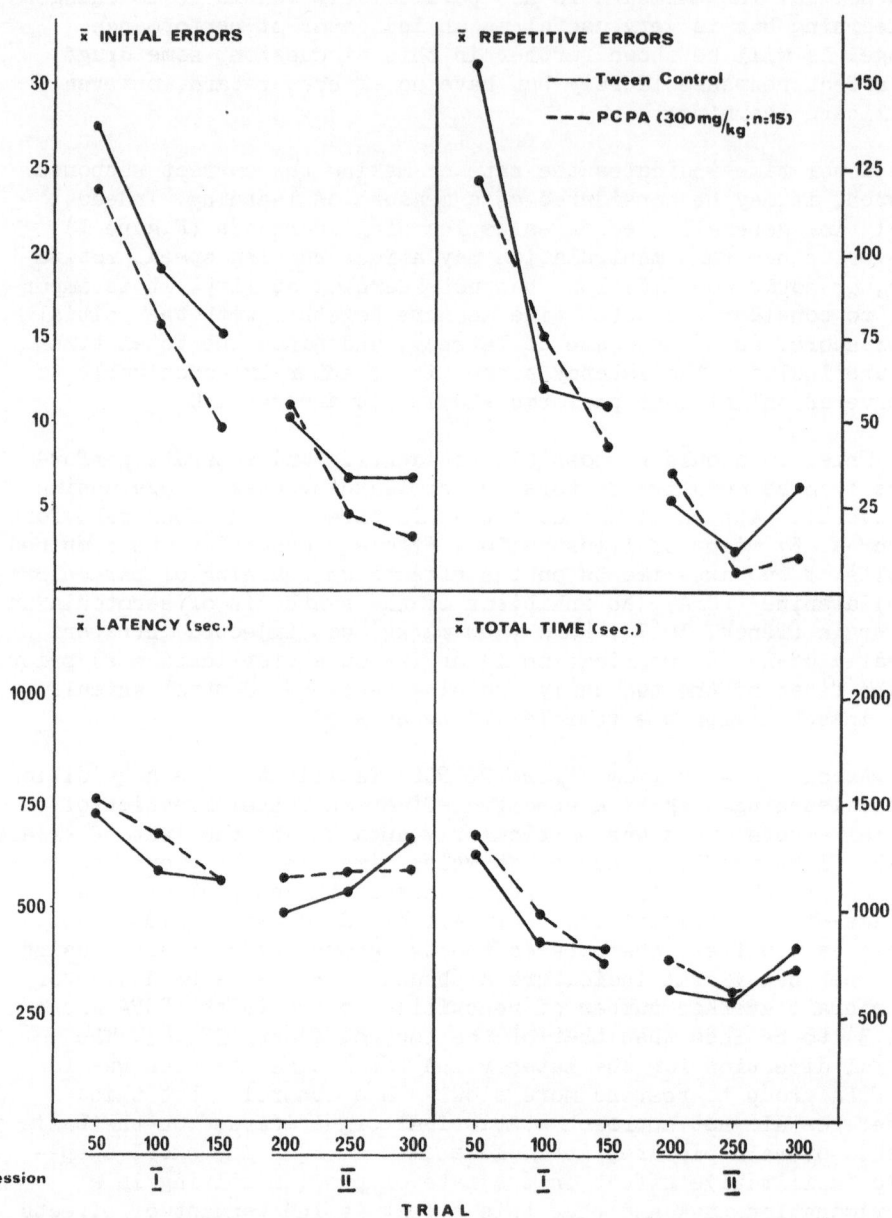

Fig. 2. Effects of PCPA (300 mg/kg) on a visual discrimination
         problem.

sophisticated screening procedure for the evaluation of prospective drugs that might facilitate cognitive function in the mood disorders, schizophrenia and in other learning disabilities of organic origin. Related to this aim is the goal of being able to validate the mechanism for the effect by determining the specific functional process on which the compound may act. Thus we have found that the impairment in acquisition caused by acute administration of the major tranquilizer chlorpromazine and the minor tranquilizer oxazepam is linked to a more general depressant effect of these drugs on performance. On the other hand we have observed facilitation of performance in animals being trained under the influence of non-contingent background brain stimulation in the medial forebrain bundle. Although this facilitation may relate neural reward mechanisms to the learning process (Stein, 1974), our data indicate that rewarding brain stimulation also affects response latency and total time. Thus an action of brain stimulation on arousal may be part of the cause of the acquisition facilitation in the present case and must be considered in the evaluation of results.

We have also observed that chronic administration of drugs produces a different behavioral profile on learning from that which is found in acute administration (Wise, et al., 1972). Specific facilitation of learning as measured by initial error scores, has been observed in animals that had received 21 consecutive days of chlorpromazine (3 mg/kg) as opposed to the deficit in performance observed after the acute dose. Similarly, in the case of oxazepam, the first administration of the compound impaired performance on all behavioral measures. By the second administration, however, the impairment was restricted to the inital error and the repetitive error measures suggesting a more specific effect of the compound on associative processes or possibly on a system controlling response inhibition.

These examples of drug effects, taken together with others from the literature, point to the necessity of a systematic evaluation based on several behavioral parameters before a meaningful statement can be made of the effects of drugs on learning and memory, and certainly before significant progress can be made toward the development of clinical tools to aid in the treatment of diseases of cognitive function in man.

REFERENCES

DAWSON, R.C. AND Mc GAUGH, J.L.: Drug facilitation of learning and memory. In: Deutsh J.A., The Physiological Basis of Memory, Academic Press, New York, 1973.

MILLER, N.: The analysis of motivational effects illustrated by
        experiments on amylobarbitone sodium. In: Steinberg, H.
        et al., eds., _Animal Behavior and Drug Action_. J. and A.
        Churchill, 1964.

STEIN, L.: Norepinephrine reward pathways: Role in self-stimulation,
        memory consolidation, and schizophrenia. _Nebraska Symposium
        on Motivation_, 22, 1974.

TENEN, S.S.: The effects of p-chlorophenylalanine, a serotonin
        depletor on avoidance acquisition, pain sensitivity, and
        related behavior in the rat. _Psychopharmacologia_ 10,
        204-219, 1967.

WISE, C.D., BERGER, B.D., AND STEIN, L.: Benzodiazepines: Anxiety-
        reducing activity by reduction of serotonin turnover in
        the brain. _Science_, 177, 180-183, 1972.

GENETIC ASPECTS OF SCHIZOPHRENIA: OBSERVATIONS ON THE BIOLOGICAL AND ADOPTIVE RELATIVES OF ADOPTEES WHO BECAME SCHIZOPHRENIC[*]

Seymour S. Kety

Department of Psychiatry
Massachusetts General Hospital
Boston, Massachusetts, U.S.A.

The mental illness (or illnesses) that we call schizophrenia constitute a major social problem in terms of suffering, the loss of human potential, and sheer public cost. Its gravity is matched by our ignorance regarding its causes. It is not surprising, therefore, that hypotheses have taken the place of knowledge, nor that these hypotheses have grown into doctrines and dogmas. The syndrome was first described at a time when the new sciences of microbiology and pathology were making important contributions to medicine and the natural assumption was made that schizophrenia was a simple disease of the brain that the neuropathologists would soon characterize. That did not happen convincingly and meanwhile Freud brought a new dimension into psychiatry in the recognition of the importance of life experience, the interaction of a child with its parents, especially its mother, and a new doctrine developed which postulated the overriding importance of "schizophrenogenic" parents in the development of schizophrenia. More recently, a doctrine has emerged which insists that schizophrenia is not a disease of the brain but is a myth devised by the psychiatric establishment which uses it to label what is a creative adaptation to a sick society. Although the belief in one or another of these doctrines is often very strong, the evidence on which they depend is quite weak.

* This report is based on work done in collaboration with David Rosenthal, Paul Wender, Fini Schulsinger and Bjørn Jacobsen and published in Genetic Research in Psychiatry, R. Fieve, D. Rosenthal, and H. Brill, Eds., John Hopkins University Press, Baltimore, 1975.

In the absence of demonstrable biological abnormalities in
schizophrenia, belief in their existence has rested on observations
which have suggested the importance of genetic determinants in
schizophrenia. But that evidence, too, has been inconclusive, and
compatible with alternative explanations which are difficult to
rule out.

Schizophrenia is known to "run in families" and a large number
of epidemiological studies attest to an approximately ten-fold
higher risk for schizophrenia in the siblings, parents and offspring
of schizophrenic individuals than in the general population. But
since a family shares not only its genetic endowment but also its
environmental influences, either or both of these could be operating
to account for the familial tendencies.

Better evidence has appeared to come from studies in twins,
and a substantial number of such studies that have been carried out
agree in the finding of a high concordance rate for schizophrenia
in monozygotic twins, while the concordance in dizygotic or fraternal
twins is no greater than that in siblings (1). Although these observations are compatible with genetic theory, they depend on an assumption that monozygotic twins differ from dizygotic only in the degree
of their genetic congruence. If monozygotic twins also share more of
their environmental influences than dizygotic twins, it is difficult
to determine how much of the discrepancy between monozygotic and
dizygotic twin concordance is genetic and how much accounted for by
environmental factors.

Studies with adopted individuals offer a means of minimizing
these sources of error. Since an adopted individual receives his
genetic endowment from one family but his life experience as a
member of another, it may be possible to disentangle genetic and
environmental factors by studies based upon such individuals and
their biological and adoptive families. If a total population of
adopted individuals can be surveyed, in which the occurrence of
schizophrenia in the biological relatives occurs after the time of
adoption and is not a basis for the transfer, where the mental status of the biological relatives and the adoptees are largely unknown
to each other and where independent diagnoses in each population can
be made without that information, it should be possible to reduce to
a minimum many types of selective, ascertainment and diagnostic bias.

In 1963, my colleagues, David Rosenthal, Paul Wender, Fini
Schulsinger and I began to collect a total sample of adults legally
adopted at an early age by individuals not biologically related to
them. We began with all of the legal adoptions granted in the city
and county of Copenhagen from the beginning of 1924 to the end of
1947, rejecting those who had been adopted by biological relatives,
yielding a total of 5483 adoptees. For the purposes of the study we

had included as "definite schizophrenia" three subtypes defined in
the diagnostic manual of the American Psychiatric Association:
chronic schizophrenia, latent (ambulatory or borderline) schizophrenia, and acute schizophrenic reaction. Thirty-three schizophrenic
"index" adoptees were selected by independent review of the abstracts
of the institutional records of the 507 adoptees who had ever been
admitted to a mental institution. Unanimous agreement on diagnosis
of chronic, latent or acute schizophrenia was arrived at among four
raters (FS, DR, PW, SK). A control group was selected from the
adoptees who had never been admitted to a psychiatric facility by
matching with each index case on the basis of age, sex, socioeconomic
class of the rearing family, time spent with biological relatives,
child-care institutions, or foster home before transfer to the
adopting family.

Our first report of prevalence and type of mental illness in
the relatives was based simply on an examination of institutional
records which were available for the biological and adoptive parents,
siblings and half-siblings, of the index and control adoptees. These
were identified through the adoption records and the Folkeregister.
Abstracts of the hospital records were made, translated into English,
edited to remove any information which would suggest whether a subject was related to an index case or to a control or was a biological or adoptive relative, and then independent diagnoses were made
by each of the four raters. A consensus diagnosis was arrived at by
conference among the raters.

We had previously developed the hypothesis of a "schizophrenia
spectrum" of disorders presumably related to schizophrenia and including, besides the three forms of schizophrenia we had accepted
in the selection of index cases, a category of "uncertain schizophrenia" where schizophrenia was the best diagnosis that could be
made although from the information we had we could not be certain,
and a category of "schizoid or inadequate personality" which appeared
to have some of the characteristics of schizophrenia but to a considerably milder extent. A statistically significant concentration
of "schizophrenia spectrum" disorders was found among the biological
relatives of index cases as compared with those of the controls,
while the adoptive relatives showed a low incidence of schizophrenia
spectrum disorders for both the index and the control group with no
difference between them (2). The number of these illnesses which we
found in the relatives was too small to permit a further breakdown
of the schizophrenia spectrum. Furthermore, we had secured little
information about the environment of the probands other than the
presence or absence of mental illness in their adopted relatives.
One of our other studies (3) had also suggested that there were
many more schizophrenics and individuals within the schizophrenia
spectrum than those who had ever been hospitalized.

        For these reasons we felt that it would be important to carry
out complete psychiatric interviews with these relatives which might
permit a more exhaustive survey of the population with regard to
schizophrenia and other psychiatric diagnoses and more information
about life experience. We secured the collaboration of Dr. Bjørn
Jacobsen, a Danish psychiatrist, who agreed to carry out the interviews and spent the greater part of the next two years in doing so.

        A total of 512 relatives were identified through the population
records. Of these, 119 had died and 29 had emigrated or disappeared.
There was an interesting and highly significant difference in the
death rate between the biological relatives of index cases (of whom
35 had died by February 1973 as compared with only 13 dead among
the biological relatives of controls, $p = 0.0004$). That difference
is accounted for by suicide, accidental and other traumatic deaths.
Of the remaining 364 relatives, more than 90 per cent participated
in an exhaustive psychiatric interview conducted by Dr. Jacobsen,
who had not known the relationship of any subject to a proband. In
practically all of the biological relatives, the subject himself did
not know of that relationship and did not inform Dr. Jacobsen. Extensive summaries of these interviews were then prepared, edited to
remove any clues that would permit a guess of the relationship of
the subject to a proband, and were then read independently by each
of three raters (DR, PW and SK). Each rater independently recorded
his best psychiatric diagnosis for each subject from a list of
possible diagnoses covering the entire range listed in the diagnostic
manual (DSM-II) of the American Psychiatric Association, ranging
from no mental disorder to chronic schizophrenia. After that a
consensus was arrived at among the three raters, the code was broken
and the subjects were allocated to their respective four groups:
biological or adoptive relatives of schizophrenic index adoptees
and biological or adoptive relatives of control adoptees.

        Of these four populations, one is different from the rest in
being genetically related to a schizophrenic with whom they have
not lived, i.e., the biological relatives of the index cases. With
regard to mental illness other than schizophrenia these relatives
do not differ from the rest (Table 1). Thus this study provides no
support for a genetic relationship between organic, neurotic, affective or personality disorders and schizophrenia.

        In the case of the schizophrenia spectrum of disorders and for
the individual components with the single exception of "schizoid or
inadequate personality", however, there is a concentration in the
biological relatives of index cases in contrast to the persons who
are not genetically related to a schizophrenic. For chronic schizophrenia, the prevalence in the biological relatives of index cases
is 2.9 per cent compared with 0.6 per cent in the other three groups;
for latent schizophrenia it is 3.5 per cent compared with 1.2 per
cent; and for uncertain schizophrenia it is 7.5 per cent compared

TABLE I.   Concordance rates for schizophrenia in studies of
            monozygotic and dizygotic twins*

Author	Date	Monozygotic Pairs		Dizygotic Pairs	
		N	% concordant	N	% concordant
Luxenberger	1928	19	58	13	0
Rosanoff et al.	1934	41	61	53	13
Essen-Möller	1941	11	64	27	15
Kallman	1946	174	69	296	11
Slater	1953	37	65	58	14
Inouye	1961	55	60	11	18
Tienari	1963	16	6-36	20	5-14
Kringlen	1964	55	25-38	90	4-10
Gottesman & Shields	1966	24	42	33	9
Fischer et al.	1969	21	24-48	41	10-19
Pollin et al.	1969	80	14-35	146	4-10
Gottesman & Shields	1972+	20	40	31	10

*   From the compilation by Gottesman & Shields (1972).

+   Same sample as 1966 study but now based on blind consensus of
    6 judges.

with 2 per cent. For any of these diagnoses of schizophrenic illness,
the prevalence in those genetically related to the schizophrenic
index cases is 13.9 per cent compared to 2.7 per cent in their
adoptive relatives or 3.8 per cent in all subjects not genetically
related to an index case (Table II). The difference between the
group genetically related to the schizophrenic index cases and those
not so related is highly significant statistically and speaks for
the operation of genetic factors in the transmission of schizophrenia.

The evidence thus far presented is compatible with a genetic
transmission in schizophrenia, but is not entirely conclusive,
since there are possible environmental factors such as in utero
influences, birth trauma, and early mothering experiences which
have not been ruled out. However, there are 127 biological paternal
half-siblings of index cases and controls among these relatives who
can help to settle that question, since the biological paternal half-
siblings did not share the same mother, neonatal mothering experience
or postnatal environment with their adopted half-siblings. The only
thing they shared was the same father and a certain amount of genetic
overlap. The number of paternal half-siblings is almost identical for
index cases and controls, but the number of those who were diagnosed

TABLE II.   Status (as of February 1973) of the biological and
            adoptive relatives (parents, siblings, half-siblings)
            of the index and control probands

	BIOLOGICAL RELATIVES		ADOPTIVE RELATIVES		TOTAL RELATIVES
	INDEX	CONTROL	INDEX	CONTROL	
TOTAL IDENTIFIED	173	174	74	91	512
DIED*	35	13	35	36	119
LEFT DENMARK, SWEDEN OR NORWAY	13	11	0	2	26
DISAPPEARED	1	1	0	1	3
ALIVE AND ACCESSIBLE	124	149	39	52	364
AGREED TO INTERVIEW	112	138	34	45	329
REFUSED INTERVIEW	12	11	5	7	35
REFUSED BUT ADEQUATE INFORMATION	6	2	1	3	12
REFUSED AND INADEQUATE INFORMATION	6	9	4	4	23
INTERVIEW OR ADEQUATE INFORMATION OBTAINED	118	140	35	48	341

* The only significant differences between the groups are the
  number of deaths being significantly higher for the index biological relatives vs. control (p = 0.0004) and for control
  adoptive vs. control biological relatives (p < 0.0001); the
  latter is undoubtedly a reflection of the age differences. The
  percentage of interviews granted or refused in the accessible
  populations are not significantly different.

TABLE III. Psychiatric diagnoses outside the schizophrenia spectrum made by a consensus of 3 raters

	BIOLOGICAL RELATIVES				ADOPTIVE RELATIVES			
	INDEX	PREVALENCE %*	CONTROL	PREVALENCE %*	INDEX	PREVALENCE %*	CONTROL	PREVALENCE %*
TOTAL IDENTIFIED	173		174		74		91	
ADEQUATE INTERVIEWS	118		140		35		48	
INTERVIEWS WITHOUT SPECTRUM DIAGNOSIS	82		121		31		41	
NORMAL	30	36.6	49	40.5	11	35.5	11	26.8
ORGANIC	7	8.5	6	5.0	5	16.1	6	14.6
NEUROSIS	4	4.9	6	5.0	3	9.7	2	4.9
AFFECTIVE DISORDER	2	2.4	11[+]	9.0	1	3.2	3	7.3
PERSONALITY DISORDER	27	32.9	39	32.2	8	25.8	15	36.6
OTHER THAN SCHIZOPHRENIA SPECTRUM	40	48.8	62	51.2	17	54.8	26	63.4

* Calculated as % of interviewed relatives excluding those with schizophrenia spectrum diagnosis.
+ Prevalence of affective disorder is lower in index biological relatives than in the control biological relatives (p = 0.049); for none of the other diagnostic categories is the prevalence significantly different between index relatives and their respective controls.

TABLE IV. Prevalence of schizophrenia spectrum disorders in biological and adoptive relatives

TYPE OF RELATIVES	NUMBER IDENTIFIED	NUMBER INTERVIEWED	SCHIZOPHRENIA SPECTRUM %*	CHRONIC B1%*	LATENT B3%*	UNCERTAIN D1,D2,D3%*	SCHIZOID + INADEQUATE %*
BIOLOGICAL INDEX	173	118	21.4	2.9	3.5	7.5	7.5
ALL BIOLOGICAL CONTROLS	174	140	10.9	0	1.7	1.7	7.5
SCREENED BIO-LOGICAL CONTROL+	113	86	6.4	0	0.9	0	8.8
p (ALL INDEX VS. ALL CONTROLS)	N.S.	N.S.	0.006	0.03	0.25	0.009	N.S.
p (ALL INDEX VS. SCREENED CONTROLS)	N.S.	N.S.	0.007	0.08	0.16	0.001	N.S.
ADOPTIVE INDEX	74	35	5.4	1.4	0	1.4	2.7
ALL ADOPTIVE CONTROLS	91	48	7.7	1.1	1.1	3.3	2.2
SCREENED ADOPTIVE CONTROLS+	64	34	4.7	0	0	1.6	3.1

Subgroup p values for all index vs. all controls and for all index vs. screened controls are all N.S.

* In each instance % is calculated as N/identified relatives

+ Relatives of the 23 "screened" controls (interviewed and found to be free of illness).

TABLE V. Schizophrenic illness in the biological paternal half-
          siblings of schizophrenic index cases and controls (as
          obtained by consensus diagnoses based upon institutional
          records or interviews)

PROBANDS (N)	NUMBER OF BIOLOGICAL PATERNAL HALF-SIBS	NUMBER WITH DIAGNOSIS OF SCHIZOPHRENIA		
		DEFINITE	UNCERTAIN	TOTAL
		N (%)	N (%)	N (%)
SCHIZOPHRENIC INDEX (33)	63	8 (12.7)	6 (9.5)	14 (22.2)
CONTROL (34)	64	1 (1.6)	1 (1.6)	2 (3.1)
p (INDEX VS. CONTROL)	N.S.	0.015	0.055	0.001
SCREENED CONTROLS (23)	42	0 (0)	0 (0)	0 (0)
p (INDEX VS. SCREENED CONTROL)	N.S.	0.014	0.042	0.0004

TABLE VI. Schizophrenic illness in the biological and adoptive families of schizophrenic index cases and controls (ascertained by consensus diagnoses based upon institutional records or interviews)

PROBANDS	NUMBER OF FAMILIES	NUMBER OF FAMILIES WITH ONE OR MORE MEMBERS DIAGNOSED AS SCHIZOPHRENIC							
		BIOLOGICAL				ADOPTIVE			
		DEFINITE		DEFINITE OR UNCERTAIN		DEFINITE		DEFINITE OR UNCERTAIN	
		N	%	N	%	N	%	N	%
SCHIZOPHRENIC INDEX	33	14	(42.4)	17	(51.5)	1	(3.0)	3	(9.0)
CONTROL	34	3	(8.8)	5	(14.7)	3	(8.8)	5	(14.7)
p INDEX VS. CONTROL		0.002		0.001		N.S.		N.S.	
SCREENED CONTROL	23	1	(4.3)	1	(4.3)	1	(4.3)	2	(8.7)
p INDEX VS. SCREENED CONTROL		0.001		0.0001		N.S.		N.S.	

as having definite or uncertain schizophrenia is markedly different, with 14 among the half-siblings of the index cases and only 2 among the half-siblings of controls (p = 0.0001). There is a similar concentration if we restrict the diagnosis to definite schizophrenia (Table III). We regard this as the most compelling evidence we have obtained that genetic factors operate significantly in the transmission of schizophrenia.

These data do not permit the conclusion that schizophrenia is a unitary disorder, since they are equally compatible with a syndrome of multiple etiologies and different modes of genetic transmission. Although the 24 diagnoses of definite or uncertain schizophrneia were distributed among the biological relatives of 17 of the index probands, there were 16 who had no diagnosis of schizophrenic illness in their biological relatives. The possibility that there are at least two forms of schizophrenia in one of which there is a strong genetic basis which is weak or absent in the other would be compatible with our data.

These data do not imply that genetic factors and the biological processes involved in their expression are the only important influences in the etiology and pathogenesis of schizophrenia. We are currently engaged in analyzing these interviews with respect to experiential factors and their possible interaction with biological vulnerability to make possible or prevent the development of schizophrenia.

REFERENCES

1. GOTTESMAN, I.I. and SHIELDS, J.: Schizophrenia and Genetics: A Twin Study Vantage Point. New York and London: Academic Press, 1972.

2. KETY, S.S.: Biochemical theories of schizophrenia. Science 129, 1528-1532; 1590-1596, 1959.

3. KETY, S.S., ROSENTHAL, D., WENDER, P.H. and SCHULSINGER, F.: The types and prevalence of mental illness in the biological and adoptive families of adopted schizophrenics. In: The Transmission of Schizophrenia, eds. D. Rosenthal and S.S. Kety. Oxford: Pergamon Press, pp.345-362, 1968.

4. KETY, S.S., ROSENTHAL, D., WENDER, P.H., SCHULSINGER, F. and JACOBSEN, B.: Mental illness in the biological and adoptive families of adopted individuals who have become schizophrenic: A preliminary report based upon psychiatric interviews. In: Genetic Research in Psychiatry, eds. R. Fieve, D. Rosenthal and H. Brill. Baltimore

and London: The Johns Hopkins University Press, pp. 147-165, 1975.

5.   ROSENTHAL, D.: Problems of sampling and diagnosis in the major twin studies of schizophrenia. _Journal of Psychiatric Research_ 1, 116-134, 1962.

6.   ROSENTHAL, D., WENDER, P.H., KETY, S.S., WELNER, J. and SCHULSINGER, F.: The adopted away offspring of schizophrneics. _American Journal of Psychiatry_ 128(3), 307-311, 1971.

7.   WNEDER, P.H., ROSENTHAL, D., KETY, S.S., SCHULSINGER, F. and WELNER, J.: Crossfostering: A research strategy for clarifying the role of genetic and experimental factors in the etiology of schizophrenia. _Archives of General Psychiatry_ 30, 121-128, 1974.

GENETIC AND BIOLOGIC STUDIES OF AFFECTIVE ILLNESS

Elliot S. Gershon

National Institute of Mental Health

Bethesda, Maryland 20014

INTRODUCTION

The overall goal of our studies for some years has been to identify biological characteristics that are genetically transmitted factors in the affective disorders, mania and depression. Formidable obstacles to this goal are presented on the one hand by the unresolved issues in the genetics of these disorders, and on the other hand by the quantitative (as opposed to qualitative) biologic findings that have been found to distinguish persons with these disorders from normal controls. For a given patient or relative, there is always a degree of uncertainty both about the genotype underlying his psychiatric state and the genotype indicated by an enzyme activity or other quantitative variable. The question of whether the same genetic factor is producing both the biologic and the psychiatric findings in a given person becomes a complicated one, although still one that is subject to investigation. In this paper I shall discuss these issues, and review some of the strategies we have used in studying them in the Jewish population of Jerusalem, Israel.

CLINICAL ISSUES: PENETRANCE, MULTIPLE MANIFESTATIONS, HETEROGENEITY

The evidence suggesting that a genetic factor is generally present in affective illness consists of twin and family studies of ill persons. The pooled concordance for major affective illness in monozygotic (MZ) twins in six studies was 69.2%, whereas in dizygotic (DZ) twins it was 13.3% as reviewed elsewhere. (1) In a compilation of case reports of MZ twins reared apart, 67% were

---

concordant, suggesting that the rearing environment is not a factor (2).

The lack of 100% concordance suggests that there is incomplete penetrance of the genetic diathesis for these disorders. In the MZ twin data, correction for age of onset enhances the observed concordance to nearly 100%. In study of more distant relatives it has been repeatedly reported that even with age correction the prevalences in relatives are not as high as would be expected in simple Mendelian traits, (3-7) although not all investigators find this (8,9).

Mechanisms of variable penetrance or of multiple gene effects, or postulation of phenocopies, must therefore by introduced into proposed genetic hypotheses of these disorders. Variable age-of-onset is perhaps the most easily understood factor in penetrance, but in the data of most investigators it is clearly not the only factor, since age correction does not produce Mendelian ratios in relatives. It is not clear why low prevalence in relatives has been noted by some investigators (5,4,3) but not others (8,9) even when large numbers of relatives are studied and systematic diagnostic criteria are applied.

The multiple forms of affective illness present problems for genetic analyses. Leonhard (11,12) subdivided the affective disorders into unipolar (UP) and bipolar (BP) forms, where patients with mania and depression are bipolar and patients with depression only are unipolar. Leonhard found the two forms to be separable in the prevalence of psychiatric illness in relatives. From this, he hypothesized that the two forms may be clinically and genetically distinct entities. Studies of MZ twins revealed that 86% of concordant twin pairs were concordant for polarity, but in 14% one twin was BP and the other UP (13). In all but one family study of patients with bipolar illness there is a considerable prevalence of unipolar illness in relatives (3,5-9). In the one study (4) "other depressions and suicide" were found in relatives of bipolar patients, but these were not called unipolar because of the distinctive criteria used. These data suggest that there is a genetic component in polarity, but that the same genetic diathesis can be clinically expressed as either unipolar or bipolar illness. However, the general question of the genetic distinctness of unipolar and bipolar illness is not settled by the twin and family data. Unipolar and bipolar illness might be different forms of the same genetic illness, that is, pleiotropic effects of a single genetic diathesis, as one possibility. As another possibility, there might be two biologically and genetically separate illnesses, but a small proportion of persons with one illness have a clinical picture indistinguishable from the other illness. In this case, biological or pharmacologic studies of afflicted families would be needed to demonstrate that an apparently unipolar person should be considered biologically bipolar.

Besides unipolar and bipolar affective illness, previous
family studies suggested that a spectrum of affective and related
disturbances may exist in the families of patients with major
affective illness, including moderate depressions, cyclothymic
personality, unexplained suicides, alcoholism and sociopathy (10).
If these related disorders are produced as pleiotropic manifestations of the same genetic factors that produce the major affective
illness in these families, they must be taken into account by
genetic hypotheses of the mode of transmission of these disorders.

Clinical Genetic Findings: The Jerusalem Study

Since some of the differences between family study investigations may represent population differences, we decided to
develop a comprehensive set of data on affective illness in the
Jewish population of Jerusalem, Israel. No previous study of
affective disorders had produced a comprehensive epidemiologic
and genetic study of a single population, to which genetic models
could be applied. In our study, we gathered epidemiologic data
from a central registry, and did a family study of psychiatric
disorders in relatives of patients with unipolar illness, bipolar
illness, and normal controls. Data on inbreeding and assortative
mating in this population was also collected. The study is more
completely described elsewhere (5).

It should perhaps be emphasized that although these data
were collected to test genetic hypothesis, they are of epidemiologic interest even without assuming there is a genetic factor.
Questions which may be settled by such data include: (a) whether
there is a concentration of affective disorders within a relatively
limited number of families in the population; (b) what clinical
syndromes are inherited in the affective disorders, can the concept of a spectrum of disorders be usefully incorporated into
genetic studies; (c) is there overlap in the types of illnesses
found in the families of unipolar and bipolar patients.

At the time of this study (1971-1973) there were approximately 301,300 people in Jerusalem, of whom 222,200 were Jews (14).
For Jews, the lifetime prevalence of hospitalization for affective
illness was 2.4%. Of those hospitalized, 45% were bipolar and 55%
were unipolar. This is a higher proportion of BP illness than was
found in Sweden (4), although in Iraq a similar percentage was
reported in Arabs (15), which may reflect different gene pools
in Mediterranean and Northern European populations.

A striking concentration of affective illness in a limited
number of families is evident in this population. The overall
prevalence of major affective disorders in first degree relatives

TABLE 1. Psychiatric Illness in Parents, Children, and
Sibs (from Gershon et al., in press (5))

	Diagnosis of probands			
	Bipolar (BP) (I + II)*	Unipolar (UP)	All affective disorders (BP + UP)	Normal Controls
No. of relatives at risk				
Bipolar†	340·54	95·75	436·28	517·63
Unipolar†	264·41	77·32	341·73	410·50
Over age 15	411	113	524	619
Major affective disorders				
Bipolar I	12		12	1
Bipolar II	1	2	3	
Unipolar	23	11	34	3
Related affective disturbances				
Moderate depression	10	2	12	4
Cyclothymic personality	9	2	11	
Undiagnosed major psychiatric illness‡	7		7	1
Unrelated affective disturbances				
Chronic depression	1		1	6
Post partum	1	1	2	1
Cyclic depressive personality	3	1	4	2
Psychoses				
Schizophrenia	1		1	2
Schizo-affective	3		3	
Other psychoses		1	1	1
Other neurotic and personality orders				
Hysteria	1	1	2	2
Alcoholism and/or drug abuse	3	1	4	1
Sociopathic	4	2	6	4
Other neuroses	5	1	6	3
Other personality disorders	5	3	8	3
Suicide				
With diagnosis of major affective disorder	3	2	5	
With other diagnosis or normal	1		1	

*BP I = Bipolar I (history of mania and depression); BP II = Bipolar II (history of hypomania
 and depression).
†Corrected for age.
‡In 5/7 cases a single acute psychotic or confusional episode.

of psychiatrically normal controls was about one tenth the prevalence in the relatives of UP and BP patients (Table 1). (First
degree relatives are parents, offspring, and full siblings). To
define a spectrum of affective disturbances that are transmitted
together within families, we included any diagnosable entity which
was significantly more prevalent in the relatives of patients with
major affective illness, as compared with relatives of normal
controls. The diagnostic criteria for each entity are defined
elsewhere (5). These comparisons allow us to describe a spectrum
of affective illness which includes the BP and UP forms of major
affective illness, moderate episodic depression, cyclothymic
personality, and a history of a single episode of acute psychosis.
Some affective distubances were clearly not in the spectrum,
including chronic mild depression and depressive personality.
Clearly not includable in the spectrum were alcoholism and sociopathy; this is in contrast to findings reported in the U.S. (16),
and underscores the variability of clinical manifestations between
populations. Because of the small number of relatives of UP patients,
we did not investigate whether there are different spectrums for
BP and UP illness.

Bipolar patients were more likely to have bipolar relatives,
suggesting that polarity is transmitted familially. However, there
is an overlap of illnesses in relatives of each type of patient,
in that bipolar patients had some unipolar relatives and unipolar
patients has some bipolar relatives (Table 1). It therefore
appeared worthwhile to consider genetic hypotheses in which UP and
BP illness and the spectrum of related disorders are all produced
by the same underlying genetic diathesis. It appears necessary to
introduce variable penetrance or multiple gene effects in any
genetic hypotheses applied to this data, since we found the age
corrected prevalence of affective + spectrum disorders in sibs
is 33/204.7, less than the minimum expectation of 25% for a completely penetrant single autosomal locus.

STRATEGIES OF GENETIC ANALYSIS

Strategies for elucidating the genetics of a disorder with
multiple manifestations and variable penetrance include application of appropriate genetic models, identification of biologic
markers of vulnerability to the disorder, and demonstration of
linkage to known chromosomal markers.

GENETIC MODELS

Only recently have testable genetic models been developed for disorders with variable penetrance (17-19). A genetic model is a set of hypotheses that predicts the genotype and phenotypic status of persons of interest from variables known as parameters and from a hypothesized mode of transmission. To be tested against observed data, it is required that a model be determinate, that is, that there be more degrees of freedom in the data than the number of parameters of the model. If a model is indeterminate it will not be possible to test its predictive ability. It can be demonstrated that models of multifactorial or single locus autosomal trans- mission of an all-or-none trait with variable penetrance (such as the presence or absence of psychiatric illness) are indeterminate, and cannot be tested with family study data (17,20).

When there is more than one form of illness, and one form can be associated with a heavier loading of the genetic diathesis than the other, a testable model can be produced (17). One such model for BP and UP illness is illustrated in the figure (Fig. 1). This model postulates a continuous scale of liability to illness. Persons whose liability is greater than a threshold value will have an illness. There can be multiple threshold values, associated with the multiple forms of illness. In the depicted model there is a single autosomal locus with two alleles, and each genotype pro- duces a different mean liability to illness. Environmental factors produce a normally distributed variation in liability for each genotype, so that there is a finite probability of each illness (penetrance) associated with each genotype. Similar models may be constructed for multifactorial (MF) and X-chromosome modes of in- heritance.

The goodness-of-fit of a model to a given set of family study data is tested by iteratively searching the parameter space for the parameters that provide the closest fit of the model to the family study and population prevalence data. If there is a signi- ficant difference between the predicted and observed prevalences, using a chi-square test, the model may be rejected. The utility of model fitting lies in this capacity to reject certain genetic hypotheses. An acceptable fit for a given model is simply a con- firmation of the null hypothesis, and does not imply that it must be the correct model. However, further and more rigorous testing of various genetic models should eventually rule out those that are incorrect for a given trait. In the current context, a genetic hypothesis is more rigorously tested when there are a greater number of thresholds, more observed relatives, or both.

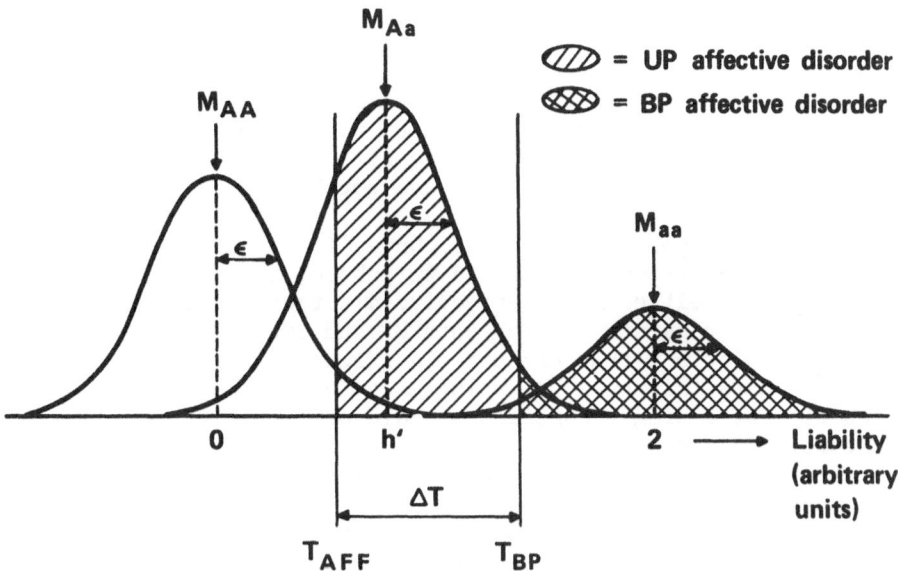

Fig. 1.   Parameters of single major locus model as
defined by Kidd (adapted from Kidd et al)(21).
Horizontal axis is a scale of liability to a disorder, which is a function of genetic and independent (random or environmental) components. Thresholds shown are for affective disorders, in which
T_{AFF} = threshold for all affective illness, and
T_{BP} = threshold for bipolar illness. M_{AA}, M_{Aa} and
M_{aa} are the mean liability values for each genotype.
ε is the square root of the independent (random
or environmental variance of liability which in the
model shown has the same value for each genotype.
h' is the liability value for the heterozygote Aa;
the liability values for the homozygotes are set
at arbitrary values of 0 and 2. For each genotype,
the hatched and cross-hatched areas represent the
proportion of persons with that genotype who will
have unipolar (UP) or bipolar (BP) affective disorder. In this model the parameters are T_{AFF} T_{BP}
h', ε^2 and q, the gene frequency of the a allele.
(From Gershon et al, in press (47).)

In our study, two-threshold autosomal transmission models of
UP and BP illness give an acceptably good fit for single major
locus (SML) and MF inheritance as described elsewhere (47). The
differences in family history between bipolar and unipolar patients,
which are confirmed in this study (5) and in several others (3,4)
thus need not imply genetically distinct entities. A single genetic
diathesis responsible for both illnesses, with bipolar illness
representing a more severe liability to affective disorder, cannot
be ruled out for our observed family and population data.

The related disorders can be accounted for in threshold liability models by introducing a third threshold, lower on the liability scale than either major affective disorders or bipolar illness. The best-fit parameters for both MF and SML models of inheritance give predictions that are not significantly different from
the observed data (Tables 2,3). This lends further support to the
applicability of a single continuous scale of liability to all of
the affective disorders in this population. The goodness-of-fit
of the three threshold models appears to be not as good as for
the two threshold models. For the SML models the parameters are
noticeably different for the two-threshold and three-threshold
solutions. The discrepancies between the two and three threshold
solutions may reflect the large portion of the parameter spaces
that give acceptable solutions. Also, separate thresholds for
each of the related disorders may be required. Both of these issues
might be settled with an order of magnitude larger sample of
patients and relatives, including patients with the related disorders.

The biological implication of a single genetic diathesis for
all the affective disorders is that for some important biological
abnormalities, UP and BP patients will either share the abnormality, or will differ quantitatively where the direction of the
difference is predicted by the liability thresholds. That is,
one would expect BP patients to differ from normals in the same
direction as UP patients, and where there is a BP-UP difference
the BP patients should be more deviant than the UP patients.
Similarily, one would anticipate biological findings where UP
and normals were similar but BP patients were different, but not
findings where BP and normals were similar and UP patients were
different. Some biological studies to test these implications are
presented below.

X-chromosome transmission can be tested in a threshold model
with a single threshold, unlike autosomal transmission hypothesis.
(22) We could therefore test the current hypothesis that major
affective illness (BP + UP) in the families of BP patients is
transmitted as a single locus on the X-chromosome (23,24). This
hypothesis was tested with a single threshold for all major
affective illness in the relatives and with separate thresholds

TABLE 2. Multifactorial (Polygenic) Multiple Threshold Genetic Models

Description of Parameter	Parameter	Two Thresholds	Three Thresholds
Population Prevalence (UP+BP)	K_{pw}	1.8%	1.6%
Population Prevalence (BP)	K_{pn}	0.4%	0.4%
Population Prevalence (UP+BP + Spectrum)	K_{pxw}	–	3.1%
Correlation Between Parents-Offspring	R_{po}	0.31	0.39
Correlation Between Sibs	R_{sibs}	0.37	0.35
Goodness of Fit			
x^2		11.46	23.13
		$0.4 > p > 0.3$	$0.1 > p > 0.05$
DF		10	15

TABLE 3. Single Major Locus Multiple Threshold Genetic Models

Description of Parameter	Parameter	Two Threshold	Three Threshold
Gene Frequency	Q	0.21	0.05
Independent Variance	ϵ^2	0.14	0.28
Dominance	H	0	1.42
Threshold (UP + BP)	T_{AFF}	2.1	1.9
Threshold (BP)	T_{BP}	2.4	2.3
Threshold (UP + BP + Spectrum)	$T_{Related}$	-	1.7
Goodness of Fit	χ^2	8.03	18.29
		$0.7 > p > 0.5$	$0.2 > p > 0.1$
	DF	9	14

for BP and UP illness in the relative. Neither hypothesis gave an
acceptable fit for the present data (22). It also did not appear
that a significant subgroup in this data might be X-chromosome
transmitted, since the prevalence in male parents and offspring
of male BP probands was slightly higher than the prevalence in
female parents and offspring (Table 4). If there were a significant subgroup with X-chromosome transmission one would expect
some excess of female-to-male (and male-to-female) over male-to-
male transmissions in the family study data, assuming a dominant
gene.

BIOLOGIC STUDIES

Genetic modeling studies indicated that the transmission of
these disorders in the Jerusalem population is autosomal, and may
be related to a single underlying diathesis, but could not definitely specify the number of genes involved or other genetic
parameters. To determine whether a biologic phenomenon is implicated in the transmission of affective illness in this population,
we developed criteria which would be applicable in either of the
autosomal transmission models that fit the clinical data.

We consider a biological variable to be implicated in the
transmission of a psychiatric disorder if: (a) The characteristic
distinguishes persons with affective disorders from normals;
(b) It is a stable characteristic of the individual studied, and
can be evaluated in well relatives; (c) It is heritable in first-
degree relatives; (d) Independent assortment of the marker and
of affective disorder is not present. That is, within a pedigree
the persons who have affective illness have different measurements
on the marker than the persons who are well. The use of these
criteria will distinguish phenomena that segregate along with the
illness from phenomena that are simply associated with the illness
(for example if both are more concentrated in population subgroups).
These criteria are applicable to quantitatively variable traits,
such as enzyme activities, which are known to be heritable but
whose mode of transmission is not precisely established.

We applied these criteria to two biologic variables that had
previously been found to distinguish patients with affective illness from normal controls - erythrocyte catechol-0-methyl transferase (COMT) and the amplitude-intensity function of the visual
average evoked response (AER).

COMT in affective illness was studied in collaboration with
Dr. W.Z. Jonas (25). COMT is the enzyme responsible for the initial
enzymatic inactivation of released catecholamines (26,27). The
enzyme is found in erythrocytes (28) and in other tissues in both
membrane bound and soluble states. Evidence has been presented

TABLE 4.   Parents and Offspring of Male Bipolar Probands

Sex of Parents and Offspring	Bipolar	Unipolar	Related Disorders	Other (Including Normal)
Male	1	2	2	22.9
Female	0	1	5	20.2

that the soluble and membrane bound enzymes are identical immunologically and by electrophoretic mobility (29) but not all investigators are in agreement that the two forms are identical (30,31). Data are presented here on the soluble fraction of erythrocyte COMT.

Erythrocyte soluble COMT activity was measured using the method of Jonas and Gershon (32). In that method, an acid substrate (dihydroxyphenylacetic acid) is used, which gives a greatly enhanced yield of methylated product, and avoids methanol formation during the incubation with the enzyme.

Results: The order of presentation of results will correspond to our criteria for a genetic marker. Male controls had significantly higher COMT activity than female controls but the difference between male and female patients was not significant. A two-way analysis of variance (33) was performed to determine if the patients had significantly different activity from controls, after controlling for the effect of sex. This analysis revealed two significant main effects: males had higher activity than females ($p < .05$) and persons with affective disorder had higher activity than controls ($p < .05$). The interaction between illness and sex was not significant (Table 5).

Comparisons between unipolar and bipolar patients could be made only for females, because only one unipolar male was studied. There was not a significant difference between unipolar and bipolar females in erythrocyte COMT activity; the mean for the 10 unipolar females was higher ($5.32 \pm .56$) than the mean for the 28 bipolar females ($4.64 \pm .23$).

Our finding of increased activity is apparently discrepant from reports in which women but not men with primary affective disorder had lower activity than normal controls (34,35). Other investigators have also reported non-confirmation (36,37) of the

TABLE 5.   Erythrocyte Catechol-O-Methyl Transferase (COMT) Activity* in Patients with Primary Affective Disorder and in Controls

	Men		Women	
	N	Activity	N	Activity
Primary affective disorder	15	$5.27 \pm .36$	38	$4.82 \pm .23$
Controls	17	$4.97 \pm .38$	21	$3.73 \pm .33$

Analysis of Variance

Source	Sum of Squares	df	Variance	F
Illness	9.59	1	9.59	4.22†
Sex	14.28	1	14.28	6.29†
Interaction	3.19	1	3.19	1.40
Within	197.55	87	2.27	....

* Activity expressed as nanomols of homovanillic acid formed per milliliter packed red blood cells per hour, $\pm$ SE.

† $p < .05$

initial report of reduced activity. These apparent discrepancies may be due to differences between populations studied, to variations due to the method of assay used, to different enzyme substrate preferences, or to other causes.

COMT is heritable in first degree relatives. The sib-sib correlation was 0.53 (p < .05) and the mid-parent to mid-offspring correlation was 0.49 (NS). Other studies have demonstrated the heritability (40,39) and stability of this enzyme activity within individuals (38).

As a test for independent assortment, we compared the mean COMT activity for ill persons in a family with the mean for well persons in the same family. Persons were considered ill if they had affective or related disorders, and well if they had any other diagnosis. "Family" includes proband and parents, siblings or children.

Within families, erythrocyte COMT activity distinguished healthy relatives from probands and ill relatives. COMT activity in the affectively ill persons within a family was significantly higher than in the healthy persons(p < .05) (Table 6). This was true for the 23 families where the ill persons had erythrocyte COMT activity greater than the control mean (p < .001), but not for the 11 families where the ill persons had reduced activity. Thus, in the families where affective illness is associated with elevated COMT activity, the psychiatric disorder and the enzyme activity do not show independent assortment. With the demonstration of non-independent assortment the criteria outlined above are satisfied, suggesting that COMT is a marker of genetically determined vulnerability to affective illness.

AER. Several studies have now indicated that patients with affective disorders show greater rates of increase in visual AER amplitude with increasing stimulus intensity for component P100-N140 (augmenting) than do matched normal controls (41,42). In collaboration with Dr. Monte Buchsbaum, we have studied this AER function to determine if it also serves as a marker of genetic vulnerability to affective illness (42).

Results: Patients with primary affective disorders had greater increases in AER amplitude with increasing intensity (augmentation of AER slope) than controls (Table 7). Thus our AER measure meets the first criterion of distinguishing persons with affective illness from normal controls. No significant differences between men and women were observed; nor did we find a significant sex by diagnostic group interaction. Across the entire group, the correlation between AER slope and age was 0.097 (N.S). There was

TABLE 6.   <u>COMT Activity Distinguishes Well and Ill</u>

<u>Persons Within Families</u>

	Well Persons	Persons with Affective and Related Disorders
Mean of Family Means	0.16 ± 0.27	0.75 ± 0.25

Mean difference = 0.58

Paired t = 2.40, df = 33, p < .05

Each enzyme measurement expressed as deviation of activity from control mean for its sex.

no difference between BP and UP patients, which parallels the findings with COMT.

A sib-sib correlation of 0.30 (p < .05) for the AER slope was found in this data, suggesting that AER slope is heritable. As with COMT, a precise estimate of heritability cannot be made because of the skewed sample. Heritability of this AER measure was previously reported by Buchsbaum (45).

AER slope did not differ between ill and well persons within families, suggesting that a single genetic factor was not responsible for assortment of the clinical and the biologic findings within in families.

Even though AER slope and affective disorders do not appear to be transmitted by a single genetic factor, the AER may still be related to genetic vulnerability. This is suggested by the finding that the well relatives of probands with affective illness had significantly higher amplitude/intensity slopes (mean = 0.33) than normal controls (mean = 0.11, difference significant by t test, p < .005). This was true both of well family members from families of bipolar probands (mean = 0.32) and of unipolar probands (mean = 0.04), and both comparisons were significantly different from normal (p < 0.01).

A POPULATION GENETIC VIEWPOINT ON BIPOLAR AND UNIPOLAR ILLNESS

The provocative hypothesis that biologic-genetic differences between populations may be found in the affective disorders is

TABLE 7.   <u>AER Amplitude - Intensity Slope In Affective Disorders</u>

	Male			Female		
	AER Slope		N	AER Slope		N
Primary Affective Disorder	.31 $\pm$ .07		17	.30 $\pm$ .09		34
Normal Controls	.14 $\pm$ .07		23	.08 $\pm$ .06		31

<u>Analysis of Variance:</u>

	Sum of Squares	df	Mean Square	F
Diagnosis	0.941	1	0.941	5.84*
Sex	0.031	1	0.031	0.19
Interaction	0.011	1	0.011	0.07
Within cells	16.261	101	0.161	

* $p < 0.05$

suggested by comparative analysis of studies in Israel and in the United States. Bipolar-unipolar differences in erythrocyte COMT activity and in AER augmenting have been reported in NIMH patients in Bethesda, Maryland (38,41,42) but were not present in Jewish patients in Jerusalem, even though these biologic variables distinguished patients with affective illness from controls in both locations.Bipolar illness is apparently more often found in the relatives of unipolar patients in Jerusalem than either in Sweden (4) or Bethesda (46).

It is agreed by nearly all investigators that unipolar illness (or other depression) is found in increased frequency in the relatives of bipolar patients, and that these UP relatives share the same underlying biologic affliction as the BP proband. A large proportion of all UP illness in Jerusalem may be biologically related to BP disorder in this way, as suggested by our genetic modeling results, and this may produce the appreciable prevalence

of BP illness in the relatives of UP patients, and the lack of
BP-UP biologic differences. This speculation is compatible with
the relatively large proportion of persons hospitalized for affective illness who are bipolar (45%) which is considerably higher
than reported by Perris in Sweden (20%), even though his criteria
for UP illness are more exclusive, since he requires three depressive
episodes.

One implication of this speculation is that affective illness
is biologically more homogeneous in Jerusalem than in other populations. A second implication is that UP patients in Jerusalem are
more like BP than like UP patients from other populations, as we
have noted for AER augmentation.

Activity in blood cells of enzymes catabolizing monoamines
also may vary between patients in Jerusalem and in Bethesda because
of population differences. Platelet MAO activity is decreased in BP
patients studied in Bethesda, Maryland as reported by Murphy and
Weiss, (48) and as recently replicated at the same center with a
new series of patients by Leckman et al (49). In Jerusalem, however
using the same diagnostic and laboratory techniques, Belmaker et al
have found that bipolar patients have significantly higher platelet
MAO activity than normal controls (50). In a partially overlapping
patient sample, we have found that erythrocyte COMT activity is also
increased in Jerusalem. In BP and UP patients, erythrocyte COMT had
higher activity in affective illness than in normal controls or in
the patients' well relatives. In Bethesda patients, women with
affective illness were reported to show decreased COMT activity (38).
If these differences in enzyme activity of COMT and MAO in affective
illness in fact represent population differences, one interpretation
would be that either increased or decreased peripheral enzyme activity may be associated with affective illness. These peripheral
findings might represent epiphenomena or adaptational adjustments
associated with perturbations of a monoamine-related system in the
CNS, where several types of perturbation of this central system may
result in affective illness.

The discrepant data on X-chromosome transmission in different
populations may also reflect population differences. As an index
of the degree of X-chromosome dominant transmission of affective
illness in a population we would use the relative amount of father-
son vs. mother-son ill pairs, since autosomal modes of inheritance
would generally not be expected to produce an excess of one over
the other, whereas to the extent that there is X-chromosome dominant
transmission an excess of mother-son pairs will be found. (This
statement is true assuming there is no significant sex-effect in
autosomal transmission, as discussed elsewhere (1)). Given this
criterion, X-chromosome transmission would be generally present
in the St. Louis population studied by Winokur, where father-son
transmission is absent (8). In the population sampled by the Lithium

clinic of the New York State Psychiatric Institute, X-chromosome
transmission may be common but not generally present, since some
excess of mother-son transmission has been found (9). [However, in
a later study in the same clinic no excess of mother-son transmission
was found (39)]. In Jerusalem, we find no excess in mother-son transmission, which suggests that X-chromosome transmission, if it exists
at all in this population, is uncommon. Here again, the Jerusalem
population may be more homogeneous than other populations studied.

The present series of studies underscores the value of cross-
national comparative biologic and population genetic studies. The
need for definition of the clinical spectrum of related disorders
in each new population studied is also evident. It appears that the
Jewish population of Jerusalem represents a uniquely homogeneous and
possibly biologically distinct resource for future biologic and
genetic studies of the major affective disorders.

REFERENCES

1.   GERSHON, E.S., BUNNEY, W.E., Jr., LECKMAN, J.F., VAN EERDEWEGH,
     M., DEBAUCHE, B.A.: The inheritance of affective disorders:
          a review of the data and hypotheses. Beh Genet, in press
          1976.

2.   PRICE, J.: The genetics of depressive behavior, in recent
          developments in affective disorders edited by Coppen,
          A., Walk, A., Br. J. Psychiatry, Special Publication
          No. 2, 37-54,1968.

3.   ANGST, J: Zur atiologie und nosolgie endogener depressiver
          psychosen in Monographien aus dem Neurologie und Psychiatrie,
          Berlin, Springer-Verlag, No. 112, 1-118, 1966.

4.   PERRIC, C.: A study of bipolar (manic-depressive) and unipolar
          recurrent depressive psychoses. Acta Psychiat. Neurol.
          Scand. 42: (suppl) 194, 1966.

5.   GERSHON, E.S., MARK, A., COHEN, M., BELIZON, N., BARON, M.,
     KNOBE, K.E.: Transmitted factors in the morbid risk of affective
          disorders: A controlled study. J. Psychiat. Res, in press

6.   JAMES, N.M., CHAPMAN, C.J.: A genetic study of bipolar affec-
          tive disorder. Brit. J. Psych., 126:449-456, 1975.

7.   HELZER, J., WINOKUR, G.: A family interview study of male
          manic-depressives. Arch. Gen. Psychiat. 31: 73-77, 1974.

8. WINOKUR, G., CLAYTON, P.: Family history studies I. two types
    of affective disorders separated according to genetic and
    clinical factors, in Recent Advances in Biologic Psychiatry,
    edited by Wortis, I.J., New York, Plenum Press, 9:35-50,
    1967.

9. MENDLEWICZ, J., RAINER, J.D.: Morbidity risk and genetic trans-
    mission in manic-depressive illness. Amer. J. of Hum. Gen,
    26:692-701, 1974.

10. GERSHON, E.S., DUNNER, D.L. and GOODWIN, F.K.: Toward a biology
    of affective disorders: genetic contributions. Arch. Gen.
    Psychiat, 25: 1-15, 1971.

11. LEONHARD, K., KORFF, I., SCHULZ, H.: Die temperamente in den
    familien der monopolaren und bipolaren phasischen psychosen.
    Psychiatry Neurol., 143:416-434, 1962.

12. LEONHARD, K.: Aufteilung der Endogenen Psychosen, First ed.
    Berlin, Akademie Verlag, 1957.

13. PERRIS, C.: The genetics of affective disorders, Biological
    Psychiatry, edited by Mendels, J., New York, John Wiley &
    Sons, 385-415, 1973.

14. GERSHON, E.S., LIEBOWITZ, J.H.: Sociocultural and demographic
    correlates of affective disorder in Jerusalem, J. Psychiat.
    Res., 12:37-50, 1975.

15. BAZZOUI, W.: Affective disorders in Iraq, Br. J. Psychiat. 117,
    195, 1970.

16. WINOKUR, G., CADORET, R., BAKER, M.: Depressive disease.
    Arch. of Gen. Psychiat. 24: 135-144, 1971.

17. REICH,T., JAMES, J.W., MORRIS, C.A.: The use of multiple
    thresholds in determining the mode of transmission of
    semi-continuous traits. Ann. Hum. Genet. 36:163, 1974.

18. ELSTON, R.C., STEWART, J.: A general model for the genetic
    analysis of pedigree data. Human Heredity, 21:523-542,
    1971.

19. MORTON, N.E., MACLEAN, C.J.: Analysis of family resemblance.
    III. Complex segregation of quantitative traits, Am. J.
    Hum. Gen., 26:489-503, 1974.

20. JAMES, J.W.: Frequency in relatives for an all-or-none trait.
     Ann. Hum. Gen. 35: 47, 1971.

21. KIDD, K.K., REICH, T., KESSLER, S.: Sex effect and the single
     gene. Submitted for publication.

22. VAN EERDEWEGH, M., GERSHON, E.S., VAN EERDEWEGH, P.:
     X-Chromosome models of bipolar illness. To be presented
     at 1976 annual meeting of American Psychiatric Association.

23. WINOKUR, G., CLAYTON, R.J., REICH, T.: Manic-Depressive
     Illness. C.V. Mosby Co., St. Louis, Mo., 1969.

24. MENDLEWICZ, J., FLEISS, J.L.: Linkage studies with X-chromo-
     some markers in bipolar (manic-depressive) and unipolar
     (depressive) illnesses. Biol Psychiat, 9:261-294, 1974.

25. GERSHON, E.S., JONAS, W.Z.: A clinical and genetic study of
     erythrocyte soluble catechol-0-methyltransferase activity
     in primary affective disorder. Arch. Gen. Psychiat.,
     32: 1351-1356, 1975.

26. AXELROD, J.: Methylation reactions in the formation and
     metabolism of catecholamines and other biogenic amines.
     Pharmacol. Rev., 18:95-113, 1966.

27. HERTTING, G., AXELROD, J.: Fate of tritiated norepinephrine
     at the sympathetic nerve-ending. Nature 192:172-173, 1961.

28. AXELROD, J., COHN, C.K.: Methyltransferase enzymes in red
     blood cells, J. Pharmacol. Exp. Ther. 176: 650-654, 1971.

29. CREVELING, C.R., BORCHARDT, R.T., ISERSKY, C.: Immunological
     characterization of catechol-0-methyltransferase, Frontiers
     in Catecholamine Research, Usdin, E., Snyder, S. (eds),
     New York, Pergamon Press, 117-119, 1973.

30. BOHUON, C., ASSICOT, M.: Catechol-0-methyltransferase,
     Frontiers in Catecholamine Research, Usdin, E., Snyder, S.
     (eds), New York, Pergamon Press, 107-112, 1973.

31. ROFFMAN, M., REIGLE, T.G., ORSULAK, P.J., et al: Comparative
     properties of soluble and particulate catechol-0-methyl
     transferases from rat red blood cells. Adv. Biochem.
     Psychopharmacol. 12:189-194, 1974.

32. JONAS, W.Z., GERSHON, E.S.: A method for determination of
     catechol-0-methyltransferase activity in red blood cells.
     Clin. Chim. Acta, 54:391-394, 1974.

33. WINER, B.J.: <u>Statistical Principles in Experimental Design</u>.
    New York, McGraw Hill Book Co. Inc., 1962.

34. COHN, C.K., DUNNER, D.L., AXELROD, J.: Reduced catechol-O-
    methyltransferase activity in red blood cells of women
    with primary affective disorder. <u>Science</u> 170:1323-1324,
    1970.

35. BRIGGS, M.H., BRIGGS, M.: Hormonal influences on erythrocyte
    catechol-O-methyltransferase activity in humans. <u>Experientia</u>
    29:278, 1973.

36. MATTSSON, B., MJORNDAL, T., ORELAND, L., et al: Monoamine
    oxidase and catechol-O-methyltransferase in affective
    disturbances. <u>Nord Psykiatr. Tidsskr</u>, 26:359-360, 1972.

37. SHULMAN, R., GRIFFITH, J.: Unpublished data.

38. DUNNER, D.L., COHN, C.K., GERSHON, E.S., et al: Differential
    catechol-O-methyltransferase activity in unipolar and
    bipolar affective illness. <u>Arch. Gen. Psychiatry</u>.
    25:348-353, 1971.

39. WEINSHILBOUM, R.M., RAYMOND, F.A., ELVEBACK, L.R., et al:
    Correlation of erythrocyte catechol-O-methyltransferase
    (COMT) activity between siblings. <u>Nature</u> 252:490-491, 1974.

40. GRUNHAUS, L., EBSTEIN, R., BELMAKER, R.H., JONAS, W.Z.:
    Erythrocyte COMT activity in MZ and DZ twins, submitted
    for publication.

41. BUCHSBAUM M., GOODWIN, F.K., MURPHY, D.L., BORGE, G.F.:
    AER in affective disorders. <u>Am. J. Psychiat</u>. 1971.

42. BORGE, G.F.: Perceptual modulation and variability in psychia-
    tric patients. <u>Arch. Gen. Psychiat</u>. 29:760-763, 1973.

43. DUNNER, D.L., FIEVER, R.R.: Psychiatric illness in fathers
    of men with bipolar primary affective disorder. <u>Arch. Gen.
    Psychiat</u>. 32:1134-1137, 1975.

44. GERSHON, E.S., BUCHSBAUM, M.: A genetic study of average evoked
    response augmenting/reducing in affective disorders. To be
    presented at American Psychopathological Association 1976
    Meeting.

45. BUCHSBAUM, M.: Average evoked response and stimulus intensity
    in identical and fraternal twins. <u>Physiological Psychology</u>.
    2:365-370.

46. GERSHON, E.S., DUNNER, D.L., STURT, L., GOODWIN, F.K.:
     Assortive mating in the affective disorders: a preliminary
     report. Biol. Psychiat. 7:63-74, 1973.

47. GERSHON, E.S., BARON, M., LECKMAN, J.F.: Genetic models of the
     transmission of affective disorders. J. Psychiat. Res.,
     in press.

48. MURPHY,D.L., WEISS, R.: Reduced monoamine oxidase activity
     in blood platelets from bipolar depressed patients.
     Am. J. Psychiat., 128:11 1351-1357, 1972.

49. LECKMAN, J.F., GERSHON, E.S., MURPHY, D.L., NICHOLS, A.S.:
     Reduced platelet monoamine oxidase activity in first
     degree relatives of individuals with bipolar affective
     disorders: A preliminary report. To be presented at the
     1976 annual meeting of American Psychiatric Association.

50. BELMAKER, R.H., EBBESEN, K., EBSTEIN, R., RIMON, R.:
     Platelet monoamine oxidase in schizophrenia and manic
     depressive illness. in press, Brit. J. Psychiat. 1976.

GENETIC STUDIES IN SCHIZOAFFECTIVE ILLNESS

J. Mendlewicz

New York State Psychiatric Institute

New York, N.Y. 10032 U.S.A.

The group of schizoaffective illnesses raises some important nosological problems in defining the eventual relationship between schizophrenic and manic depressive illnesses.

Schizoaffective illness is usually defined as a syndrome combining schizophrenic-like symptoms and affective episodes either of a manic or of a depressive nature.

However, psychotic symptoms such as hallucinations and paranoid delusions are not rare in manic patients and depression as well as hyperactivity is also found in the course of schizophrenia.

In the last edition of the American Psychiatric Association manual, schizoaffective illness is classified as a subtype of schizophrenia. This hypothesis is not confirmed however by any clinical or biological study.

The aim of the present investigation is to review our current knowledge on the genetics of schizoaffective syndromes and present some additional data to study this syndrome in relation to schizophrenia and affective illness.

Most investigators today agree that schizophrenia and manic-depression represent two distinct genetic disorders.

The incidence of schizophrenia in the first degree relatives of affectively ill probands is no greater than in the general population (1). This is not true however for involutional melancholia. Kallmann has shown, in his New York State family study, the risk for schizophrenia in first degree relatives of involutional depressives to be three to four times greater than in the general population (2).

This observation is rather unexpected if one considers that involutional depression is a late onset disorder while schizophrenia
usually starts earlier in life.

Furthermore, the risk for schizophrenia in children of bipolar
manic-depressive parents is estimated to be 3-4%, while the risk
for manic-depressive psychosis in the families of schizophrenia is
no greater than in the general population. Another argument in
favor of a genetic distinction between schizophrenia and manic-
depression is the absence of reported pairs of monozygotic twins
where one brother is schizophrenic and the other manic-depressive.
In Slater's twin study on manic-depression, there is no single case
of schizophrenia in the relatives and/of co-twins of identical twins
(3).

Thus, there seems to be no genetic overlap between schizophrenia and manic-depression, which makes it unlikely that the heredity
of schizoaffective syndromes results from a combination of schizophrenic and affective genes. A natural genetic inbreeding experiment
is further provided by assortative mating between schizophrenic
and manic-depressive parents. If schizoaffective individuals possess
both schizophrenic and manic genes, one would expect such matings
to generate schizoaffective offsprings. Most of the studies descri-
bing such matings indicate that this is not the case: the affected
children are either schizophrenic or manic-depressive, but rarely
schizoaffective (4). These observations confirm the fact that the
schizoaffective phenotype is not determined by an interaction between schizophrenic and affective genotypes.

More recent studies done in the U.S. and in Japan suggest the
existence of a genetic link between schizoaffective syndromes and
affective psychoses. Asano, from Mitsuda's group in Japan, has
shown manic-depression to be frequent in the families of "atypical
manic probands", i.e. patients presenting both manic and schizo-
phrneic-like symptoms (5). Clayton et al, from Winokur's group,
have obtained similar results in a family study of 39 schizoaffective
probands (6). These authors have also shown that schizophrenia and
schizoaffective illness are rarely diagnosed in these families.
Recently, Cohen et al. have provided some interesting twin data
collected from 15,909 charts of twins hospitalised in the V.A.
hospitals (7). These investigators examined 420 twin pairs characte-
rised by one twin being psychotic.

Concordance rates in monozygotic twins are greater than in
dizygotic twins for each diagnostic category. These data underline
the importance of genetic factors in schizophrenia, manic-depression
and schizoaffective illness. Unexpectedly, the highest concordance
rates are found for schizoaffective twins, and these rates are
closer to the one found in manic-depressive psychosis than schizo-

TABLE 1.   CONCORDANCE RATES IN MONO AND DIZYGOTIC TWINS[*]

DIAGNOSIS	% CONCORDANCE MZ	% CONCORDANCE DZ
SCHIZOAFFECTIVE	50	0
MANIC-DEPRESSIVE	38.5	0
SCHIZOPHRENIC	23.5	5.3

[*] From Cohen et al. Arch. Gen. Psychiat., 26, 539, 1972.

affective illness is more comparable to the heritability of manic-depression than schizophrenia, an additional argument in favor of a genetic link between schizoaffective syndromes and affective psychoses.

The present study is part of an overall investigation of genetic factors in psychiatric illnesses. The probands are all from a population of 326 patients consecutively admitted from January 1971 until July 1973 in an outpatient (236 patients) and inpatient (90 patients) clinic treating patients with affective disorders at the New York State Psychiatric Institute. The sample consisted of 70 unipolar patients, 126 bipolar patients, 50 schizo-affective patients and 80 schizophrenic patients. All patients, their spouses, and their available first-degree, second degree, and third degree relatives on both the maternal and paternal sides were personally examined. When interviewing a proband's relative, the examiner was not informed as to whether the proband was unipolar, bipolar or schizoaffective. A modified version of the Current and Past Psychopathology Scales (8) and a clinical semistructured interview were used for the evaluation of psychopathology. Details on diagnosis and methodology are provided elsewhere (9). The diagnoses of bipolar and unipolar illness were based on criteria similar to those of Winokur et al (1) and according to the concept of "primary affective disorders" (10). The diagnosis of schizophrenia was based on Feighner's criteria (11). The diagnosis of schizoaffective illness required the presence of episodic affective syndromes of a manic or depressive type, as well as the presence of at least one schizophrenic .episode not concurrent to an affective syndrome. The duration of schizophrenic episodes varied from 6 weeks to 12 years. From this sample, 45 schizoaffective probands were matched for age and sex to 45 schizophrenics, 45 bipolar and 45 unipolar patients.

TABLE 2.   MORBIDITY RISKS IN FIRST-DEGREE RELATIVES

PROBAND	ALL AFFECTIVE ILLNESS in %	SCHIZOPHRENIA in %
BIPOLAR (N = 45)	41 ± 4	1.4 ± 1
UNIPOLAR (N = 45)	29 ± 6	3 ± 2
SCHIZOAFFECTIVE (N = 45)	36 ± 5	11 ± 4
SCHIZOPHRENIA (N = 45)	9 ± 4	17 ± 2

The age match was within three years.

Table II summarises the morbidity risks for affective illnesses and schizophrenia in the first degree relatives of affectively ill probands (bipolar and unipolar) versus schizoaffective
and schizophrenic probands. The risks tabulated are age corrected
estimates according to the Weinberg method (12). The risk period
has been adopted to be between 15 and 70 years for all illnesses.
The highest risks observed in relatives for all illnesses are for
bipolar and schizoaffective illnesses. The risks for all affective
illnesses in these relatives are also greater than in the relatives
of schizophrenic and unipolar probands. On the other hand, the risks
for schizophrenia in the relatives of bipolar and unipolar patients
are much lower than in the relatives of schizophrenic and schizoaffective patients where these risks are far from being negligible.
The risks for schizoaffective illness in all groups were too low
to be tabulated.

Table III illustrates the risks for unipolar versus bipolar
illness in the first-degree relatives of the probands. Here again,
the risks for both conditions are quite comparable in the relatives
of bipolar versus schizoaffective probands, although the risk for
bipolar illness is slightly more elevated in the relatives of bipolar patients. In previous observations, bipolar illness was rarely
found in relatives of unipolar and schizophrenic probands (13,14).
The risks for unipolar illness in the relatives of schizophrenic
patients are apparently higher than the one expected in the general
population.

The above family risk data indicate that both bipolar and unipolar illness are as common in the relatives of bipolar patients
as compared to schizoaffective patients. This may suggest some

TABLE 3. RISKS FOR BIPOLAR AND UNIPOLAR ILLNESS IN FIRST-DEGREE
RELATIVES

PROBAND	BIPOLAR in %	UNIPOLAR in %
BIPOLAR (N = 45)	18.6 ± 4.1	20.4 ± 2.8
UNIPOLAR (N = 45)	2.4 ± 3.1	27.2 ± 4.8
SCHIZOAFFECTIVE (N = 45)	13.7 ± 3.9	22.6 ± 4.1
SCHIZOPHRENIA (N = 45)	1.9 ± 2.4	7.3 ± 3.3

genetic overlap between the two psychoses. Schizophrenia, however,
is also present in a number of schizoaffective families, an observation indicating the presence of a possible genetic relationship
between schizoaffective and schizophrenic psychoses. But perhaps,
the most striking finding is the rarity of schizoaffective illness
in the relatives of schizoaffective probands. From the genetic point
of view, these observations make it very unlikely that schizoaffective illness represents a distinct genetic syndrome. More
conceivable, however, is the hypothesis that some schizoaffective
syndromes share some common genes with affective disorders, while
others may share genes with schizophrenia. In light of recent
genetic studies showing the presence of an X-linked dominant gene
in the transmission of manic-depression in a number of families (1),
we have been carrying linkage studies with X-linked chromosome
markers in various psychiatric conditions such as bipolar and unipolar illness (15) and more recently schizoaffective illness (14).

The description of methods and sampling have been published
in the above studies. In summary, the psychiatric interviews of
the relatives were always performed before the color vision examin-
ations, and by investigators who were blind to the psychiatric
status of the proband.

Figure 1 presents the pedigree of an informative family (L)
for the analysis of linkage between protanopia (an X-linked recessive color vision deficiency) and some psychiatric conditions including schizoaffective illness. The mother I (2) is unipolar and
heterozygous for protanopia, and according to the phenotype of her
brother I (3) who is bipolar, but not color blind, she is carrying
the traits for affective illness and color blindness in repulsion.
The proband II (1) is schizoaffective and has normal color vision,

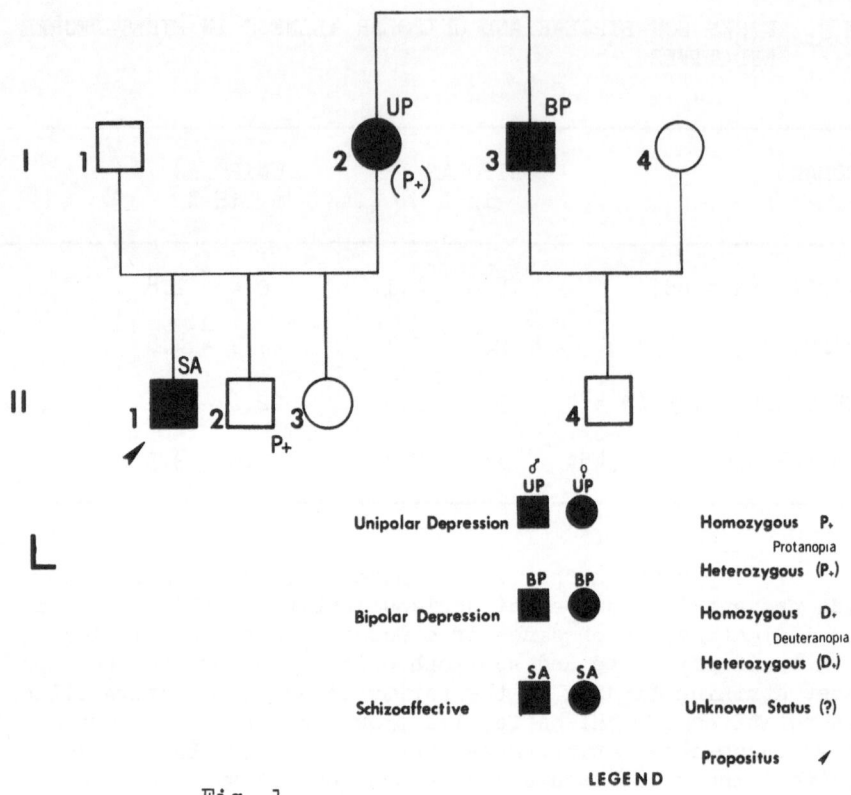

Fig. 1

while his younger brother II (2) is normal and color blind. Therefore II (1) and II (2) can be counted as two non-recombinants.

Figure 2 presents an informative pedigree (M), where deuteranopia and some mental disorders appear to assort in coupling. The
proband II (3) is schizoaffective and heterozygous for deuteranopia.
Her older brother II (2) is not color blind and normal, while the
youngest sister II (4) is bipolar and carries the gene for color
blindness. The proband's older sons III (1) and III (2), are both
bipolar and color blind, and the younger son III (3), is normal
and does not present any color vision anomaly. They have two first
cousins, III (5) and III (6), who have either both traits together,
III (6), or none of them, III (5).

In the next pedigree(T) (Figure 3), the proband II (3) carries
the genes for schizoaffective illness and deuteranopia in coupling,
as evidenced by her brother's phenotype II (2) and her father's
phenotype I (1). III (1), the older son is unipolar and color blind,
while the youngest son III (2) has none of these traits. Therefore,
III (1) and III (2) can be counted as two non recombinants.

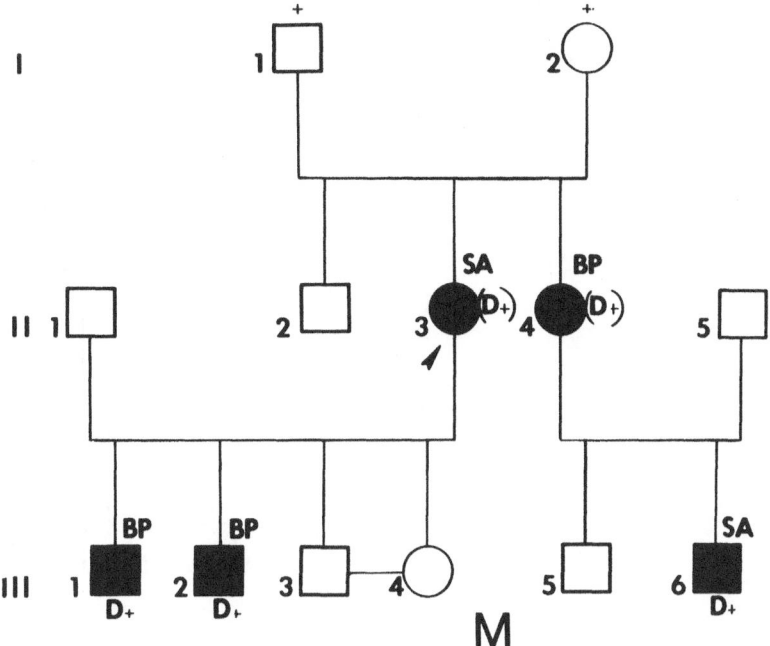

Fig. 2.   Same legend as Fig. 1.

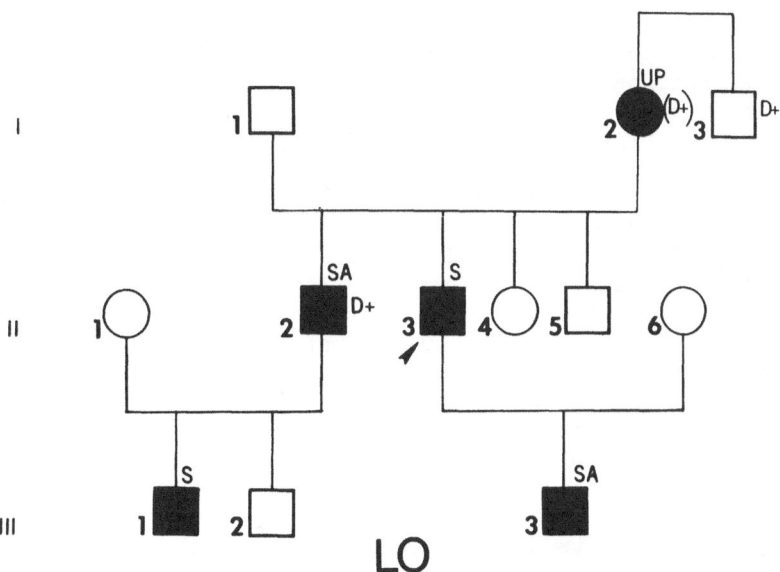

Fig. 3.   Same legend as Fig. 1.

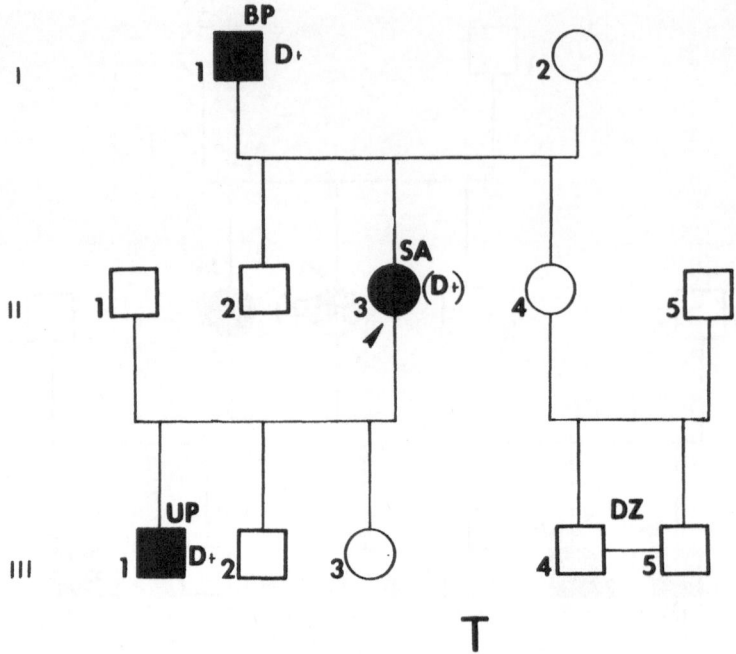

Fig. 4.   Same legend as Fig. 1.

Figure 4 illustrates an informative family (LO), where the
proband II (3) is schizophrenic. The proband's motherI (2) is
unipolar and heterozygous for deuteranopia. She carries the traits
in repulsion according to her brother's phenotype I (3), who is
normal and color-blind. The proband II (3) is schizophrenic but
not color-blind, while his older brother II (2), is schizoaffective
and color-blind, and his younger brother II (5), is normal and not
color-blind. Family LO also shows the presence of male to male
transmission in two instances: II (2) to II (1) and II (3) to III
(3). In both instances, the mothers II (1) and II (6) are not affected and there is no evidence of psychiatric disorder on the mother's
side of the family. Thus, it is clear that X-linkage can be ruled
out in family LO. This family also differs from the previous ones
in that schizophrenia is present in some relatives while bipolar
illness seems to be absent. It is too premature to say that the
presence of schizophrenia in a family together with other affective
psychosis is an indication that we are not dealing with an X-linked
form of disease. This is because of the rather limited number of
families studied to date and in light of the recent report of such
a family assorting for various affective illnesses (including
schizoaffective illness), schizophrenia, and the Xg blood group(16).

TABLE IV

FAMILY	Psychiatrically-ill and color-blind or well and normal vision	Psychiatrically-well and color-blind or ill and normal vision
L	0	2
M (proband's children)	3	0
(sister's children)	2	0
T	2	0
LO	2	1

In this report, data were consistent with X-linkage.

Table IV summarizes the results of the four informative families. The data are consistent with X-linkage in three of the four families. This table shows that in all but one of the sibships that there was consistency of the phase of color blindness and of psychiatric illness. This finding is compatible with X-linkage. These linkage studies are still in a preliminary stage and more families have to be ascertained before one can make more definite conclusions. Our family studies, although dealing with limited samples, enable through the matching process to compare on a more reliable basis, homogenous groups of psychiatric patients.

At this point, we can say that, at least on the basis of genetic studies, there is no evidence that schizoaffective illness represents a separate genetic entity. The definition and diagnostic criteria remain unclear however, and there are no longitudinal investigations to study the clinical outcome of this syndrome. One other hypothesis would be to consider a schizoaffective patient as someone who carries two different psychiatric disorders. Indeed, we have no biological reason to believe that the presence of schizophrenia in one individual would make this individual immune against manic-depressive illness, and vice-versa. This association, however, would be difficult to comprehend from the psychodynamic point of view. Furthermore, if one takes 1 of 10,000 as the gene frequency for manic-depression or

individual would be 1 out of 100,000,000 $(1/10^8)$, thus quite
improbable.

In conclusion, family and twin studies as well as linkage
studies with chromosome markers are suggestive of a main genetic
relationship between schizoaffective syndromes and affective
psychoses. Our studies also indicate that some schizoaffective
syndrome may be transmitted through the X-chromosome, as has been
demonstrated for some families with bipolar manic-depressive illness. It is thus conceivable that some schizoaffective phenotype
may express an allelic form of bipolar illness. Nevertheless, a
higher than expected incidence of schizophrenia is also reported
in the relatives of schizoaffective probands, and at least one
informative family assorting for schizoaffective and other illnesses
demonstrates a pattern clearly inconsistent with X-linkage. Those
preliminary observations indicate that at least one type of schizoaffective illness may be genetically related to schizophrenia.
Schizoaffective illness is thus to be considered as an heterogenous
condition encompassing different genetic forms, some of which are
related to affective psychoses while others are related to schizophrenia.

Current investigation pertaining to clinical outcome and long
term treatment response in various schizoaffective syndromes in
relation to genetic history are in progress.

REFERENCES

1.   WINOKUR, G., CLAYTON, P. and REICH, T.: Manic-depressive
         illness. C.V. Mosby, St. Louis, Missouri, 1969.

2.   KALLMANN, F.J.: Genetic principles in manic-depressive psycho-
         ses. In: Depression, eds. Hoch and Zubin, Grune &
         Stratton, New York, 1954.

3.   SLATER, E.: Psychotic and neurotic illnesses in twins. Spec.
         Ser. Med. Res. Coun., 278 Her Maj. Stat. Office, London,
         1953.

4.   SCHULZ, B.: Kinder von Elternsaaren mit einem schizophrenen
         und einem affektpsychotischen Partner. Z. Ges. Neurol.
         Psychiat., 170, 1940.

5.   ASANO, N.: Clinico-genetic study of manic-depressive psychoses.
         In: Clinical genetics in psychiatry, ed. Mitsuda H.,
         Osaka, 1967.

6.   CLAYTON, P.J., RODIN, L. and WINOKUR, G.: Family history studies
     III. Schizoaffective disorders, clinical and genetic
     factors including a one to two year follow-up. Compr.
     Psychiat., 9, 31, 1968.

7.   COHEN, S.M., ALLEN, M.G., POLLIN, W., HRUBEC, Z.: Relationship
     of schizoaffective psychosis to manic-depressive
     psychosis and schizophrenia. Arch. Gen. Psychiat.
     26, 539, 1972.

8.   ENDICOTT, J. and SPITZER, R.L.: Current and past psychopathology
     scales: rationale, reliability and validity. Arch. Gen.
     Psychiat., 27, 678, 1972.

9.   MENDLEWICZ, J., FLEISS, J.L., CATALDO, M., RAINER, J.D.:
     The accuracy of the family history method in family
     studies of affective illness. Arch. Gen. Psychiat.,
     32, 309-314, 1975.

10. ROBINS, E. and GUZE, S.B.: Classification of affective disorders;
     the primary-secondary, the endo-genous-reactive, and the
     neurotic-psychotic concepts. In: Recent Advances in
     Psychobiology of the Depressive Illness. Williams, T.A.
     Katz, M.M., and Shield, J.A. (Eds). Dept. of Health,
     Education and Welfare Publ. No. (HSM), 10-9053.

11. FEIGHNER, J.P., ROBINS, E., GUZE, S.B., WOODRUFF, R.A., Jr.
     WINOKUR, G., MUNOZ, R.: Diagnostic criteria for use in
     psychiatric research. Arch. Gen. Psychiat. 26, 57-63,
     1972.

12. WEINBERG, W.: Zur Vererbung bei manisch-depressiven Irresein.
     Z. fuer Ang. Anat. und Konst. Lehre, 6, 380-388, 1920.

13. ANGST, J. and PERRIS, C.: Zur nosologie endogener Depression.
     Vergleich der Ergebnisse der Untersuchungen. Arch.
     Psychiat. Z. Neurol., 210, 373, 1966.

14. MENDLEWICZ, J.: Donnees genetiques sur les schizophrenies
     dysthymiques. Symposium sur les troubles thymiques
     dans les schizophrenies. Clinique des Maladies Mentales
     et de l'Encephale. U.E.R. Cochin-Port-Royal. Publication
     Roche, 34-40, 1975.

15. MENDLEWICZ, J., FLEISS, J.L.: Linkage studies with X-chromosome
     markers in bipolar (manic-depressive) and unipolar
     (depressive) illnesses. Biol. Psychiat., 9, 261-294,
     1974.

16. BELMAKER, R.H., WYATT, R.J.: Possible X-linkage in a family
        with varied psychoses. <u>Israel Annals of Psychiatry</u>,
        in press.

THE SEARCH FOR GENETIC POLYMORPHISMS OF HUMAN BIOGENIC-AMINE RELATED ENZYMES

Robert H. Belmaker and Richard P. Ebstein

Jerusalem Mental Health Center

P.O.B. 140, Jerusalem, Israel

Genetic studies have provided some of the most convincing evidence of biological contributions to the etiology of severe mental illness (1). Both manic-depressive illness and schizophrenia appear to have large genetic components in their etiology, though nongenetic factors are clearly important too (2,3). As the role of genetic factors becomes increasingly clear and scientifically well-founded, the next challenge becomes the elucidation of the mechanism of genetic transmission. Some aspect of physiology or biochemistry must be altered in an individual who carries the genetic predisposition to a mental illness. This genetically-based alteration, if identified, could conceivably someday serve as a "genetic marker" for mental illness, and allow medicine to concentrate its preventive efforts on those individuals who are genetically at risk. An analogy can be found in the disease favism, caused by a defect in the enzyme glucose-6-phosphate dehydrogenase (G6PD) (4). The enzyme is often assayed in screening programs of populations at risk, and affected individuals are advised on proper dietary avoidances. Favism provides an analogy for another important point relating to schizophrenia and manic-depressive illness, in that not all individuals with the abnormal gene for favism develop symptoms of the illness (5). The gene for favism is inherited as a simple X-linked recessive, but ingestion of special foods or other environmental circumstances are necessary to provoke the symptoms of hemolytic anemia in an individual carrying the gene. It is clear that not all individuals genetically at risk for schizophrenia or manic-depressive illness develop these illnesses (1,2). A third to two-thirds of monozygotic cotwins of schizophrenics are not schizophrenic (2,6), though they are of course genetically identical in every way to their siblings. The search for genetic markers of

241

schizophrenia and manic-depressive illness does not contradict
the importance of environmental factors in enhancing or inhibiting
the expression of abnormal genes.

The "central dogma" of modern molecular biology states that
genes express themselves through proteins, often enzyme proteins
(7). The gene is a DNA structure that serves as a code or template
for the synthesis (or translation) of RNA, which carries the genetic
message to the cytoplasmic ribosomes. On the basis of the RNA code
or template, the synthesis (or transcription) of proteins is accomplished. Each set of three nucleotide base pairs in DNA codes for
a particular amino acid in a protein (though in some cases the DNA
code is redundant and other sets of base pairs code for nonstructural
"instructions"). Alterations in a DNA base pair (a mutation) usually
results in the replacement of a particular amino acid in a particular
protein by another amino acid (7). If this amino acid change occurs
in an unimportant part of the protein structure, no obvious change
in physiology or biochemistry may occur. If, however, the active
site or a regulatory site in an enzyme protein is altered, biochemical and physiological repercussions of the DNA mutation may be
evident. If the amino acid substitution occurred in a subtle
regulatory site whose function is dependent on specific environmental circumstances, the repercussions of the DNA mutation may
be apparent only under those specific environmental circumstances(7).

Rare gene mutants account for the enzyme abnormalities seen in
diseases such as phenylketonuria (4), Tay-Sachs disease (8), or
homocystinuria (9). However, other enzyme or protein variants are
much more common, such as G6PD mutants (10) or sickle cell hemo-
globin (4). G6PD deficiency occurs in almost 50% of the population
of Kurdish Jewish males (11) in Israel, and perhaps 40% of individuals in some parts of Africa have one allele for sickle cell hemo-
globin (4). It has been proposed that these polymorphisms, or
common variant forms, have been selected for because of some natural
advantage in specific environments. Harris, however, has found that
a third of the enzymes studied have demonstrated polymorphic genetic
forms in human populations (4). Surveys of enzymes in fruit flys
and mice have also revealed extensive natural variation in enzyme
structure (12). Table 1 suggests the large number of as yet undis-
covered human polymorphisms. The evolutionary or physiological
function of this polymorphism is unknown. Johnson (13) has suggested
that polymorphism of enzymes occurs most commonly at regulatory sites
in metabolism, where the existence of heterozygosity allows for a
doubled range of enzyme "abilities". He suggests also that enzymes
utilizing substrates from the external environment are often polymorphic, allowing a species to adjust easily to changes in the
chemical environment. Zouros, (12) on the other hand, suggests that
most enzyme polymorphism is evolutionarily neutral and related to
genetic shift or random, nonsignificant DNA mutations. Yoshida (10)
has emphasized with regard to the over 80 known forms of G6PD enzyme

TABLE 1   Estimate of Number of Protein Polymorphisms in Man[*]

Total nucleotide pairs in haploid human chromosome set	3 billion
Maximum number of genes (1 gene per 1000 nucleotide pairs)	3 million
Probable number of structural genes (2% of DNA)	60,000
Probable number of polymorphic genes (30% of structural genes)	20,000
Number of human polyphormisms known:	50
Percent of polymorphic genes discovered (50/20,000)	.25

[*]   Reprinted with permission from reference 14.

in man, that some forms are associated with pathology but many other forms seem physiologically neutral.

The above discussion has attempted to introduce the idea that particular genetic forms of some human proteins or enzymes may represent the biological basis of the genetic predisposition to schizophrenia or manic-depressive illness. Just which of the 60,000-odd proteins in human metabolism (14) should be studied in mental illness is to some extent an educated guess. The known biogenic-amine neurotransmitters are synthesized and metabolized by less than a dozen enzymes, (15) and careful but not exclusive attention to these enzymes is perhaps justified by the importance of their associated neurotransmitters. A Utopian, simple model of manic-depressive illness, for example, might hypothesize a genetic alteration in tyrosine hydroxylase that damages its regulatory feedback site for norepinephrine binding. Such an enzyme, which in vivo is indeed rate-limiting in the synthesis of catecholamines, (15) might function normally under average circumstances. A stimulus to increase catecholamine synthesis, however, might not be checked by appropriate feedback inhibition and thereby lead to extreme catecholamine excess ("mania") (16).Or a stimulus to decrease catecholamine synthesis might not be checked by appropriate release of feedback inhibition, thereby leading to extreme catecholamine depletion ("depression") (16). The role of environmental triggers is clearly apparent in this speculative model.

Unfortunately, tyrosine hydroxylase is not obtainable peripherally in a convenient manner in psychiatric patients. Study of this enzyme from autopsy brain material in psychiatric patients might be most worthwhile. Several other catecholamine-related enzymes are available in human blood, however. The present review will discuss our findings with catechol-O-methyltransferase (COMT) and monoamine oxidase (MAO), the two catabolic enzymes of biogenic amine metabolism. Studies of enzyme activity will serve as an introduction to electrophoretic studies that have attempted to discover mutant or polymorphic forms

of these enzymes, i.e. genetically based amino acid substitutions in
these enzymes.

COMT is one of the two principal enzymes responsible for the
catabolism of catecholamines (17). O-methylation serves to terminate
the action of that fraction of neuronally-released catecholamines
which is not removed from the synaptic cleft either by the high
affinity uptake system or by simple diffusion away from the receptor.
The presence of soluble COMT activity in human red blood cells (RBC)
was first reported by Axelrod and Cohn (18). Some of the parameters
important in the regulation of COMT activity in RBC have been identified (19,20,21). Most importantly, Weinshilboum et al (22) have
reported a significant sibling-sibling correlation for soluble RBC
COMT activity, suggesting a major role of heredity in determining
the levels of activity of this enzyme. These results were corroborated by a recent twin study from our laboratory by Grunhaus et
al (23).

Cohn et al (24) reported in 1970 that total RBC COMT activity
was significantly reduced in female patients with affective disorders.
The reduced COMT activity in the affectively-ill patients was not
related to the phase of the illness, drugs or hospitalization (25,26).
These results were confirmed by Briggs and Briggs (19) who also
reported decreased activity of RBC COMT in affectively-ill patients.
However, Gershon and Jonas (27) at the Jerusalem Mental Health Center
observed a significant increase in RBC COMT activity in manic-depressive patients. It is important to note that Cohn et al (24) used
norepinephrine as substrate whereas Gershon and Jonas (27) used
dihydroxphenylacetic acid (DOPAC). The failure of Gershon and Jonas
(27) to corroborate the findings of Cohn et al (24) could be due to
the existence of different molecular forms of COMT with different
substrate specificities. This, in addition to the large degree of
genetic control over RBC COMT activity (22,23) suggested the possibility that the reduced COMT levels in patients with affective disorders might reflect an underlying genetic difference in the COMT
molecule in affective illness (28). Several reports have suggested
possible involvement of COMT in schizophrenia as well as affective
illness. Matthyse and Baldessarini (29) observed a small increase
in RBC COMT activity in schizophrenic patients. Although Poitou
et al (30) found no such increase for soluble RBC COMT, they did
observe a significant increase in the activity of the membrane-bound
COMT in schizophrenic patients. Furthermore, Shopsin et al (31)
reported a higher Michaelis constant for RBC COMT obtained from
paranoid schizophrenic patients.

We therefore decided to examine RBC COMT from schizophrenic
patients and manic-depressive patients for possible amino acid substitutions. We chose the technique of polyacrilamide gel electrophoresis (PAGE) because of its sensitivity and its success in detecting

variant forms of other enzymes (4). In the PAGE system the enzyme is placed at the end of a prepared gel of specific pore size and the gel is placed in an electric field (32,33). Most proteins are negatively charged and thus migrate toward the anode. The rate of migration is determined at least partly by the specific electric charge of the specific protein, and thus PAGE sensitively separates different proteins. The algebraic sum of the exposed charged amino acids containing free COO^- or NH_3^+ groups determines the charge of the protein (7). Thus a mutation with an amino acid substitution that changes the charge of a protein will change the protein's migration rate in PAGE. It is important to note that the charge of a protein depends also on pH, since free H^+ radicals in acid solutions neutralize the charge of carboxyl groups, and the yielding of H^+ by NH_3 groups in basic solutions eliminates their charge (7). Under some pH conditions an amino acid substitution may well not be revealed, and the mutant enzyme may migrate identically with the normal form. If a mutant form is present with a different charge and thus a different migration rate, PAGE can often separate the mutant form from the native enzyme form. Another aspect of PAGE is its ability to separate natural isozymes, or different protein molecules that in the same individual perform similar biochemical catalyses (4). The five different isozymes of lactate dehydrogenase (LDH) or the two different isozymes hexosaminodase are examples (4,8). In Tay-Sachs disease only one hexosaminodase isozyme is absent (8), presumably because of a mutation that totally abolishes this isozyme's activity. Thus in PAGE the investigator searches both for migration rate differences between individuals and for changes in isozymic forms in enzymes that have isozyme subtypes.

For PAGE of COMT a 7.5% polyacrilamide gel was used. Twenty-five microliter samples of packed human RBC, diluted 1:4 in water, was optimal to give adequate enzyme activity for detection and acceptable sharpness of electrophoretic pattern. Electrophoresis was run at 5°C at pH 8.3 for approximately 90 minutes, the exact time being determined by the running time of a bromphenol blue dye marker. Gels were sliced by hand into 2mm segments and each segment was assayed for COMT activity with a specific radioactive assay as described in detail elsewhere (34). Stains for enzyme activity were not found sensitive enough for the detection of the small amounts of COMT activity in individual RBC samples (35), or (see below) the small amounts of MAO activity in individual platelet or plasma samples (36). About 35% of the COMT (or MAO) activity applied to a gel column could be recovered after electrophoresis.

Fig. 1 shows the COMT pattern after PAGE from 15 controls, 14 schizophrenic and 12 manic-depressive individuals. Two peaks of enzyme activity are detectable, but there are no differences in the rate of migration of either band in any of the groups examined. No individual person was observed to have a band of COMT activity

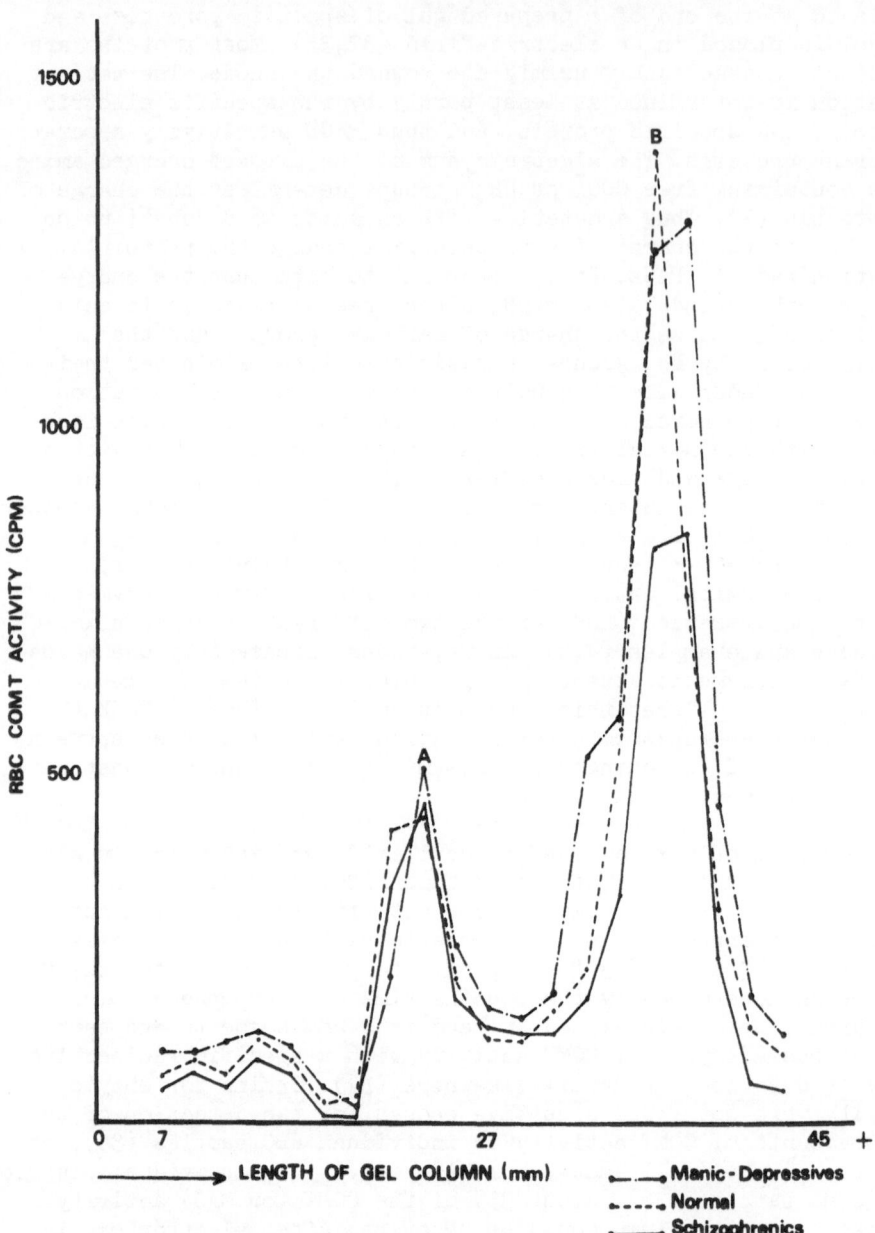

Fig. 1. Mean electrophoretic pattern of RBC COMT
         from schizophrenic, manic-depressive and
         control individuals.

with an abnormal rate of migration at the pH 8.3 used, or a total absence of either COMT band. Re-examination of total RBC COMT activity before PAGE of this group of individuals confirmed the previous report from the Jeruslaem Mental Health Center to the effect that manic-depressive patients have higher RBC COMT activity (27,34).

White and Wu (35) have also reported two PAGE bands of COMT from human brain and human liver during electrophoresis at higher pH levels. The brain and liver enzymes showed identical electrophoretic mobility, suggesting that peripheral COMT enzyme is indeed the same protein as that in brain. That the peripheral enzymes are identical to those in brain is indeed a critical assumption of the research strategy presented here. Some human genetic diseases, such as Tay-Sachs (8) or homocystinuria (9), provide fruitful examples of the correctness of such an assumption in some enzyme systems. Tay-Sachs disease and homocystinuria primarily affect the brain, yet the etiologic enzyme abnormality can be detected in peripheral tissues. Enzymes in the glycolytic pathway (14), however, may be examples of marked tissue differences between brain and periphery in the nature of enzyme proteins.

Monoamine oxidase (MAO) is the other important enzyme in the catabolism of brain biogenic amines (37,38). Human platelets contain an intramitochondrial MAO that is similar in many physiochemical properties to brain MAO (39). There are large differences between human individuals in levels of activity of the platelet MAO enzyme, and these individual differences seem to be largely genetic in origin (40). Schizophrenic (41) and manic-depressive (42) patients have been reported as having low platelet MAO. Reduced platelet MAO activity has been felt to be a possible genetic marker in schizophrenia (43), because of the results of a study of monozygotic twins discordant for schizophrenia. In this study of monozygotic discordant twins Wyatt et al (43) found that both the schizophrenic twin and his healthy co-twin had reduced platelet MAO activity, indicating that the finding is not due to hospitalization, psychoactive drugs or other secondary effects of illness (44).

Fig. 2 shows the distribution of platelet MAO activity in a series of schizophrenic patients and controls from Bethesda, Maryland (39). It is clear that mean enzyme activity is reduced in the patient group but that considerable overlap of enzyme activiity exists between the two groups. No bimodality of enzyme activity is suggested, either in the patient or control group. The report of Cohn et al (24) of reduced COMT activity in affective disorder was also characterized by overlap between patients and controls and absence of bimodality. It has been discussed elsewhere that overlap between ill and control groups is an expected, perhaps essential, feature of genetic findings in psychiatry (39). Monozygotic twin discordance rates imply that

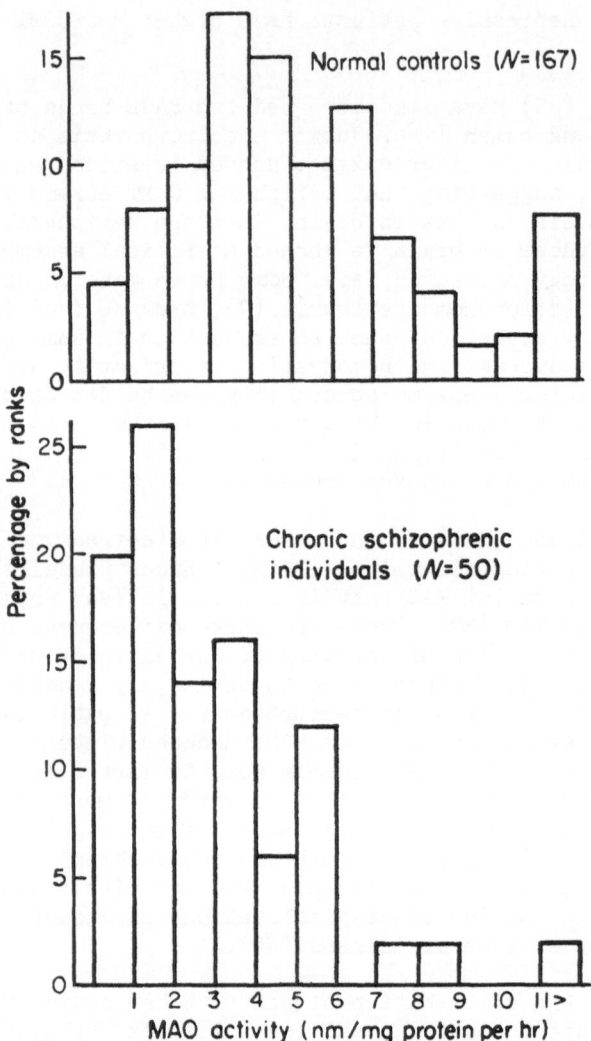

Fig. 2.   Distribution of platelet MAO activity in
          a series of schizophrenic and control
          individuals from Bethesda, Maryland.
          Reproduced with permission from reference 39.

many normal individuals carry the unexpressed genetic predisposition
for mental illness. These individuals will show the same "genetic
markers" as ill patients (39). It is also true that qualitative
enzyme abnormalities, such as mutant forms, need not result in a
bimodal distribution of enzyme activity (4). Fig. 3 shows the
enzyme activity in a population containing three qualitatively
different alleles of acid phosphatase. These alleles are electrophoretically distinguishable, but the distribution of human RBC
acid phosphatase activity is unimodal and almost normally distributed (4).

The finding of low platelet MAO in schizophrenia was confirmed
by Meltzer and Stahl (45) in chronic patients, but was not found
by Carpenter et al (46) in a group of acute schizophrenic patients.
Friedman et al (47) using newly admitted patients with recurrent
schizophrenia, could not demonstrate reduced platelet MAO activity.
A recent study at the Jerusalem Mental Health Center (48) could
not demonstrate a reduction in platelet MAO of chronic schizophrenic
patients, but found manic-depressive patients to have significantly
higher (!) platelet MAO activities than controls. Unlike the situation with COMT, this directly opposite result was found despite the
use of identical substrates (benzylamine and tryptamine) in the
Jerusalem study (48) and the Bethesda studies (39). E.S. Gershon
in this volume has commented on possible relevant population
differences between Bethesda and Jerusalem, in attempting to understand why both COMT and MAO may be reduced in manic-depressive
patients in Bethesda and elevated in manic-depressive patients in
Jerusalem. It struck us that enzyme activity may not be an etio-
pathologic factor in itself, but merely a reflection of mutant
enzyme forms. The different mutant forms of MAO, both associated
with manic-depressive illness, could conceivably be associated in
one case with reduced and in the other case with elevated enzyme
activity. Examples of this sort of phenomenon occur among G6PD
mutant types (10). If such a model were true, a different mutant
form might be prevalent in Bethesda than in Jerusalem, much as
sickle cell disease is a major cause of anemia in Africa and
thalassemia a major cause of anemia in Greece (4).

Again, we turned to PAGE to attempt to find mutant forms of
platelet MAO. PAGE of MAO is more difficult than PAGE of COMT,
because MAO is a much larger molecule and is membrane-bound in
addition (49). The platelet MAO was solubilized for PAGE as gently
as possible, with 5 seconds of sonication in 1% Triton X-100.
PAGE with 5% gels was necessary to allow entry of the enzyme,
but no Triton was used in the gel or buffer solution itself. We
feared that an excess of Triton would coat all proteins present
and prevent the appearance of differences in migration rate due
to small charge differences. Fifty microliter samples of platelet
sonicate were placed on the gels for PAGE, and after electrophoresis
the gels were sliced and each segment assayed for MAO activity as

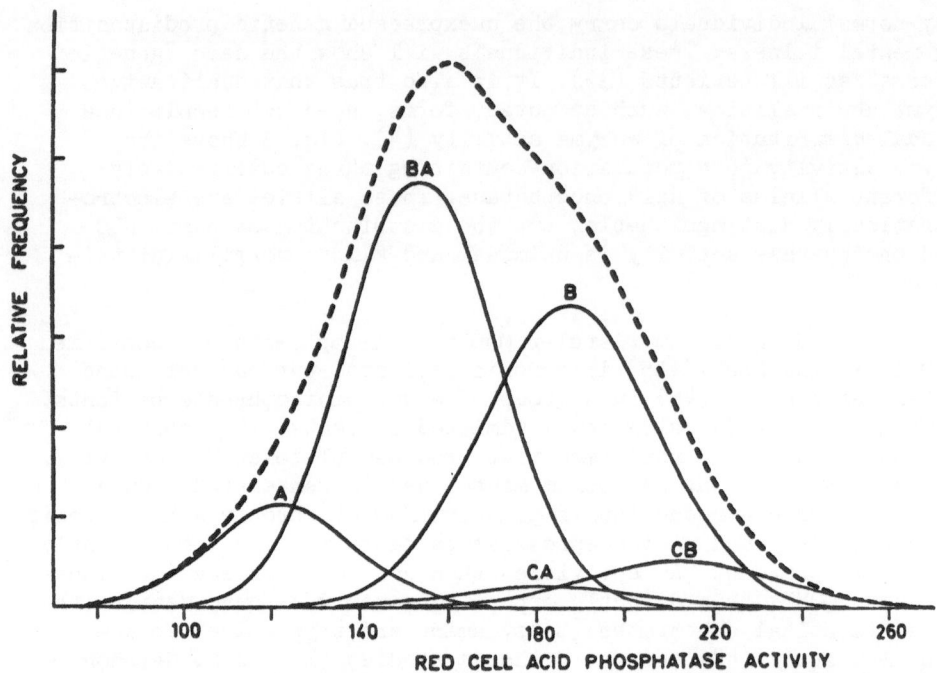

Fig. 3. Distribution of red cell acid phosphatase
activities in the general population (broken
line) and in the separate pheno-types.
Reproduced with permission from reference 4.

described elsewhere (50). The activity was confirmed to be platelet
MAO by abolition of activity with $10^{-4}M$ pargyline.

Fig. 4 shows the platelet MAO pattern after PAGE from 11 control, 12 schizophrenic, and 10 manic-depressive individuals. Two
peaks are apparent, confirming the recent study of Edwards and
Chang (51). A previous report (49) that found platelet MAO to be
electrophoretically homogenous used purified enzyme that may have
undergone changes in physiochemical properties. Edwards and Chang
(51) suggest that the slower peak of platelet MAO may represent
an aggregrate, though we did not find differences in the two peaks
with varying amounts of sonication.

No rate variations were found between the clinical groups in
platelet MAO electrophoresis. The increased platelet MAO activity
of manic-depressive patients in Jerusalem (48) is clearly apparent
in Fig. 4 even after the enzyme has been subjected to PAGE. However,
no individual patients were noted to have an absence of either
electrophoretic band, and no individual was found with a peak
in a reproducibly altered position on the gel at the pH 8.3 used.

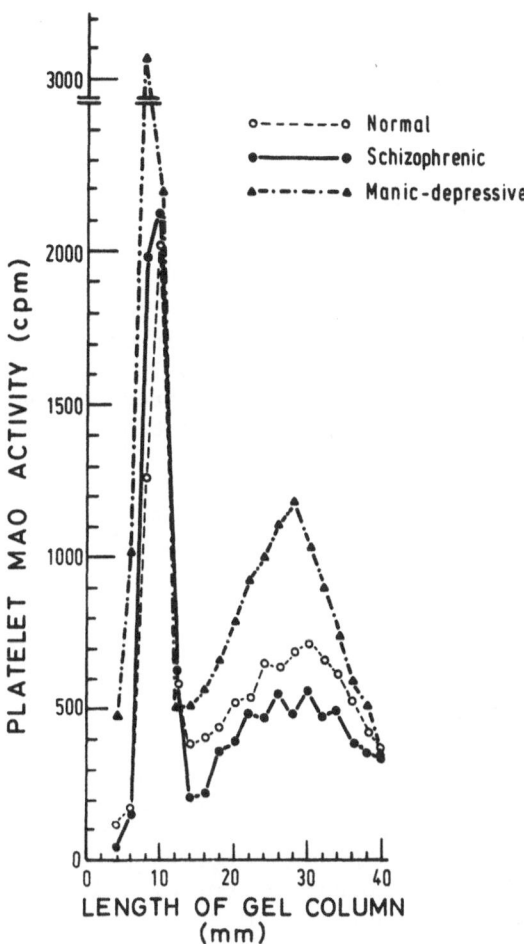

Fig. 4. Mean electrophoretic pattern of platelet MAO from schizophrenic, manic-depressive and control individuals.

The relationship of platelet and brain MAO has been a subject of considerable controversy (39). Multiple electrophoretic forms of MAO have been reported in brain (52), which suggested that platelet MAO characteristics could scarcely have general relevance for brain MAO. Tipton (53) et al, however, have reported that the multiple electrophoretic forms of brain MAO can be reduced to one by treatment with perchloric acid, an agent that presumably strips varying types of lipid attachment. This implied that perhaps one MAO gene product exists, one MAO protein, whose properties are partially determined by lipid attachments. Others have divided MAO into Type A and Type B, according to inhibition sensitivity with clorgyline or deprenyl (54). Platelet MAO is a B Type enzyme in this classification whereas "brain-specific" MAO is Type A (55). Inhibitor sensitivity, however, may also be affected by lipid attachments, as perchlorate treatment abolishes differences in response to clogyline (53). Three recent studies of brain MAO from schizophrenic patients did not reveal reduced enzyme activity compared to controls (56,57,58) but interpretation of these studies is complicated by the technical problems of human post-mortem studies (58). The present lack of success in finding polymorphic forms of platelet MAO should not be accepted as conclusive. Additional pH levels should be used for further electrophoretic screening. Additionally, biochemical methods need to be developed to "clean" MAO of its lipid attachments without coating the enzyme with Triton-like detergents. Electrophoresis of such a clean enzyme might yield more information about the enzyme's characteristics, including possible mutant forms.

Plasma MAO is an entirely different enzyme than platelet MAO and is probably much further from brain MAO than is the platelet enzyme (39). Plasma MAO is soluble rather than mitochondrial, uses pyridoxal rather than FAD as a cofactor, and is much less sensitive to pargyline inhibition than the mitochondrial MAO's (39). Nevertheless, plasma MAO has been reported as reduced in schizophrenic patients (59) and elevated in depressed patients (60). Nies et al (40) found a high degree of genetic control over levels of plasma as well as platelet MAO, and Robinson et al (61) reported that plasma, platelet and brain MAO all rise with age in a parallel manner. In order to examine whether possible mutant forms of the plasma MAO exist, we carried out PAGE of plasma MAO from 10 schizophrenic patients, 10 manic-depressive patients, 5 unipolar depressive patients and 8 normal controls. Electrophoresis was run on 7.5% gels at pH 8.3 using 50 microliter plasma samples. The plasma MAO inhibitor isoniazid at 10^{-2}M was capable of abolishing 100% of the activity on the gel after PAGE. Further details of the procedure are reported elsewhere (62). Fig. 5 shows PAGE patterns of the clinical groups. The enzyme is homogenous with a single peak. Again, no pattern differences were observed between clinical groups and no reproducible individual differences were observed for any subject. This is in contrast to the preliminary report of Shih and Eiduson (63), who found multiple bands of plasma MAO that varied in depression. These authors, however, used staining technique which have been criticized as productive of artifacts, (36) and which were not reliable in our hands. Studies at the Jerusalem Mental Health Center could also find no changes in the enzyme activity of plasma MAO in affective disorder (64) or schizophrenia (48).

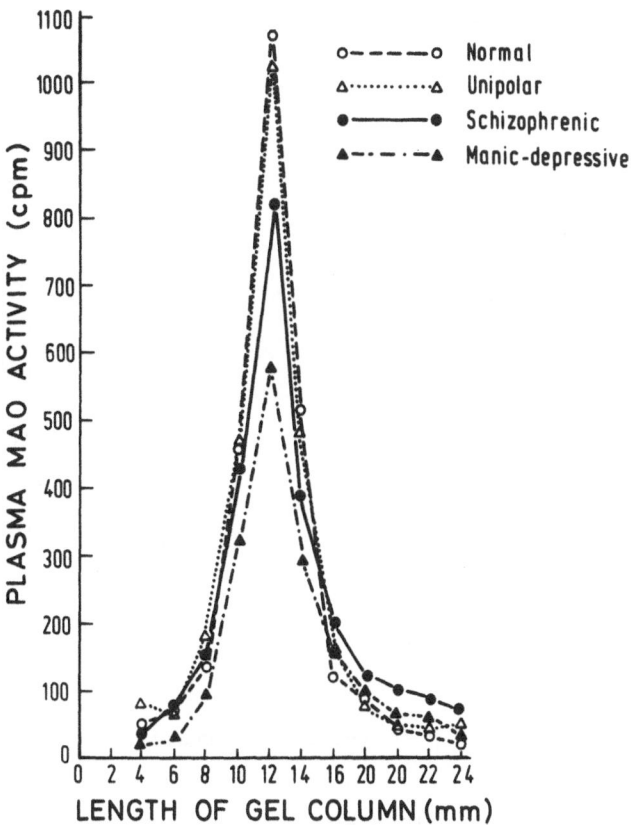

Fig. 5.   Mean electrophoretic pattern of plasma MAO
          from schizophrenic, manic-depressive, uni-
          polar depressive and control individuals.

A summary statement of the present state of catecholamine
enzymes and psychiatric disorder should convey both the modesty
of the findings and the excitement of the field. COMT is elevated
in manic-depressive illness in Jerusalem but reduced in Bethesda.
Platelet MAO is markedly reduced in schizophrenia in Bethesda but
is normal in Jerusalem schizophrenic patients. No mutant forms of
RBC COMT or platelet or plasma MAO have been identified, despite
the general findings by others (4) that a third of enzymes studied
have variants. Studies by Omenn and Motulsky (14) on enzymes in
the glycolytic pathway in the brain (Table 2.) were also surprisingly
negative, in that mutant forms were extremely rare. It may be that
brain and even more specifically catecholamine systems are highly
conservative evolutionarily, and highly restricted in polymorphism.
On the other hand, schizophrenia and manic-depressive illness are

TABLE 2. Electrophoretic Screening of Glycolytic Enzymes in Human
          Brain Tissue[*]

Enzyme	No. variant/Total alleles
Hexokinase	0/300
Phosphohexoseisomerase	0/300
Phosphofructokinase	0/240
Aldolase	0/600 (2 loci)
Triosephosphate isomerase	0/300
Glyceraldehyde-3-phosphate dehydrogenase	0/240
Phosphoglycerate kinase	1/203
Phosphoglycerate mutase	0/300
Enolase	1/300
Pyruvate kinase	0/300
Lactate dehydrogenase	0/600 (2 loci)

*   Reprinted with permission from reference 14.

partially genetic illnesses and modern genetics is largely biochemical genetics. Peripheral MAO and COMT may provide windows
into the genes that control catecholamine enzymes. Much further
study of these enzymes is justified, including electrophoretic
screening at different pH levels in psychiatric patients and
determination of the biochemical relationship between the enzyme
activities in different tissues and brain.

REFERENCES

1. ROSENTHAL, D.: Genetic Theory and Abnormal Behavior,
   McGraw-Hill Book Co., New York, 1970.

2. POLLIN, W.: The pathogenesis of schizophrenia, Arch. Gen.
   Psychiat, 27:29,1972.

3. GERSHON, E.S., DUNNER, D.L. and GOODWIN, F.K.: Toward a biology
   of affective disorders: genetic contributions. Arch. Gen.
   Psychiat., 25:1-15, 1971.

4. HARRIS, H.: The Principles of Human Biochemical Genetics.
   North-Holland Publishing Co., Amsterdam, 1975, Second Ed.

5. WINTROBE, M.M., THORN, G.W., ADAMS, R.D., BENNET, I.L. jr.,
   BRAUNWALD, E., ISSELBACHER, K.J., PETERSDORF, R.G. (eds),
   Harrison's Principles of Internal Medicine, Vol. II, Sixth
   Ed. 1970, McGraw-Hill p. 1621

6. BELMAKER, R., POLLIN, W., WYATT, R.J., COHEN, S.: A follow-up
   of monozygotic twins disordant for schizophrenia, Arch. Gen.
   Psychiat., 30:219, 1974.

7. WATSON, J.D.: The Molecular Biology of the Gene, W.A. Benjamin,
   New York, 1965.

8. OKADA, S. and O'BRIAN, J.S.,: Tay-Sachs disease: Generalized
   absence of a B-D-N-acetylhexosaminidase component. Science,
   165:698, 1969.

9. UHLENDORF, W.B. and MUDD, H.S.: Cystathionine Synthase in tissue
   culture derived from human skin: enzyme defect in homocystinuria. Science, 160:1007-1009, 1968.

10. YOSHIDA, A.: Hemolytic anemia and G6PD deficiency. Science,
    179-532, 1973.

11. SZEINBERG, A.: Investigation of genetic polymorphic traits in
    Jews. Israel J. Med. Sci., 9:1171, 1973, (Supplement).

12. ZOUROS, E.: Electrophoretic variation in allelozymes related
    to function or structure? Nature, 254:446, 1975.

13. JOHNSON, G.B.: Enzyme polymorphism and metabolism, Science,
    184:28, 1974.

14. OMENN, G.S. and MOTULSKY, A.G.: Biochemical genetics and the
    evolution of human behavior, Genetics, Environment and
    Behavior. Ehrman.L.. Omenn. G.S. and Caspari, E. (eds),

15. SPECTOR, S., GORDON, R., SJOERDSMA, A. and UDENFRIEND, S.: End-product inhibition of tyrosine hydroxylase as a possible mechanism for regulation of norepinephrine synthesis. Molec. Pharmac., 3:549, 1967.

16. SCHILDKRAUT, J.J.: The catecholamine hypothesis of affective disorders: A review of supporting evidence. Amer. J. Psychiat. 122:509, 1965.

17. AXELROD, J.: Methylation reactions in the formation and metabolism of catecholamines and other biogenic amines. Pharmacol. Rev., 18:95, 1966.

18. AXELROD, J. and COHN, C.K.: Methyltransferase enzymes in red blood cells. J. Pharmacol. Exp. Ther., 176:650, 1971.

19. BRIGGS, M.H. and BRIGGS, M.: Hormonal influences on erythrocyte catechol-0-methyltransferase activity in humans. Experientia, 29:278,;973.

20. WEISS, J.L., COHN, C.K. and CHASE, T.N.: Reduction of catechol-0-methyltransferase activity by chronic L-dopa therapy. Nature, 234:218, 1971.

21. GUSTAVSON, K.H., WETTERBERG, L., BACKSTROM, M. and ROSS, S.B.: Catechol-0-methyltransferase activity in erythrocytes in Down's syndrome. Clin. Gen., 4:279, 1973.

22. WEINSHILBOUM, R.M., RAYMOND, F.S., ELEVEBACK, L.R. and WEIDMAN, W. H.: Red blood cell catechol-0-methyltransferase activity: sibling-sibling correlation. Nature, 252-490, 1974.

23. GRUNHAUS, L., EBSTEIN, R., BELMAKER, R.H., SANDLER, S.G. and JONAS, W.: A twin study of human red blood cell catechol-0-methyltransferase. Brit. J. Psychiat., 128, 494-98, 1976

24. COHN, C.K., DUNNER,D.L. and AXELROD, J.: Reduced catechol-0-methyltransferase activity in red blood cells of women with primary affective disorders. Science, 170:1323, 1970.

25. DUNNER, D.L., COHN, C.K., GERSHON, E.S. and GOODWIN, F.K.: Differential catechol-0-methyltransferase activity in unipolar and bipolar affective illness. Arch. Gen. Psychiat., 25:348, 1971.

26. WEINSHILBOUM, R.M., RAYMOND, F.A., ELEVEBACK, L.R. and WEIDMAN, W.H.: Red blood cell catechol-0-methyltransferase activity: sibling-sibling correlation, Pharmacologist, 16:236, 1974.

27. GERSHON, E.S. and JONAS, W.Z.: Erythrocyte soluble catechol-O-
    methytransferase activity in primary affective disorder.
    Arch. Gen. Psychiat., 32:1351, 1975.

28. MURPHY, D.L.: Technical strategies for the study of catechol-
    amines in man, Frontiers in Catecholamine Research, Usdin,
    E. and Snyder, S. H. (eds), Pergamon Press, p. 1077, 1973.

29. MATTYSSE, S and BALDESSARINI, R.J.: S-adenosylmethionine and
    catechol-O-methyltransferase in schizophrenia. Amer. J.
    Psychiat., 128:10,1972.

30. POITOU, P., ASSICOT, M. and BOHUON, C.: Soluble and membrane
    catechol-O-methyltransferase in red blood cells of schizo-
    phrenic patients. Biomedicine, 21:91-93, 1974.

31. SHOPSIN,B., WILK, S., GERSHON, S., ROFFMAN, M. and GOLDSTEIN,
    M.: Collaborative psychopharmacologic studies exploring cate-
    cholamine metabolism in psychiatric disorders, Frontiers
    in Catecholamine Research, Usdin, E. and Snyder, S.H. (eds),
    Pergamon Press, p. 1173, 1973.

32. ORNSTEIN, L.: Disc electrophoresis, Part I. Ann. NY Acad. Sci.,
    121:321, 1964.

33. DAVIS, B.: Disc electrophoresis-II: Method and application to
    human serum proteins. Ann. NY Acad. Sci., 121:404, 1964.

34. EBSTEIN, R., BELMAKER, R.H., BENBENISTY, D. and RIMON, R.:
    Electrophoretic pattern of red blood cell catechol-O-
    methyltransferase in schizophrenia and manic-depressive
    illness. J. Biol. Psychiat., in press.

35. WHITE, H.L. and WU, J.C.: Properties of catechol-O-methy-
    transferase from brain and liver of rat and human.
    Biochem. J., 145:135, 1975.

36. YOUDIM, M.B.H. and LAGNADO, J.R.: Limitation in the use of
    tetrazolium salts for the detection of multiple forms of
    monoamine oxidase. Costa, E. and Greengard, P. (eds),
    Advances in Biochemical Psychopharmacology, 5:289, New York,
    Raven Press 1972.

37. KOPIN, I.J.: Storage and metabolism of catecholamines: The role
    of monoamine oxidase. Pharmac. Rev.,16:179, 1964.

38. WEINER, N. and BJUR,R.: The role of intraneuronal monoamine
    oxidase in the regulation of norepinephrine synstesis.
    Monoamine Oxidases - New Vistas, Costa, E. and Sandler, M.
    (eds). Raven Press, New York, p. 409, 1972.

39. MURPHY, D.L., BELMAKER, R.H. and WYATT, R.J.: Monoamine oxidase
    in schizophrenia and other behavioral disorders. J. Psychiat.
    Res.,11:221-247, 1974.

40. NIES, A., ROBINSON, D.S., LAMBORN, K.R. and LAMPERT, R.P.:
    Genetic control of platelet and plasma monoamine oxidase
    activity. Arch. Gen. Psychiat., 28:834, 1973.

41. MURPHY, D.L. and WYATT, R.J.: Reduced MAO activity in blood
    platelets from schizophrenic patients. Nature, 238:225, 1972.

42. MURPHY, D.L. and WEISS,R.L.:Reduced monoamine oxidase activity
    in blood platelets from bipolar depressed patients. Am. J.
    Psychiat., 128:11, 1972.

43. WYATT, R.J., MURPHY, D.L., BELMAKER, R.H., COHEN, S., DONNELLY,
    C.H. and POLLIN, W.: Reduced monoamine oxidase in platelets:
    A possible genetic marker for vulnerability to schizophrenia.
    Science,179:916, 1973.

44. WYATT, R.J., BELMAKER, R.H., and MURPHY, D.L.: Low platelet
    monoamine oxidase and vulnerability to schizophrenia.
    Modern Problems in Pharmacopsychiatry, Mendlewicz, J., (ed),
    Karger, Vol. 10, Basel 1975.

45. MELTZER, H.Y. and STAHL, S.M.: Platelet monoamine oxidase activity
    and substrate preferences in schizophrenic patients. Res. Comm.
    in Chem. Path. and Pharmacol., 7:419, 1974.

46. CARPENTER, W.T. jr., MURPHY, D.L. and WYATT, R.J.: Platelet mono-
    amine oxidase activity in acute schizophrenia. Am. J. Psychiat.
    132:438, 1975.

47. FRIEDMAN, E., SHOPSIN, B., SATHANANTHAN, G. and GERSHON, S.:
    Blood platelet monoamine oxidase activity in psychiatric
    patients. Am. J. Psychiat., 131:1392, 1974.

48. BELMAKER, R.H., ELBESEN, K., EBSTEIN, R. and RIMON, R.:
    Platelet monoamine oxidase in schizophrenia and manic-
    depressive illness. Brit. J. Psychiat., in press.

49. COLLINS, G.G.S. and SANDLER, M.: Human blood platelet monoamine
    oxidase. Biochem. Pharmac., 20:289, 1971.

50. BELMAKER, R., EBSTEIN, R., RIMON, R.: Electrophoresis of platelet
    monoamine oxidase in schizophrenia and manic-depressive ill-
    ness, Acta Psychiat. Scand. in press.

51. EDWARDS, D.J. and CHANG, S.S.: Evidence for interacting cata-
    lytic sites of human platelet monoamine oxidase. Biochem.
    Biophys. Res. Comm., 65:1018, 1975.

52. YOUDIM, M.B.H.: Multiple forms of mitochondrial monoamine oxidase.
    Brit. Med. Bull. 29:120, 1973.

53. TIPTON, K.F., HOUSLAY, M.D. and GARRETT, N.J.: Allotopic
    properties of human brain monoamine oxidase. Nature New
    Biology, 246:213, 1973.

54. NEFF, N.H. and GORIDIS, C.: Neuronal monoamine oxidase: Specific
    enzyme types and their rates of formation. Advances in
    Biochemical Psychopharmacology. Costa, E. and Greengard, P.
    (eds), 5:307, N.Y. 1972.

55. MURPHY, D.L. and DONNELLY, C.H.: Monoamine oxidase in man:
    enzyme characteristics in platelets, plasma and other
    human tissues. Advances in Biochemical Psychopharmacology,
    E. Usdin, ed. Raven Press, N.Y., Vol. 5, 1974.

56. DOMINO, E.F., KRAUSE, R.R. and BOWERS, J.: Various enzymes
    involved with putative transmitters. Arch. Gen. Psychiat.,
    29:195, 1973.

57. WISE, C.D., BADEN, M.M. and STEIN, L.: Post-mortem measurement
    of enzymes in human brain: Evidence of a central noradrenic
    deficit in schizophrenia. J. Psychiat. Res., 11:185, 1974.

58. SCHWARTZ, M., AIKENS, A.M. and WYATT, R.J.: Monoamine oxidase
    in brains from schizophrenic and mentally normal individuals.
    Psychopharmacologia, 38:319, 1974.

59. EHRENSVARD, G., LIIJEVIST, J. and NILSSON, M.T.: Studies of
    human serum constituents in relation to schizophrenia.
    Molecular Basis of Some Aspects of Mental Activity.
    Walaas, O. (ed), Academic Press, New York, 2:231, 1967.

60. KLAIBER, E.L., BROVERMAN, D.M., VOGEL, W., KOBAYASHI, Y. and
    MORIATRY, D.: Effects of estrogen therapy on plasma MAO activity
    and EEG driving responses of depressed woman. Am. J. Psychiat.,
    128:1492, 1972.

61. ROBINSON, D.S., DAVIS, M.M., NIES, A., RAVARIS, C.L. and
    SYLVESTER, D.: Relation of sex and aging to monoamine oxidase
    activity of human brain plasma and platelets. Arch. Gen.
    Psychiat., 24:536, 1971.

62. BELMAKER, R.H., EBSTEIN, R. and BENBENISTY, D.: Electrophoretic
    pattern of plasma MAO in schizophrenia and affective illness.
    J. Psychiat. Res., in press.

63. SHIH, J.H.C. and EIDUSON, S.: Multiple forms of monoamine
    oxidase in developing tissue: The implications for mental
    health. Ho, B. and McIsaac, W. (eds), Brain Chemistry and
    Mental Diseases, Plenum Publishers, pp. 3-20, 1971.

64. GERSHON, E., BELMAKER, R. and EBSTEIN, R.: Plasma monoamine
    oxidase in patients with affective disorder and their
    families. Submitted for publication.

TWIN STUDIES AND DIAGNOSTIC ISSUES IN SCHIZOPHRENIA

Margit Fischer

Department of Psychiatry

University of Aarhus, Denmark

Twin studies (Luxenburger, 1928; Rosanoff et al., 1934; Essen-Möller, 1941; Kallmann, 1946; Slater, 1953; Inoye, 1961; Tienari, 1963; Kringlen, 1968; Gottesman & Shields, 1972; Fischer 1973; Pollin et al., 1969) and fostering and adoption studies (Karlsson, 1966; Heston, 1966; Rosenthal et al., 1968; Kety et al., 1968), show that genetic factors play a major role in the etiology, but other, environmental, factors are important as well. That statement is generally accepted so I will summarize some of the questions which come into my mind regarding schizophrenia and genetics:

1. Is the syndrome we call schizophrenia a disease which can be identified in countries with different social and cultural background?

Ans. 1. Yes. One of the reasons for my Yes is the results obtained in The International Pilot Study of Schizophrenia (World Health Organization, 1973). This is a study initiated by WHO where 9 countries participated: Colombia, Czechoslovakia, Denmark, India, Nigeria, Russia, Taiwan, United Kingdom and United States.

These centres represented both developing and developed countries and a variety of social and cultural background. I will briefly outline the methodology and one of the results: In all 9 centres, all admissions of patients aged 15-44 coming from a defined catchment area were screened during a one-year period. Patients included in the study should present at least one of 10 specified psychotic symptoms, but were not included if they were "chronic", had an organic disorder or drug or alcohol abuse.

A total of 1202 patients were included in the study. All these patients were examined in a standardized way with similar interview schedules translated into the different languages. The interviews contained a Present State Examination (Wing, 1970; Sartorius et al., 1970), a Psychiatric History, a Social Description and a Physical Examination.

It was possible to develop a diagnostic computer programme (Fischer, 1973), (called DIAX) based on symptoms rated present at admission. I used 4 different ways of testing the computer diagnosis called DIAX.

1. I compared with the clinical diagnosis.
   It appeared that there was a rather high degree of agreement though detailed analysis showed that there were differences in the level of agreement. In Russia and United States the clinical criteria for schizophrenia appeared to be broader than in most other centres, and in some centres the diagnosis of manic-depressive psychosis was used very seldom.
2. Using only the Aarhus patients I found a high degree of correlation between the computer diagnosis and outcome rated at the 2 year follow-up.
3. I compared the DIAX diagnosis made at the initial examination with the one made at the 2 year follow-up.

   The hypothesis was, that if the DIAX diagnosis was valid the patients who had not completely recovered at the follow-up examination should fall into the same main diagnostic group as they did at the initial examination. "Severe disagreement", such as being diagnosed manic-depressive at one examination and schizophrenic at the other examination, appeared only in approximately 10% of the cases, and these cases may well represent the "schizo-affective" psychoses.

4. The last way to test the validity was to examine what kind of mental disorder appeared in first degree relatives of probands with a DIAX diagnosis of definite schizophrenia and bipolar manic-depressive psychoses. After age-correction it appeared that in the first group there were 6% schizophrenics and in the second group 17% with affective disorder. Thus it seems possible to use standardized criteria for the two major psychoses, and it seems possible to separate them and recognize at least a core group of each in very different populations.

2.   The next question is whether the syndrome we call schizophrenia consists of one or several nosological enitities. Even if we use rather strict criteria for the diagnosis, is it likely that in some patients the disease is mainly genetically determined, while in other patients the etiology is mainly determined by environmental factors?

<u>Ans. 2</u>. In order to try to answer this question I will describe one aspect of the twin study I performed (Fischer et al., 1969; Fischer, 1971; Fischer, 1973). We have in Denmark a twin register collected by Harvald and Hauge (Hauge et al., 1968). This twin register was established from birth register and comprises all twin births during the period 1870-1920. We also have a Central Psychiatric Register which was started during the 1930's. By comparing these two registers we established what we call the Psychiatric Twin Register. A total of 395 same-sexed pairs were found in whom one or both twins had been admitted to a mental hospital. Out of these 395 pairs I found 78 probands from 70 pairs which I diagnosed as having schizophrenia, and the diagnostic criteria I applied would correlate with what is generally accepted as process-schizophrenia. The zygosity of these pairs established independently of the psychiatric diagnosis by examination of blood- and serum groups whenever possible. Twenty-five probands from 21 pairs were found to be MZ and the concordance rate was 56%. Approximately half of the MZ twins were concordant, the other half were discordant. I wanted to test whether genetic factors played a minor or perhaps no role in the etiology of the schizophrenia in the discordant MZ twins.

I therefore examined the offspring of the MZ twins. They were divided into two groups: one where one of the parents was a schizophrenic MZ twin and the other group where one of the parents was a normal MZ co-twin to a schizophrenic twin.

The first group had a total of 44 offspring, the second group had 27 offspring; Table 3 shows the total number after age correction (31 and 23) and the number and percentage with schizophrenia in both groups (3 = 10% and 3 = 13%).

The result should be taken with some reservation, because of the relatively small number, but with this reservation it shows two things: In both groups the risk figures are similar to what would be expected in the offspring of one schizophrenic parent. It shows that there is no reason to believe that the discordant schizophrenic MZ twins are phenocopies. Schizophrenia appears as frequent in the offspring of these twins as in the offspring of the concordant MZ twins. It also shows that for this group of offspring it did not seem to be of any significance whether you were brought up by a schizophrenic parent or not. At the moment I can not think of any way to determine clinically how to separate subgroups of schizophrenia which might have different etiology.

3. The next question is, what model of inheritance fits the results best?

<u>Ans. 3</u>. The risk figures from family studies indicate very clearly that it is not a simple recessive or dominant Mendelian way of

TABLE 1. Comparison of clinical diagnoses and DIAX diagnoses

D I A X diagnosis	Clinical diagnosis (at episode of inclusion)										
	paranoid	non-paranoid	residual	schizo-affective	paranoid psychosis	paranoid + schiz. pers.	Mania + mixed	Psychotic dep.	non-psychotic dep. + hypo-mania	Other diagnoses	Total
Schizo. paranoid	169	95	3	36	16	–	4	1	–	2	326
Schizo. non-paranoid	59	131	5	26	8	–	8	8	1	9	255
Schizo. residual	1	17	–	–	–	1	1	2	–	3	25
Schizo. schizo-affective	19	24	–	11	7	–	14	3	2	–	80
Paranoid psychosis	30	16	–	2	15	–	2	1	–	3	69
Paranoid + schizoid personality disorder	3	8	–	5	2	–	–	3	10	11	42
Affective disorder Mania + mixed	24	29	1	14	11	–	52	14	16	10	171
Affective disorder psychotic depression	9	20	1	16	7	–	2	52	41	9	157
Affective disorder non-psychotic depression + hypomania	1	7	1	1	2	–	4	2	4	9	31
Other diagnoses	7	14	2	1	7	–	2	2	1	10	46
Total	322	361	13	75	75	1	89	88	75	66	1202

Reference: (Table from M. Fischer, 1974)

TABLE 2. Relationship between DIAX diagnosis and prognosis. Number of patients in total material and first admissions. (Aarhus patients)

DIAX DIAGNOSIS	CLINICAL OUTCOME GROUPS			TOTAL
	No abnormality 1 + 2	Slight impairment 3	Moderate + severe impairment 4 + 5	
Affective psychoses				
All	15	13	7	35
First admissions	8	3	3	14
Schizophrenia				
All	6	10	46	62
First admissions	3	4	18	25
Paranoid psychoses				
All	1	3	5	9
First admissions	–	3	3	6
All other diagnoses				
All	3	6	11	20
First admissions	2	1	2	5
Total				
All	25	32	69	126
First admissions	13	11	28	50

Reference: (Table from M. Fischer, 1974).

TABLE 3. Schizophrenia and schizophrenia-like psychosis, and suicide in present offspring material. Distribution by zygosity and diagnosis of one parent (MZ twin) and diagnosis of offspring

Parents	Offspring									Suicide
	Total N	Total after age correction			Schizophrenia and schizophrenia-like pschosis					Number
					Number			%		
	M + F	M	F	M + F	M	F	M + F	M + F		F
Group 1: One parent:schizophrenic MZ twin	44	17.0	14.2	31.2	1	2	3	9.6		1
Group 2: One parent:normal MZ co-twin	27	13.6	9.5	23.1	0	3	3	12.9*		0
Total	71	30.6	23.7	54.3	1	5	6	-		1

* Fischer test: p = 0.30822 (difference not significant).

Reference: (Table from M. Fischer, 1971)

environmental factors, but so far I have not seen results from
methodologically good studies which could indicate what kind of
environmental factors are important or how the interaction with
the genetic factors function.

My own hypothesis is that one or two genes play a major role
in the majority of the patients we diagnose as having schizophrenia,
and that a few, say 3 or 4, other genes can influence the major
genes in such a way that the person's vulnerability to environmental factors may be weaker or stronger. Whether some combination
of some genes facilitates what sometimes is described as the schizo-
phrenia-spectrum disorder is an unsolved question.

During the past couple of years Professor Gottesman and I
have examined the offspring of dual matings in the hope that we
will be able to answer at least a few of the questions. The parents
were found in the Danish Central Psychiatric Register. We have
about 150 couples with at least one child. Together they have
approximately 400 offspring which now have a mean age of 35. There
are all kinds of matings, schizophrenia + schizophrenia, manic-
depression + schizophrenia, manic-depression + sociopath, schizophrenia + neuroses, etc.

We hope to see which matings produce which offspring and to
look into the environment and personality of the rather large
number of offspring who in spite of genetic loading and chaotic
upbringing seem to have developed into mentally normal persons.

I looked at the title of this symposium: "The Impact of
Biology on Modern Psychiatry". "Biology", comes from Greek: "Bios",
meaning "life" and "logos" meaning "knowledge of". As I was not
quite satisfied with this translation, I went to the Oxford and
Webster's Dictionaries. The definition given there was:
    "The science of physical life dealing with organized
beings, their morphology, physiology, origin, development and
distribution". In that broad definition of the word is included
practically everything and the symposium here is only dealing with
a very limited part of biology.

"Modern psychiatry". Modern, compared to what? Psychiatry,
would that include both actual treatment and research and would
it include non-psychotic behaviour disorders as well as the major
psychoses?

My hope is that the impact of biology will serve to make
modern psychiatry more balanced between its two extremes. We
as psychiatrists should keep in mind that we are dealing with
highly complex matters: the brain, its function and structure,
the mutual influence and interdependency of the brain and the

other part of the body. There is no dichotomy between body and
soul. Everything that happens with or within a human being has
a biochemical level, whether he is using a muscle or whether he
is trying to solve a problem or whether he has auditory hallucinations. However, it is also evident that no matter how detailed
our knowledge about biochemistry becomes, there will continue to
be certain phenomena which can only be explained and understood
in psychological terms. We must recognize that we can not in biochemical terms describe, for instance, the image we have when we
think that the sky is blue. Our patients as well will translate
what is going on "on the biochemical level" into language and
pictures.

Interpretations and reactions from the outside world will
raise emotions within a person, emotions that have both a biochemical level and a psychological level which may continue to
influence each other. I want to stress the complexity of the
problems when we are dealing with psychoses in human beings. I
want to stress the difficulty in translating results from animals
to human beings because one of the major symptoms is a disorder
in abstract thinking and the ability for abstract thinking and
language is probably the most impressive difference between
animals and human beings.

REFERENCES

ESSEN-MÖLLER, E.: Empirische Ähnlichkeitsdiagnose bei Zwillingen.
        Hereditas, Genetiskt Arkiv. 27, 1-50, (a) 1941.

ESSEN-MÖLLER, E.: Psychiatrische Untersuchungen an einer Serie
        von Zwillingen. Acta Psychiatrics et Neurologica Scand-
        inavica, Suppl. 23. (b). 1941.

FISCHER, M., HARVALD B. AND HAUGE, M.: A Danish twin study of
        schizophrenia. Brit. J. Psychiat. 115, 981-990, 1969.

FISCHER, M.: Psychoses in the offspring of schizophrenia mono-
        zygotic twins and their normal co-twins. Brit. J. Psychiat.
        118, 43-52, 1971.

FISCHER, M.: Genetic and Environmental factors in schizophrenia.
        A study of schizophrenic twins and their families.
        Munksgaard, Copenhagen, 1973.

FISCHER, M.: Development and validity of a computerized method
        for diagnoses of functional psychoses (DIAX). Acta psychiat.
        Scand., 50, 243-288, 1974.

GOTTESMAN, I.I. AND JAMES SHIELDS.: Schizophrenia and Genetics.
        A twin study vantage point. Academic Press, New York and
        London, 1972.

HARE, E.H. AND WING. J.K.: Psychiatric epidemiology. London,
        Oxford University Press, 1970.

HAUGE, M., B. HARVALD, M. FISCHER, K. GOTLIEB-JENSEN, N. JUEL-
        Nielsen, I. RAEBILD, R. SHAPIRO AND T. VIDEBECH: A Danish
        Twin Register. Acta genet. med. (Roma) 17, 315-332, 1968.

HESTON, L.L.: Psychiatric disorders in foster home reared children
        of schizophrenic mothers. Brit. J. of Pyschiat. 112,
        819-825, 1966.

INOUYE, E.: Similarity and dissimilarity of schizophrenia in twins.
        Proceedings of the Third World Congress on Psychiatry.
        Vol. 1, pp. 524-530. Montreal: University of Toronto Press,
        1961.

INTERNATIONAL Pilot Study of Schizophrenia. World Health Organi-
        zation, Geneva, 1973.

KALLMANN, F.J.: The genetic theory of schizophrenia: An analysis
        of 691 schizophrenic twin index families. American Journal
        of Psychiatry. 103, 309-322, 1946.

KARLSSON, J.L.: The biologic basis of schizophrenia. Springfield.
        Illinois: Thomas, 1966.

KETY, S.S., ROSENTHAL, D., WENDER, P.H., AND SCHULSINGER, F.: The
        types and prevalence of mental illness in the biological
        and adiptive families of adopted schizophrenics. In:
        D. Rosenthal and S.S. Kety (Eds.), The Transmission of
        Schizophrenia . Oxford Pergamon, pp.345-362, 1968.

KRINGLEN, E.: An epidemiological-clinical twin study on schizo-
        phrenia. In: D. Rosenthal and S.S. Kety (Eds.) The Trans-
        mission of Schizophrenia Oxford, Pergamon, pp. 49-63, 1968.

LUXENBURGER, H.: Vorläufiger Bericht über psychiatrische Serien-
        untersuchungen an Zwillingen. Zeitschrift für die gesamte
        Neurologie und Psychiatrie, 116, 297-326, 1928.

POLLIN, W., ALLEN, M.G., HOFFER, A., STABENAU, J.R. AND HRUBEC, Z.:
        Psychopathology in 15,909 pairs of veteran twins: Evidence
        for a genetic factor in the pathogenesis of schizophrenia
        and its relative absence in psychoneurosis. The American .
        Journal of Psychiatry , 126, 597-610, 1969.

ROSANOFF, A.J., HANDY, L.M., PLESSET, I.R. AND BRUSH, S.: The
        Etiology of so-called schizophrenic psychoses with special
        reference to their occurrence in twins. American Journal
        of Psychiatry, 91, 247-286, 1934.

ROSENTHAL, D., WENDER, P.H.,KETY, S.S., SCHULSINGER, F., WELNER, J.
        AND L. ØSTERGAARD.: Schizophrenics' offspring reared in
        adoptive homes. IN: D. Rosenthal and S.S. Kety (Eds.)
        The Transmission of Schizophrenia. Oxford: Pergamon,
        pp. 377-391, 1968.

SARTORIUS, N., BROOKE E.M. AND LIN. T.Y.,: Reliability of psy-
        chiatric assessment in international research. In: E.H.
        Hare and J.K. Wing (Eds.), Psychiatric epidemiology,
        London, Oxford University Press, 1970.

SLATER, E.: (with the assistance of J. Shields) Psychotic and
        Neurotic Illnesses in Twins. Medical Research Council
        Special Report Series No. 278. London: Her Majesty's
        Stationery Office, 1953.

TIENARI, P.: Psychiatric illnesses in identical twins. Acta
        Psychiatrica Scandinavica Suppl. 171, 1963.

WING, J.K.: A standard form of psychiatric present state examination
        (PSE) and a method for standardising the classification
        of symptoms. In. E.H. Hare and J.K. Wing (Eds.). Psychia-
        tric epidemiology, London, Oxford University Press, 1970a.

LIST OF PARTICIPANTS

DR. RUTH ASHKENAZI, Department of Physiology, Hadassah-Hebrew
    University School of Medicine, Jerusalem, Israel.

DR. ABRAHAM ATSMON, Professor of Medicine, Tel-Aviv University
    School of Medicine, Tel-Aviv, Israel.

DR. ROBERT H. BELMAKER, Director, Department of Research,
    Jerusalem Mental Health Center. P.O.B. 140, Jerusalem,
    and Lecturer, Department of Psychiatry, Hadassah-Hebrew
    University School of Medicine, Jerusalem, Israel.

DR. BARRY D. BERGER, Professor and Chairman, Department of
    Psychology, Haifa University, Haifa, Israel.

DR. SAMUEL I. COHEN, Consultant Psychiatrist, The London
    Hospital (Whitechapel) England.

DR. SHAMAI DAVIDSON, Director, Shalvata Psychiatric Center.
    Hod Hasharon, Israel.

DR. RICHARD P. EBSTEIN, Senior Neurochemist, Jerusalem Mental
    Health Center, P.O.B. 140, Jerusalem, Israel.
    and Research Associate, Department of Psychiatry,
    Hadassah-Hebrew University School of Medicine, Jerusalem,
    Israel.

DR. ELI EDELSTEIN, Associate Professor of Psychiatry,
    Hadassah-Hebrew University School of Medicine, Jerusalem,
    Israel.

DR. AVNER ELIZUR, Shalvata Psychiatric Center, Hod Hasharon,
    Israel, and Tel-Aviv University Medical School, Tel-Aviv,
    Israel.

DR. MARGIT FISCHER, Institute of Psychiatric Demography,
    Aarhus Psychiatric Hospital and Department of Psychiatry
    Aarhus University, Aarhus, Denmark.

DR. ELLIOT S. GERSHON, Chief, Unit on Psychogenetics, Adult
    Psychiatry Branch, National Institute of Mental Health
    Bethesda, Maryland 20014, U.S.A.

DR. SAMUEL GERSHON, Professor of Psychiatry, Neuropsycho-
        pharmacology Research Unit, Department of Psychiatry,
        New York University Medical Center, New York, U.S.A.

DR. RUTH GUTTMAN, Department of Psychology, Hebrew University,
        Jerusalem, Israel.

DR. SEYMOUR S. KETY, Psychiatric Research Laboratories,
        Massachusetts General Hospital, Boston, Massachusetts,
        and Professor of Psychiatry, Harvard Medical School,
        Boston, Mass. U.S.A.

DR. AMOS D. KORCZYN, Department of Physiology and Pharmacology,
        Sackler School of Medicine, Tel-Aviv University, Israel.

DR. JONATHAN MAGNES, Professor of Physiology, Hebrew University,
        Jerusalem, Israel.

DR. ARNOLD MANDELL, Professor and Co-Chairman, Department of
        Psychiatry, University of California at San Diego
        La Jolla, California 92093 U.S.A.

DR. JULIEN MENDLEWICZ, New York State Psychiatric Institute
        Department of Medical Genetics, New York, N.Y. 10032, U.S.A.
        Current Address: Institut de Psychiatrie,
                         Hopital Universitaire Brugmann
                         4, place Van Gehuchten,
                         Brussels 1020, Belgium.

DR. HERMAN M. van PRAAG, Professor and Chairman, Department of
        Biological Psychiatry, State University Groningen, Groningen,
        Netherlands.

DR. RANAN RIMON, Professor of Psychiatry, University of Kuopio,
        Finland. Currently: Staff Psychiatrist, Jerusalem Mental
        Health Center, and Visiting Professor of Psychiatry,
        Hadassah-Hebrew University School of Medicine, Jerusalem,
        Israel.

DR. MILTON ROSENBAUM, Director, Jerusalem Mental Health Center -
        Ezrath Nashim and Professor of Psychiatry, Hadassah-Hebrew
        University School of Medicine, Jerusalem, Israel.

DR. DAVID SAMUEL, Sherman Professor of Physical Chemistry,
        Isotope Department, Weizmann Institute of Science,
        Rehovot, Israel.

DR. GORAN SEDVALL, Department of Pharmacology and Psychiatry,
        (St. Goran's Hospital) The Karolinska Institutet,
        S-104 01 Stockholm, Sweden.

DR. MARTA WEINSTOCK, Department of Physiology and Pharmacology,
        Sackler School of Medicine, Tel-Aviv University,
        Tel-Aviv, Israel.

DR. ISAAC P. WITZ, Department of Microbiology, The George S.
        Wise Center, Tel-Aviv University, Tel-Aviv, Israel.

DR. SHLOMO YEHUDA, Laboratory of Psychopharmacology,
        Department of Psychology, Bar-Ilan University,
        Ramat Gan, Israel.

DR. M.B.H. YOUDIM, M.R.C. Unit and University Department of
        Clinical Pharmacology, Radcliffe Infirmary, Oxford
        OX2 6HE, England.

INDEX